Contemporary Challenges in Sudden Cardiac Death

Editors

MOHAMMAD SHENASA
N.A. MARK ESTES III
GORDON F. TOMASELLI

CARDIAC ELECTROPHYSIOLOGY CLINICS

www.cardiacEP.theclinics.com

Consulting Editors
RANJAN K. THAKUR
ANDREA NATALE

December 2017 • Volume 9 • Number 4

ELSEVIER

1600 John F. Kennedy Boulevard • Suite 1800 • Philadelphia, Pennsylvania, 19103-2899

http://www.theclinics.com

CARDIAC ELECTROPHYSIOLOGY CLINICS Volume 9, Number 4
December 2017 ISSN 1877-9182, ISBN-13: 978-0-323-55268-4

Editor: Stacy Eastman
Developmental Editor: Donald Mumford

Cardiac Electrophysiology Clinics (ISSN 1877-9182) is published quarterly by Elsevier Inc., 360 Park Avenue South, New York, NY 10010-1710. Months of issue are March, June, September, and December. Subscription prices are $215.00 per year for US individuals, $331.00 per year for US institutions, $236.00 per year for Canadian individuals, $373.00 per year for Canadian institutions, $299.00 per year for international individuals, $399.00 per year for international institutions and $100.00 per year for US, Canadian and international students/residents. To receive student/resident rate, orders must be accompanied by name of affilliated institution, date of term, and the signature of program/residency coordinator on institution letterhead. Orders will be billed at individual rate until proof of status is received. Foreign air speed delivery is included in all Clinics subscription prices. All prices are subject to change without notice. **POSTMASTER:** Send address changes to Cardiac Electrophysiology Clinics, Elsevier Health Sciences Division, Subscription Customer Service, 3251 Riverport Lane, Maryland Heights, MO 63043. **Customer Service: 1-800-654-2452 (US and Canada). From outside of the US and Canada, call 314-477-8871. Fax: 314-447-8029. E-mail: JournalsCustomerService-usa@elsevier.com (for print support); JournalsOnlineSupport-usa@elsevier.com (for online support).**

Reprints. For copies of 100 or more of articles in this publication, please contact the Commercial Reprints Department, Elsevier Inc., 360 Park Avenue South, New York, NY 10010-1710. Tel.: 212-633-3874; Fax: 212-633-3820; E-mail: reprints@elsevier.com.

Cardiac Electrophysiology Clinics is covered in *MEDLINE/PubMed (Index Medicus).*

Contributors

CONSULTING EDITORS

RANJAN K. THAKUR, MD, MPH, MBA, FHRS
Professor of Medicine, Director, Arrhythmia Service, Thoracic and Cardiovascular Institute, Sparrow Health System, Michigan State University, Lansing, Michigan, USA

ANDREA NATALE, MD, FACC, FHRS
Executive Medical Director, Texas Cardiac Arrhythmia Institute, St. David's Medical Center, Austin, Texas, USA; Consulting Professor, Division of Cardiology, Stanford University, Palo Alto, California, USA; Adjunct Professor of Medicine, Heart and Vascular Center, Case Western Reserve University, Cleveland, Ohio, USA; Director, Interventional Electrophysiology, Scripps Clinic, San Diego, California, USA; Senior Clinical Director, EP Services, California Pacific Medical Center, San Francisco

EDITORS

MOHAMMAD SHENASA, MD
Heart and Rhythm Medical Group, Department of Cardiovascular Services, O'Connor Hospital, San Jose, California, USA

N.A. MARK ESTES III, MD
Professor of Medicine, Tufts University School of Medicine, Director, New England Cardiac Arrhythmia Center, Tufts Medical Center, Boston, Massachusetts, USA

GORDON F. TOMASELLI, MD
Professor, Department of Medicine, Michel Mirowski MD Professor, Division of Cardiology, The Johns Hopkins University School of Medicine, Johns Hopkins University, Baltimore, Maryland, USA

AUTHORS

MICHAEL J. ACKERMAN, MD, PhD
Windland Smith Rice Cardiovascular Genomics Research Professor, Department of Cardiovascular Diseases, Division of Heart Rhythm Services, Department of Pediatrics, Division of Pediatric Cardiology, Department of Molecular Pharmacology and Experimental Therapeutics, Windland Smith Rice Sudden Death Genomics Laboratory, Mayo Clinic, Rochester, Minnesota, USA

GOURG ATTEYA, MD
SUNY Downstate Medical Center, Brooklyn, New York, USA

RAIMUNDO BARBOSA-BARROS, MD
Chief of Coronary Center, Hospital de Messejana Dr Carlos Alberto Studart Gomes, Fortaleza, Ceará, Brazil

CHARLES I. BERUL, MD
Division of Cardiology, Children's National Health System, Professor, Department of Pediatrics, The George Washington University School of Medicine and Health Sciences, Washington, DC, USA

WULFRAN BOUGOUIN, MD, PhD
Paris Cardiovascular Research Center–
INSERM U970 (PARCC), Paris Sudden Death
Expertise Center (SDEC), European Georges
Pompidou Hospital, Paris, France

MOHAMED BOUTJDIR, PhD
Professor of Physiology, New York University,
New York, New York, USA; Professor of
Physiology, SUNY Downstate Medical Center,
Research Scientist, VA NY Harbor Health Care
System, Brooklyn, New York, USA

NOEL G. BOYLE, MD, PhD
Professor of Medicine, Director of Cardiac EP
Labs and Fellowship Program, UCLA Cardiac
Arrhythmia Center, UCLA Health, David Geffen
School of Medicine at UCLA, Los Angeles,
California, USA

ALFRED E. BUXTON, MD
Director, Clinical Electrophysiology
Laboratory, Department of Medicine,
Cardiovascular Division, Beth Israel
Deaconess Medical Center, Professor of
Medicine, Harvard Medical School, Boston,
Massachusetts, USA

NIKOLAOS DAGRES, MD
Department of Electrophysiology, University
Leipzig Heart Center, Leipzig, Germany

DEVINDER S. DHINDSA, MD
Department of Medicine, Division of
Cardiology, Emory University School of
Medicine, Atlanta, Georgia, USA

DANNY J. EAPEN, MD
Department of Medicine, Division of
Cardiology, Emory University School of
Medicine, Atlanta, Georgia, USA

NABIL EL-SHERIF, MD
Professor of Medicine and Physiology,
SUNY Downstate Medical Center,
Distinguished Scientist, American College of
Cardiology, Chief, Cardiology Division, VA NY
Harbor Health Care System, Brooklyn,
New York, USA

**ANDREW E. EPSTEIN, MD, FAHA, FACC,
FHRS**
Professor of Medicine, Cardiovascular
Division, Hospital of the University
of Pennsylvania, Philadelphia, Pennsylvania,
USA

N.A. MARK ESTES III, MD
Professor of Medicine, Tufts University School
of Medicine, Director, New England Cardiac
Arrhythmia Center, Tufts Medical Center,
Boston, Massachusetts, USA

JEFFREY J. GOLDBERGER, MD
Chief, Cardiovascular Division, Department of
Medicine, Miller School of Medicine, University
of Miami, Miami, Florida, USA

GERHARD HINDRICKS, MD
Department of Electrophysiology, University
Leipzig Heart Center, Leipzig, Germany

MUNTHER K. HOMOUD, MD
Assistant Professor, Tufts University School of
Medicine, Co-Director, New England Cardiac
Arrhythmia Center, Division of Cardiology,
Tufts Medical Center, Boston, Massachusetts,
USA

WILLIAM A. HUANG, MD
Clinical Cardiac Electrophysiology Fellow,
UCLA Cardiac Arrhythmia Center, David
Geffen School of Medicine at UCLA,
Los Angeles, California, USA

XAVIER JOUVEN, MD, PhD
Paris Cardiovascular Research Center–
INSERM U970 (PARCC), Paris Descartes
University, Paris Sudden Death Expertise
Center (SDEC), Cardiology Department,
European Georges Pompidou Hospital, Paris,
France

NICOLE KARAM, MD, PhD
Paris Cardiovascular Research Center–
INSERM U970 (PARCC), Paris Descartes
University, Paris Sudden Death Expertise
Center (SDEC), Cardiology Department,
European Georges Pompidou Hospital, Paris,
France

JAY KHAMBHATI, MD
Department of Medicine, Division of
Cardiology, Emory University School of
Medicine, Atlanta, Georgia, USA

RACHEL LAMPERT, MD
Professor of Medicine, Yale School of
Medicine, New Haven, Connecticut, USA

WORAWAN LIMIPITIKUL, BS
Department of Biomedical Engineering, Johns
Hopkins University, Baltimore, Maryland, USA

CONSTANCIA MACATANGAY, MD
Cardiovascular Division, Department of
Medicine, Miller School of Medicine, University
of Miami, Miami, Florida, USA

CHRISTOPHER MADIAS, MD
Division of Cardiology, New England Cardiac
Arrhythmia Center, Tufts Medical Center,
Boston, Massachusetts, USA

ELOI MARIJON, MD, PhD
Paris Cardiovascular Research
Center–INSERM U970 (PARCC), Paris
Descartes University, Paris Sudden Death
Expertise Center (SDEC), Cardiology
Department, European Georges Pompidou
Hospital, Paris, France

DANIEL P. MORIN, MD, MPH
Associate Professor of Cardiology, Medical
Director, Cardiovascular Research, Ochsner
Medical Center, UQ Ochsner Clinical School,
University of Queensland Medical School, New
Orleans, Louisiana, USA

ROBERT J. MYERBURG, MD
Professor of Medicine and Physiology, Division
of Cardiology, American Heart Association
Chair in Cardiovascular Research, Miller
School of Medicine, University of Miami,
Miami, Florida, USA

KUMAR NARAYANAN, MD
Paris Cardiovascular Research Center–
INSERM U970 (PARCC), Paris, France;
Cardiology Department, Maxcure Hospitals,
Hyderabad, India

ROBERT W. NEUMAR, MD, PhD
Professor, Chair, Department of Emergency
Medicine, University of Michigan Medical
School, Ann Arbor, Michigan, USA

CHIN SIANG ONG, MBBS
Department of Medicine, Division of
Cardiology, The Johns Hopkins University
School of Medicine, Baltimore, Maryland, USA

ANDRÉS RICARDO PÉREZ-RIERA, MD, PhD
ABC School of Medicine, ABC Foundation,
Santo André, São Paulo, Brazil; Cardiologist,
Hospital do Coração, São Paulo, São Paulo,
Brazil

ROSS A. POLLACK, BS
Medical Student, The Johns Hopkins
University School of Medicine, Baltimore,
Maryland, USA

ARSHED A. QUYYUMI, MD, FACC
Professor, Department of Medicine, Division of
Cardiology, Emory University School of
Medicine, Atlanta, Georgia, USA

PRATIK B. SANDESARA, MD
Department of Medicine, Division of
Cardiology, Emory University School of
Medicine, Atlanta, Georgia, USA

PASQUALE SANTANGELI, MD, PhD
Assistant Professor of Medicine,
Cardiovascular Division, Hospital of the
University of Pennsylvania, Philadelphia,
Pennsylvania, USA

BASIL SAOUR, MD
Department of Internal Medicine, Division of
Cardiology, Northwestern University
Feinberg School of Medicine, Chicago,
Illinois, USA

PETER J. SCHWARTZ, MD
Director, Center for Cardiac Arrhythmias of
Genetic Origin, IRCCS Istituto Auxologico
Italiano, Milan, Italy

ARDALAN SHARIFZADEHGAN, MD, MPH
Paris Cardiovascular Research
Center–INSERM U970 (PARCC), Paris
Descartes University, Paris Sudden Death
Expertise Center (SDEC), Cardiology
Department, European Georges Pompidou
Hospital, Paris, France

MOHAMMAD SHENASA, MD
Heart and Rhythm Medical Group, Department
of Cardiovascular Services, O'Connor
Hospital, San Jose, California, USA

ELIZABETH D. SHERWIN, MD
Division of Cardiology, Children's National
Health System, Assistant Professor,
Department of Pediatrics, The George
Washington University School of Medicine &
Health Sciences, Washington, DC, USA

BRYAN SMITH, MD
Department of Internal Medicine, Division of
Cardiology, Northwestern University Feinberg
School of Medicine, Chicago, Illinois, USA

JAKUB SROUBEK, MD, PhD
Electrophysiology Fellow, Department of
Medicine, Cardiovascular Division, Clinical
Electrophysiology Laboratory, Beth Israel
Deaconess Medical Center, Boston,
Massachusetts, USA

POK TIN TANG, BM BCh, BA
UCLA Cardiac Arrhythmia Center, UCLA
Health, David Geffen School of Medicine at
UCLA, Los Angeles, California, USA

GORDON F. TOMASELLI, MD
Professor, Department of Medicine, Michel
Mirowski MD Professor, Division of Cardiology,
The Johns Hopkins University School of
Medicine, Johns Hopkins University,
Baltimore, Maryland, USA

GIOIA TURITTO, MD
Associate Professor, Department of
Medicine, Cornell University, New York,
New York, USA; Director, Cardiac
Electrophysiology Program, New York
Presbyterian-Brooklyn Methodist Hospital,
Brooklyn, New York, USA

MARMAR VASEGHI, MD, PhD, FHRS
Assistant Professor of Medicine, Director of
Clinical and Translational Research, UCLA
Cardiac Arrhythmia Center, David Geffen
School of Medicine at UCLA, Los Angeles,
California, USA

JUAN F. VILES-GONZALEZ, MD
Cardiovascular Division, Department of
Medicine, Miller School of Medicine, University
of Miami, Miami, Florida, USA

VICTOR WALDMANN, MD, MPH
Paris Cardiovascular Research Center–
INSERM U970 (PARCC), Paris Descartes
University, Paris Sudden Death Expertise
Center (SDEC), Cardiology Department,
European Georges Pompidou Hospital, Paris,
France, USA

JONATHAN WEINSTOCK, MD
Division of Cardiology, New England Cardiac
Arrhythmia Center, Tufts Medical Center,
Boston, Massachusetts, USA

MYRON L. WEISFELDT, MD
Professor, Department of Medicine, The Johns
Hopkins University School of Medicine,
Baltimore, Maryland, USA

ARTHUR A.M. WILDE, MD, PhD
Head, Heart Center, Academic Medical Center,
University of Amsterdam, Amsterdam, The
Netherlands; Princess Al-Jawhara Centre of
Excellence in Research of Hereditary
Disorders, Jeddah, Saudi Arabia

ANDREW L. WIT, PhD
Emeritus Professor, Department of
Pharmacology, The College of Physicians and
Surgeons, Columbia University, New York,
New York, USA

CLYDE W. YANCY, MD, Msc
Department of Internal Medicine, Division of
Cardiology, Northwestern University Feinberg
School of Medicine, Chicago, Illinois, USA

Contents

bystander use of defibrillators as the technology is applied to linking patients with shockable arrests to volunteers committed to bringing AEDs to the patients. There continues to be controversy as to the value of epinephrine, antiarrhythmic drugs, hypothermia, and mechanical chest compression in resuscitative efforts.

Regular exercise reduces cardiovascular and overall mortality. Participation in sports is an important determinant of cardiovascular health and fitness. Regular sports activity is associated with a smaller risk of sudden cardiac death (SCD). However, there is a small risk of sports-related SCD. Sports-related SCD accounts for approximately 5% of total SCD. SCD among athletes comprises only a fraction of all sports-related SCD. Sport-related SCD has a male predominance and an average age of affliction of 45 to 50 years. Survival is better than for other SCD. This article summarizes links between sports and SCD and discusses current knowledge and controversies.

Sudden cardiac death (SCD) is a rare but devastating event in children and adolescents. Etiologies include congenital heart disease, cardiomyopathies, primary arrhythmia syndromes, and miscellaneous conditions. Challenges in the diagnosis and prevention of SCD in the young are reviewed.

Sudden cardiac death (SCD) caused by ventricular arrhythmias is common in patients with genetic cardiomyopathies (CMs), including dilated CM, hypertrophic CM, and arrhythmogenic right ventricular CM (ARVC). Phenotypic features can identify individuals at high enough risk to warrant placement of an implantable cardioverter-defibrillator (ICD), although risk stratification schemes remain imperfect. Genetic testing is valuable for family cascade screening but with few exceptions (eg, LMNA mutations) do not identify higher risk for SCD. Although randomized trials are lacking, observational data suggest that ICDs can be beneficial. Vigorous exercise can exacerbate ARVC disease progression and increase likelihood of ventricular arrhythmias.

Although the electrocardiograph (ECG) was invented more than 100 years ago, it remains the most commonly used test in clinical medicine. It is easy to perform, relatively cheap, and results are readily available. Interpretation, however, needs expertise and knowledge. New data, phenomena, and syndromes are continually discovered by the ECG. It is important to differentiate between normal and abnormal ECGs first and then try to correlate the findings with clinical pathologies. Furthermore, the ECG is an integral part of the screening model for a variety of conditions, such as channelopathies, athletes, preoperative risk profile, and remains the cardiologist's best friend.

Sudden death is a major problem, with significant impact on public health. Many conditions predispose to sudden cardiac death and sudden cardiac arrest (SCA), foremost among them coronary artery disease, and an effective therapy exists in the form of the implantable cardioverter defibrillator. Risk stratification for SCA remains imperfect, especially for patients with nonischemic cardiomyopathy. Ongoing trials may make it easier to identify those at high risk, and potentially those at very low risk, in the future.

Sudden cardiac death (SCD) is a major cause of death from cardiovascular disease. Our ability to predict patients at the highest risk of developing lethal ventricular arrhythmias remains limited. Despite recent studies evaluating risk stratification tools, there is no optimal strategy. Cardiac imaging provides the opportunity to assess left ventricular ejection fraction, strain, fibrosis, and sympathetic innervation, all of which are pathophysiologically related to SCD risk. These modalities may play a role in the identification of vulnerable anatomic substrates that provide the pathophysiologic basis for SCD. Further studies are required to identify optimal imaging platform for risk assessment.

This article reviews biomarkers that have been shown to identify subjects at increased risk for cardiovascular death within the general population, in those with established coronary artery disease, and in those with heart failure. Use of biomarkers for risk stratification for sudden cardiac death continues to evolve. It seems that a multimarker strategy for risk stratification using simple measures of circulating proteins and usual clinical risk factors, particularly in patients with known coronary artery disease, can be used to identify patients at near-term risk of death. Whether similar strategies in the general population will prove to be cost-effective needs to be investigated.

Neural remodeling in the autonomic nervous system contributes to sudden cardiac death. The fabric of cardiac excitability and propagation is controlled by autonomic innervation. Heart disease predisposes to malignant ventricular arrhythmias by causing neural remodeling at the level of the myocardium, the intrinsic cardiac ganglia, extracardiac intrathoracic sympathetic ganglia, extrathoracic ganglia, spinal cord, and the brainstem, as well as the higher centers and the cortex. Therapeutic strategies at each of these levels aim to restore the balance between the sympathetic and parasympathetic branches. Understanding this complex neural network will provide important therapeutic insights into the treatment of sudden cardiac death.

Sudden cardiac death (SCD) accounts for approximately 360,000 deaths annually in the United States. Ischemic heart disease is the major cause of death in the general adult population. SCD can be due to arrhythmic or nonarrhythmic cardiac causes. Arrhythmic SCD may be caused by ventricular tachyarrhythmia or pulseless electrical activity/asystole. This article reviews the most recent pathophysiology and risk stratification strategies for SCD, emphasizing electrophysiologic surrogates of conduction disorder, dispersion of repolarization, and autonomic imbalance. Factors that modify arrhythmic death are addressed.

Ventricular arrhythmias remain a significant cause of sudden cardiac death (SCD), and knowledge of their cause and high-risk features is important. SCD occurs when the interaction between vulnerable substrates and acute triggers results in sustained ventricular tachycardia progressing to ventricular fibrillation. Here, the authors aim to review the role of ventricular arrhythmias in SCD, first by approaching the substrates that support ventricular arrhythmias, and then by exploring features of these substrates and the acute triggers that may lead to SCD.

The Centers for Diseases Control and Prevention estimates that 5.7 million adults in the United States suffer from heart failure and 1 in 9 deaths in 2009 cited heart failure as a contributing cause. Almost 50% of patients who are diagnosed with heart failure die within 5 years of diagnosis. Cardiovascular disease is a public health burden. The prognosis of patients with heart failure has improved significantly; however, the risk for death remains high. Managing sudden death risk and intervening appropriately with primary or secondary prevention strategies are of paramount importance.

Sudden cardiac death in acute coronary syndromes mostly results from complex ventricular arrhythmias. Although the incidence has fallen with contemporary management, they still pose a threat for many patients. Treatment consists of immediate termination by electrical cardioversion and prompt coronary revascularization for relief of ischemia. Beta-blockers administered prophylactically have a protective effect. For recurrent episodes, pharmacologic treatment consists of beta-blockers and amiodarone, or, in nonresponsive patients, lidocaine. Other antiarrhythmic drugs play only a marginal role. Catheter ablation performed in qualified centers can be effective in recurrent episodes of ventricular tachycardia or ventricular fibrillation triggered by premature ventricular contractions.

Cardiovascular complications of neuromuscular diseases disproportionately affect the cardiac conduction system. Cardiomyopathy and cardiac arrhythmias produce significant morbidity and mortality. Patients with neuromuscular diseases should be carefully and frequently evaluated for the presence of bradycardia, heart block, and tachyarrhythmias. Preemptive treatment with permanent pacemakers or implanted defibrillators is appropriate in patients with conduction system disease or who are at risk for ventricular arrhythmias.

Trials have demonstrated that implantable cardioverter defibrillators (ICDs) are effective in preventing sudden cardiac death (SCD). The degree of left ventricular dysfunction is the only parameter to identify primary prevention populations at higher risk of SCD in which ICDs may reduce longitudinal mortality risk. Clinical application of current stratification approaches based on left ventricular ejection fraction (LVEF) alone has failed to prevent most SCD in the general population. This lack of specificity has resulted in a significant number of potentially unnecessary ICDs. Future studies should focus on newer risk markers to improve the predictive value of LVEF and SCD prevention.

Patients with impaired left ventricular systolic function frequently die suddenly because of arrhythmic and nonarrhythmic causes. Nine trials have evaluated the utility of implantable cardioverter-defibrillators (ICDs) for primary prevention of sudden cardiac death. Individuals with stable ischemic heart disease (no recent myocardial infarction), especially those with inducible arrhythmias, seem to derive the highest mortality benefit from prophylactic ICD use. The role of ICDs in other patient populations is much less clear and even may be harmful. The use of antiarrhythmic medications has not been shown to improve survival in any patient population at risk for sudden death.

The transvenous implantable cardioverter-defibrillator (ICD) has been shown in multiple studies to be effective in the prevention of sudden cardiac death in select populations. The Achilles heel of traditional ICD technology has been the transvenous lead. The subcutaneous ICD provides effective sudden death protection while avoiding lead-related complications of traditional transvenous systems. The subcutaneous ICD is a reasonable option for patients with an ICD indication who do not need bradycardia pacing or cardiac resynchronization therapy.

There always will be a need to optimize early recognition and treatment of sudden cardiac arrest. For out-of-hospital cardiac arrest, this requires a complex system of care involving bystanders, 911 dispatchers, and emergency medical service and hospital-based providers. Optimizing this system is fundamental to improving outcomes. In addition, personnel and resources are needed to develop and sustain a research pipeline that will bring new scientific discoveries and technologies to the field. The 2015 Institute of Medicine report, *"Strategies to Improve Cardiac Arrest Survival: A Time to Act,"* provides a roadmap.

CARDIAC ELECTROPHYSIOLOGY CLINICS

THE CLINICS ARE AVAILABLE ONLINE!
Access your subscription at:
www.theclinics.com

Foreword
Sudden Cardiac Death: Back to the Future

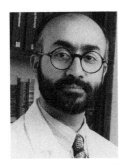
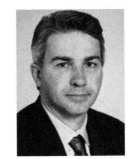

Ranjan K. Thakur, MD, MPH, MBA, FHRS   Andrea Natale, MD, FACC, FHRS

Consulting Editors

We are pleased to introduce this issue of *Cardiac Electrophysiology Clinics* on sudden cardiac death (SCD). In the 1960s and 1970s, a focus on arrhythmia mechanisms, ventricular arrhythmias, and SCD ushered in the field of cardiac electrophysiology and paved the way for adoption of the implantable cardioverter defibrillator. Befittingly, when *Cardiac Electrophysiology Clinics* was launched in December 2009, the topic chosen for a comprehensive review was SCD. Having covered myriad topics in electrophysiology over the past 8 years, we return once again, on the eighth anniversary of *Cardiac Electrophysiology Clinics*, to revisit the issue of SCD.

Despite decreasing cardiovascular mortality, including SCD mortality over the last few decades, it still remains a major public health issue, and there is much room for improvement in identifying those at risk and preventing SCD. Also, while per capita cardiovascular mortality is decreasing in the developed world, it may be increasing in much of the developing world, and therefore, it remains a prominent issue on a global scale. This issue of *Cardiac Electrophysiology Clinics* focuses on contemporary approaches and thoughts relevant to SCD.

We thank Drs Shenasa, Estes, and Tomaselli for editing this issue of *Cardiac Electrophysiology*

Clinics. They have invited expert contributors to summarize the current thinking on mechanisms of SCD, SCD in athletes and adolescents, identification of at-risk populations, and risk stratification, prevention, emergency management, and prophylaxis of SCD, to name a few topics covered in this issue. Electrophysiologists, cardiologists, and fellows in training will find these comprehensive review articles useful to bring them up to speed on contemporary ideas and controversies.

Ranjan K. Thakur, MD, MPH, MBA, FHRS
Sparrow Thoracic and Cardiovascular Institute
Michigan State University
1200 East Michigan Avenue, Suite 580
Lansing, MI 48912, USA

Andrea Natale, MD, FACC, FHRS
Texas Cardiac Arrhythmia Institute
Center for Atrial Fibrillation at
St David's Medical Center
1015 East 32nd Street, Suite 516
Austin, TX 78705, USA

E-mail addresses:
thakur@msu.edu (R.K. Thakur)
andrea.natale@stdavids.com (A. Natale)

Preface
Sudden Cardiac Death: Contemporary Challenges

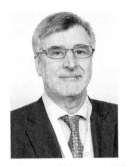 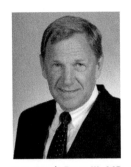 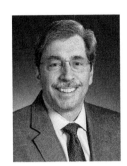

Mohammad Shenasa, MD   N.A. Mark Estes III, MD   Gordon F. Tomaselli, MD

Editors

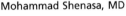

Despite the decline in mortality due to coronary artery disease over the last three decades, sudden cardiac death (SCD) remains a major health problem, claiming 250,000 to 300,000 lives annually in the United States. The annual incidence of SCD in Europe is similar to the United States, ranging from 50 to 100 per 100,000 in the general population. The overall survival rate remains poor, with only approximately 10% of individuals who experience a cardiac arrest surviving. Early defibrillation by an automated external defibrillator (AED) improves outcomes from cardiac arrest with survival rates to over 50% in some public locations. However, the majority of cardiac arrests occur in victim's homes, where AEDs have not improved survival. Based on these considerations, it is evident that identifying strategies for prediction and prevention of SCD represents an important public health priority.

Asymptomatic individuals without markers of high risk for cardiac arrest account for the majority of SCDs. Despite multiple advances in the strategies for SCD risk stratification, the current available techniques have limitations related to sensitivity, specificity, and cost-effectiveness. The goal of developing effective, low-cost, and noninvasive risk stratification tools for SCD remains elusive. While novel genetic and biological indicators of risk for SCD are being investigated, none have been integrated into clinical trials with interventions that improve overall survival.

Left ventricular ejection fraction (LVEF) remains the primary risk-stratification technique despite many limitations. Multiple prospective randomized clinical trials have shown reduction in arrhythmic death and total mortality when the patient's prior cardiac arrest is treated with implantable cardioverter-defibrillator (ICD) therapy for secondary prevention. In patients with impaired LVEF with prior myocardial infarction or dilated cardiomyopathies, pharmacologic therapy and ICDs have also been demonstrated to improve overall survival when used for primary prevention of SCD. Patients with heart failure with preserved ejection fraction represent a growing proportion of patients experiencing SCD. Risk stratification techniques and interventions that reduce arrhythmic death and improve overall mortality are being investigated.

With this background of an ongoing major public health problem of SCD and limitations of current strategies improving outcomes from cardiac arrest, we have elected to serve as editors of this issue to provide the reader with the best available science related to this important topic. In doing so, we have invited a multidisciplinary team of contributors with expertise in basic, translational, clinical, and population science. Each article not only provides a summary of the best available evidence related to sudden death, but also identifies critical knowledge gaps. Authors have also identified future research that will address these gaps and improve prediction and prevention of sudden death and patient survival.

As editors, we are grateful to the authors for providing a contemporary review of the best available science related to SCD. We also thank the

Card Electrophysiol Clin 9 (2017) xvii–xviii
https://doi.org/10.1016/j.ccep.2017.10.001
1877-9182/17/© 2017 Published by Elsevier Inc.

Elsevier staff for their guidance and professionalism. We are confident that this issue will give all who provide care to patients with cardiovascular disease the most up-to-date knowledge related to mechanisms and clinical strategies for prediction and prevention of SCD.

The Editors

Mohammad Shenasa, MD
Heart and Rhythm Medical Group
Department of Cardiovascular Services
O'Connor Hospital
San Jose, CA 95128, USA

N.A. Mark Estes III, MD
Tufts University School of Medicine
New England Cardiac Arrhythmia Center
Tufts Medical Center
Boston, MA 02111, USA

Gordon F. Tomaselli, MD
Johns Hopkins School of Medicine
Baltimore, MD 21287, USA

E-mail addresses:
mohammad.shenasa@gmail.com (M. Shenasa)
nestes@tuftsmedicalcenter.org (N.A.M. Estes)
gtomasel@jhmi.edu (G.F. Tomaselli)

Sudden Cardiac Death
Interface Between Pathophysiology and Epidemiology

Robert J. Myerburg, MD

KEYWORDS

- Sudden cardiac death • Cardiac arrest • Coronary heart disease • Population risk • Epidemiology
- Ventricular tachyarrhythmias • Asystole • Pulseless electrical activity

KEY POINTS

- Sudden cardiac death (SCD) accounts for 50% of all cardiovascular deaths; approximately 50% of all SCDs are first cardiac events; sudden cardiac arrest (SCA) accounts for up to 50% of heart disease–related years of productive life lost.
- Measures of risk of SCA and SCD can be substrate based or expression based.
- The pathophysiologic cascade for SCA includes modules of atherogenesis, plaque destabilization, onset of ischemia, and arrhythmia.
- Mechanisms of tachyarrhythmias leading to SCA differ for onset of ischemia and reperfusion of ischemic myocardium.

Sudden cardiac arrest (SCA), defined as an event characterized by an abrupt loss of blood flow caused by an unexpected cessation of cardiac mechanical function, followed by the outcome of sudden cardiac death (SCD), is a major public health problem because of its incidence and demographics. Current estimates for out-of-hospital SCDs are in the range of 390,000 per year in the United States[1,2] (**Box 1**). The number of emergency medical system (EMS)–assessed out-of-hospital SCAs (OHCAs) in the United States is estimated at 356,000, among which 347,500 are in adults more than 18 years of age.[1] An additional 200,000 in-hospital SCAs (IHCAs) occur annually.[3] The overall national survival rates following OHCA and IHCA are in the range of 10% and 26%, respectively. A perspective on the impact of SCD is provided by the so-called rule of 50s[2]: SCD accounts for 50% of all cardiovascular deaths[4]; approximately 50% of all SCDs are first (recognized) expressions of a cardiac disorder[5]; and SCA accounts for up to 50% of heart disease–related loss of years of productive life.[6] The loss of years of productive life includes both premature deaths and the consequences of persisting neurologic damage following SCA among survivors. Despite this long-recognized large public health burden attributable to SCA and SCD, prediction of risk at the individual patient level remains very limited.[2] Population studies and clinical trials have identified high-risk subgroups, but individual risk prediction, especially among the general population, awaits the identification of more powerful markers than are currently available. The exceptions are a few very-high-risk subgroups or specific causes in which individual risk prediction is adequate, but most events emerge from other segments of the population.

Four temporal elements contribute to the pathophysiologic bases of risk, expression, and outcomes of SCA: (1) prodromes, (2) onset of symptoms heralding cardiac arrest, (3) the SCA itself, and (4) consequent death versus survival.

Disclosures: None.
Division of Cardiology, University of Miami Miller School of Medicine, D-39, PO Box 016960, Miami, FL 33101, USA

Card Electrophysiol Clin 9 (2017) 515–524
http://dx.doi.org/10.1016/j.ccep.2017.07.003
1877-9182/17/© 2017 Elsevier Inc. All rights reserved.

cardiacEP.theclinics.com

Box 1

Site-specific incidence of sudden cardiac arrest (SCA). Recent incidence figures for sudden cardiac arrest in the United States are provided for out-of-hospital and in-hospital events, with subgroups according to specific sites

Out of hospital	~390,000 annually in United States
Cumulative survival ~10%	
Home/residence	~80% of events; survival 6%
Public venues (general)	~15% to 25% survival
Public venues (specific) (eg, airports, airliners, casinos)	40% to 70% survival
In hospital	~200,000 annually in United States
Cumulative survival ~24%	
SCA during procedures in electrophysiology and cardiac catheterization laboratory	Greater than 95% survival
SCA in coronary care unit or medical intensive care unit	Greater than 90% survival (ACS)
	Greater than 40% survival (transient factors)
	Less than 30% survival (heart failure; shock)
General care units	~15% to 20% survival

Because the proximate cause of SCA is an abrupt disturbance in cardiovascular function resulting in loss of consciousness caused by cessation of blood flow, the time definition must recognize the brief interval between onset of the mechanism directly responsible for initiating the cardiac arrest and the consequent loss of blood flow. The arbitrary 1-hour definition primarily refers to the duration of the heralding symptoms, and defines the interval between the onset of symptoms signaling the pathophysiologic disturbance leading to cardiac arrest and the onset of the cardiac arrest. When the pathophysiologic onset is an acute myocardial infarction or abrupt worsening of heart failure, a 1-hour definition (or longer) is appropriate, but when the heralding event is a hemodynamically significant tachyarrhythmia, the interval between onset and cardiac arrest is often a matter of seconds. Once cardiac output ceases, or central systolic blood pressure decreases to less than 60 mm Hg, loss of consciousness occurs rapidly. Human centrifuge studies during the early years of the space program identified an interval between abrupt cessation of carotid blood flow and loss of consciousness of 10 seconds or less.

Prodromes, occurring during the weeks or months before an SCA, if recognized, are general predictors of an impending event, but are not specific for SCA itself. The same premonitory signs and symptoms may be more specific for the imminent cardiac arrest when they begin abruptly. Sudden onset of chest pain, dyspnea, or palpitations and other symptoms of arrhythmias often occur within the 1-hour before the onset of the SCA. In contrast, the fourth element, biological death, may range from minutes in the absence of return of spontaneous circulation (ROSC) to a much longer delay in patients who remain biologically alive for a long period after ROSC because of failure to restore hemodynamic, metabolic, or neurologic function and stability, but ultimately leading to death. In the latter circumstance, the causative pathophysiologic and clinical event is the SCA, because the SCA is the factor responsible for the delayed biological death. Most studies link the SCD (the outcome) to the SCA (the event), rather than to a biological death that occurs during hospitalization after cardiac arrest or within 30 days. Thus, when a consequent death follows an SCA during the days or weeks of a postarrest hospitalization, it should still be defined as an SCD following an SCA. In contrast, unwitnessed deaths use the definition of SCD for persons known to be alive and functional 24 hours prior, assuming other causes, such as neurologic, hemorrhagic, traumatic, or toxicologic causes, are not identified postmortem. Not all sudden deaths that seem to be cardiac are actually cardiac in origin based on subsequent evaluation.[7] A significant proportion are associated with abrupt neurologic events or other noncardiac causes. This point emphasizes the importance of careful adjudication of events when analyzing causation data. Another caution relates to patients with unexplained SCDs, based on negative autopsy findings. Under these circumstances, postmortem genetic studies should be performed in order to identify previously undiagnosed genetic disorders, particularly among persons who are less than or equal to 40 years of age at the time of SCD.[8]

INCIDENCE OF SUDDEN CARDIAC ARREST

The incidence of SCD has long been estimated to be in the range of 1 per 1000 population per year for the middle-aged and older population.[9] Although the age at which an SCD occurs has shifted to an older age group over years, likely resulting from a combination of coronary risk factor control strategies and interventions for acute coronary syndromes, the cumulative population burden, measured as total number of SCDs, has not changed substantially but has shifted to an older age group. At the other end of the postinfancy and childhood age spectrum, specifically adolescents and young adults, the incidence of SCD is estimated at 1 per 100,000 per year, or 1% of that of the middle-aged and older population.[9] Despite these small numbers, there is specific added benefit to be gained by prediction and prevention of SCA in the younger population because the disorders that are associated with these events are those in which prevention or successful intervention is associated with much greater gains in the number of added years of quality life compared with the older population that has more comorbidities and more advanced heart disease structurally. As an example, a study of outcomes in patients with long QT who had not been diagnosed with or not undergone preventive treatment after diagnosis reported a cumulative mortality of 13% by the age of 40 years,[10] compared with less than 4% in men and less than 3% in women in the general population in that age range cited in the mortality tables for the US population. This large number of deaths for a disorder that is now treatable is an example of the value of identifying carriers in advance of cardiac events.

CAUSES AND MECHANISMS OF CARDIAC ARREST

It has long been established that coronary atherosclerosis is the most common cause of SCA and SCD in Western societies, with an increasing dominance in other areas as the world becomes more uniformly developed. The general estimates cite coronary artery disease as the cause in up to 80% of the SCDs in the United States among patients more than 35 years of age.[9] The cardiomyopathies as a group are second, accounting for approximately 10% to 20% of all SCDs, and various other disorders, such as inflammatory, infiltrative, and heart valve diseases, account for a smaller number, on the order of 5% or less. The rare diseases, such as the genetic arrhythmia syndromes, are far less common in the population more than 35 years of age, compared with a younger population, but do play a small role. Among adolescents and young adults, the pattern is different, with myocarditis and the inherited

structural diseases and arrhythmia syndromes playing important roles. In the age range between 25 and 35 years, a causation transition occurs, with increasing probability of coronary artery disease and dilated cardiomyopathy as causes during that period, compared with the other syndromes mentioned for a younger age group[9] (**Fig. 1**).

When considering the interaction between specific disease causes and mechanisms of SCA, there are 4 elements that must be taken into consideration: (1) definitions, (2) substrate-based risk, (3) expression-based risk, and (4) electrical mechanisms responsible for loss of cardiac mechanical function. As shown in **Box 2**, definitions of these components of a sudden death model should distinguish between SCA as a clinical event and SCD as the outcome. In addition, substrate and expression are separated into 2 categories, with substrate based on the anatomic (in some causes the so-called molecular anatomy) component of pathophysiology, and expression based on the dynamic components of pathophysiology. As stated earlier, coronary artery disease is the most common anatomic basis for SCA and SCD, and is defined by the pathology and pathophysiology of coronary artery disease and the anatomic and physiologic considerations of myocardial consequences of the coronary vascular disorder. A different set of substrate considerations apply to the less common anatomic causes, such as the nonischemic cardiomyopathies, infiltrative and inflammatory disorders, and cardiac valve disorders. A great deal of interest is evolving with regard to the anatomy and physiology of hypertrophied myocardium and associated myocardial scarring. These components of the anatomic substrate of SCD are increasingly suggested as risk markers and a great deal of effort is going into the definition and pathophysiology of the hypertension/hypertrophy complex and secondary scarring.

Expression-based risk considerations focus on the electrophysiologic triggering roles of transient variables based on their interaction with anatomy abnormalities. These variables include left ventricle dysfunction and heart failure, metabolic abnormalities, and autonomic fluctuations. **Fig. 2** is an algorithm showing the various components of the coronary heart disease spectrum that contributes to the risk for SCA. These components include transient ischemia, myocardial infarction, scar-related arrhythmia propensity, and the hemodynamics of ischemic cardiomyopathy.

The common denominator in cardiac arrest is loss of cardiac mechanical function, which most commonly occurs in the context of a triggering electrical event. In the past, ventricular fibrillation (VF) and pulseless ventricular tachycardia (pVT)

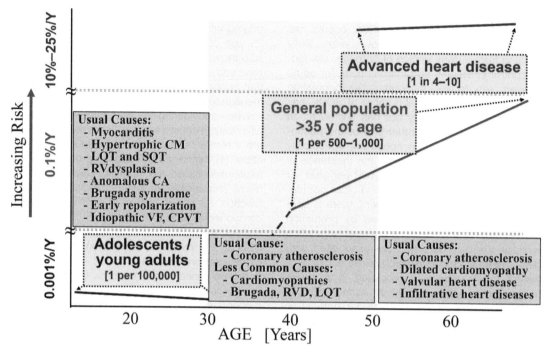

Fig. 1. Age-specific and disease-specific risk for SCD. For the general population 35 years and older, the risk for SCD is 0.1% to 0.2% per year (1 per 500–1000 population), with a wide range of subgroup risks based on the number and power of individual risk factors. Causes are dominated by coronary heart disease and nonischemic cardiomyopathy. Age-related risk for SCD increases beyond the age of 35 years. In patients older than 30 years with advanced structural heart disease and markers of high risk for cardiac arrest, the event rate may exceed 25% per year, and the age-related risk is attenuated. In adolescents and adults, the overall risk for SCD is 1 per 100,000 population or 0.001% per year, with a variety of causes such as inherited structural and electrical disorders, developmental defects, and myocarditis dominating. In the transition range from 30 to 45 years of age, the relative frequency of the uncommon disease yields to the dominance of coronary heart disease and nonischemic cardiomyopathy, but both groups of potential causes must be entertained because many of the rare disorders are expressed in that age range. CA, coronary artery; CM, cardiomyopathy; CPVT, catecholaminergic polymorphic ventricular tachycardia; LQT, long QT; RV, right ventricular; RVD, right ventricular dysplasia; SQT, short QT; VF, ventricullar fibrillation. (*Modified from* Myerburg RJ, Castellanos A. Cardiac arrest and sudden cardiac death. Chapter 39. In: Mann DL, Zipes DP, Libby P, et al, editors. Braunwald's heart disease: a textbook of cardiovascular medicine. 10th edition. Oxford (United Kingdom): Elsevier; 2015. p. 821–60; with permission.)

had been identified as the most commonly recognized initial rhythms after the onset of a cardiac arrest, but the proportion of the tachyarrhythmic mechanisms has been decreasing over the years. Tachyarrhythmic hemodynamic consequences notwithstanding, it is obvious that failure of electrical activity (asystole) or failure of mechanical activation by electrical impulses (pulseless electrical activity [PEA]) are also potential mechanisms. Recent statistics identify asystole as the most common mechanism recorded at initial contact by out-of-hospital responders, accounting for up to 50% of the initial rhythms. PEA accounts for approximately 25%, and the tachyarrhythmic patterns are now only about 25% of initial rhythms. Whether this is a direct result of changes in pathophysiologic mechanisms or a consequence of change in preventive medical therapy over the years, versus delayed response times by EMS

covering larger geographic areas, is uncertain. It is likely that both contribute to these observations. It has even been suggested in one study that the common use of β-blockers favors asystole as the initial rhythm in cardiac arrest because of the antifibrillatory potential of this class of drugs.[11]

One subtlety in definition that is often overlooked by responders is the distinction between pVT and PEA. The conventional definition of pVT is a rapid ventricular tachyarrhythmia with loss of pulse and blood flow caused by a rapid rate in a ventricle with advanced disease. In contrast, PEA is generally a slower electrical rate with failure of the electrical impulse to initiate a mechanical event. Because pVT is a shockable rhythm, which, according to some data, has a better outcome than VF, whereas PEA is a nonshockable rhythm with a poor prognosis, the emphasis of this distinction is important. It is sometimes difficult

---

Box 2
Causes and mechanisms of sudden cardiac death: interactions between disorder and pathophysiology

Definitions	SCA (event); SCD (outcome)
Substrate-based risk	Coronary heart disease
	• State of epicardial and intramyocardial vessels
	• Myocardial infarction
	Myopathy, infiltration, inflammation, valvulopathy
	Hypertrophy and scarring
Expression-based risk	Left ventricle dysfunction; heart failure; metabolic; autonomic fluctuations
	Molecular: genopathies/proteinopathies
Distribution of mechanism-based causes	Ventricular fibrillation/pulseless ventricular tachycardia, pulseless electrical activity, asystole

Modified from Myerburg RJ, Castellanos A. Cardiac arrest and sudden cardiac death. Chapter 39. In: Mann DL, Zipes DP, Libby P, et al, editors. Braunwald's heart disease: a textbook of cardiovascular medicine. 10th edition. Oxford (United Kingdom): Elsevier; 2015. p. 821–60; with permission.

---

when the rate of PEA is rapid, although typical PEA is usually at a rate slower than 100 impulses per minute. When there is doubt, based on an intermediate rate, a shock should be delivered, even though shocking classic slow PEA is futile.

In recent years, there seems to have been a shift in patterns of the anatomic basis for SCD derived from studies in unselected adult SCD populations.[12] The major observations emerging from these studies highlight the importance of hypertensive heart

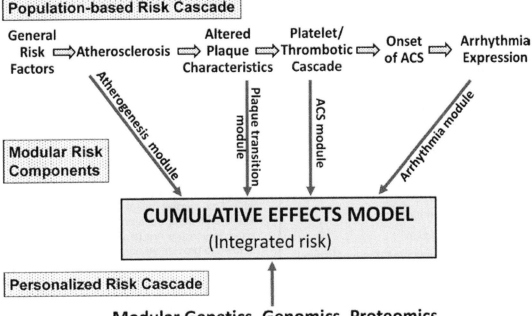

Fig. 2. Population-based and personalized risk cascades for SCA resulting from coronary artery disease. Four modules of population risk for the development and expression of coronary artery disease and its arrhythmic complications are shown. These modules each contribute to the cumulative risk for the development and expression of coronary artery disease and its arrhythmic complications. The 4 expression models may interact with the inheritance module, potentially adding power for individual risk prediction. (*From* Myerburg RJ, Junttila MJ: Sudden cardiac death caused by coronary heart disease. Circulation 125:1043, 2012; with permission.)

disease, with left ventricular hypertrophy–associated secondary myocardial scarring, and a nonspecific fibrotic heart disease pattern that has been observed in at least 1 study in a fairly young population.[13] These anatomic associations, based on postmortem studies, have reduced the proportional contribution of coronary artery disease to these events, but it still remains the most common cause.

In considering a causal association with SCAs, it is important to consider the interactions between structure-based predispositions and expression-risk modulators. The latter include left ventricular function and heart failure hemodynamics, metabolic abnormalities, and autonomic fluctuations. The notion of substrate-based risk associations and expression-based risk associations are not alternatives to one another but are interactive. As such, both can contribute to clinicians' ability to risk profile, derived from understanding of the interaction between anatomic features and pathophysiologic triggers.

MECHANISTIC TARGETS DERIVED FROM EPIDEMIOLOGIC SUBDIVISIONS

Preventive strategies targeting risk for SCA and SCD can be divided into 4 epidemiologic targets (**Box 3**). The most commonly used model from a general population perspective is conventional preventive epidemiology, targeted to primary or secondary prevention of structural heart disease

and in some cases to mechanisms of expression, such as hypertension. A second model focuses on transient risk factors as an epidemiologic category incorporating the triggering mechanisms. A commonly appreciated model of transient risk is based on the category of acute coronary syndromes and transient ischemia creating electrical instability and interacting with hemodynamic and autonomic variation. A prominent component of transient risk envisions predictors of transition from stable to unstable coronary artery plaque status, one mechanism of which may be recognizable inflammatory markers in advance of the transition. However, the limitation of this as an epidemiologic model is the short lead time between a change in the pathophysiologic state of a blood vessel or myocardium and its influence on triggering cardiac arrest.

A third model brings in the concept of individual or personalized risk based on family history, which may be driven in part by genetic determinants of risk, although cultural and lifestyle factors within families or population subsets may also contribute to these patterns. Four studies of different population sets have each come to the conclusion that a family history of SCD as the initial manifestation of previously undiagnosed or unrecognized heart disease increases the probability that subsequent generations will present SCAs in the same way. The populations studied included patients with out-of-hospital cardiac arrest,[14] a long-term prospectively followed general population of individuals who were healthy at entry into surveillance,[15] a cohort of patients presenting with ventricular tachyarrhythmias during the early phase of acute coronary syndromes,[16] and a postmortem study involving SCDs in the community.[17] The fact that the 4 different populations showed the same familial SCA clustering phenomenon supports the notion that familial clustering of SCA as a first cardiac event is likely to be correct. The limitation for each of the studies is the effect sizes, which are not large enough in any of the studies to provide stand-alone support for historical marker as a major criterion for major risk stratification. However, these observations do invite investigations into genetics of SCA expression, for which a limited amount of data currently exists. Additional studies are in progress.

The fourth model, referred to as interventional epidemiology, incorporates epidemiologic nuances derived from clinical trial data or large population subsets. It also contains a component of surveillance studies from large population databases, in an attempt to identify risk markers for SCA.

Box 3
Sudden cardiac death as a challenge for population sciences: range of epidemiologic targets

Conventional epidemiology

- Population risk and primary prevention (eg, atherogenesis)
- Secondary prevention

Transient risk prediction

- Acute coronary syndrome/transient ischemia, electrical instability, hemodynamic changes, autonomic predictors, infarction

Genetic epidemiology

- Individual (personalized) risk
- Prediction of specific expression

Interventional epidemiology

- Predictors derived from clinical trials
- Long-term surveillance observations: efficacy and safety

MECHANISMS AND PATHOPHYSIOLOGY OF SUDDEN CARDIAC ARREST IN CORONARY HEART DISEASE

SCDs caused by coronary heart disease, lethal tachyarrhythmias, or asystolic or PEA mechanisms are all the consequences of pathophysiologic cascades resulting from complex interactions between coronary vascular events, myocardial injury, variations in autonomic tone, and the metabolic and electrolyte state of the myocardium.[18,19] The general cascade, most easily viewed in the context of SCD associated with coronary heart disease, incorporates a series of modules ranging from atherogenesis, through disease development and modulation, to arrhythmogensis[18] (see **Fig. 2**). There is no single hypothesis outlining mechanisms by which these elements interact to lead to the final pathway of lethal arrhythmias. Each module is distinct with regard to contribution to risk of SCD, and all must be integrated to establish a comprehensive pathophysiologic model. **Fig. 3** shows the pathophysiologic processes, in contrast with risk modules, that may lead to SCA in coronary heart disease. These processes include the vascular,

myocardial, and functional components.[19] Risk for SCA is based on the presence of structural abnormalities that are modulated by functional variations.

Among patients with tachyarrhythmic SCAs caused by coronary atherosclerosis, the extent of chronic arterial narrowing has been well defined by multiple pathologic studies. However, the mechanisms by which these lesions associate with arrhythmogenic electrophysiologic disturbances extend beyond the consequence of steady-state reductions in regional myocardial blood flow interacting with varying oxygen demands.[20,21] A simple increase in myocardial oxygen demand, in the presence of a fixed supply, may contribute to exercise-induced arrhythmias and SCA during intense physical activity. However, the dynamic nature of the pathophysiologic mechanism of coronary events has led to the recognition that superimposed acute transitions of a chronic coronary lesions create a setting in which the metabolic or electrolyte state of the myocardium is the common circumstance leading to disturbed electrical stability. Active vascular events resulting in an acute or transient reduction in regional myocardial blood flow in the presence

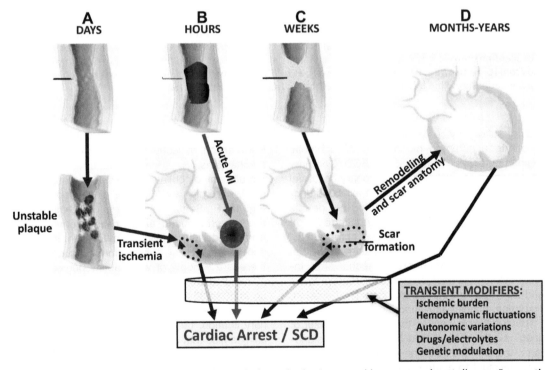

Fig. 3. Pathophysiology of life-threatening ventricular arrhythmias caused by coronary heart disease. Four pathophysiologic substrates contribute to arrhythmic risk and SCD in coronary artery disease: (*A*) transient ischemia, (*B*) acute coronary syndromes, (*C*) scar-related pathophysiology, and (*D*) ischemic cardiomyopathy. The pathophysiology, clinical implications, and long-term risk of each are described in the text. MI, myocardial infarction. (*Modified from* Myerburg RJ, Kessler KM, Mallon SM, et al. Life-threatening ventricular arrhythmias in patients with silent myocardial ischemia due to coronary artery spasm. N Engl J Med 1992;326:1451–5; with permission.)

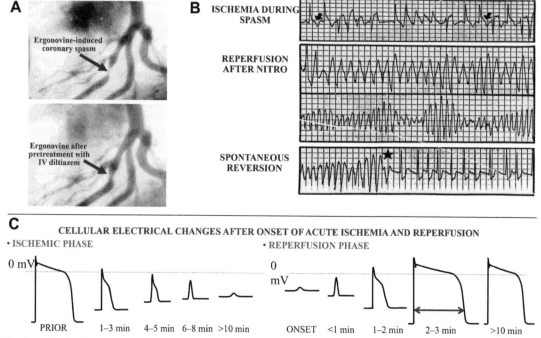

A

Ergonovine-induced coronary spasm

Ergonovine after pretreatment with IV diltiazem

B ISCHEMIA DURING SPASM

REPERFUSION AFTER NITRO

SPONTANEOUS REVERSION

C

CELLULAR ELECTRICAL CHANGES AFTER ONSET OF ACUTE ISCHEMIA AND REPERFUSION

• ISCHEMIC PHASE

• REPERFUSION PHASE

0 mV

0 mV

PRIOR　1–3 min　4–5 min　6–8 min　>10 min　　ONSET　<1 min　1–2 min　2–3 min　>10 min

Fig. 4. Arrhythmias associated with ischemia and reperfusion caused by/because of coronary artery spasm. (*A*) Induction of coronary artery spasm by ergonovine in a survivor of cardiac arrest, with blunting of the response after pretreatment with diltiazem. (*B*) Arrhythmias recorded during spasm-associated ischemia and reperfusion, the latter being a polymorphic VT with spontaneous conversion. (*C*) The cellular responses to the experimental equivalents of ischemia and reperfusion. Reperfusion was associated with induction of a transient prolongation of the time course of repolarization (*red arrow*). See text for discussion. IV, intravenous; NITRO, nitroglycerine. (*Modified from* [*A, B*] Myerburg RJ, Kessler KM, Mallon SM, et al. Life-threatening ventricular arrhythmias in patients with silent myocardial ischemia due to coronary artery spasm. N Engl J Med 1992;326:1451–5; with permission; and *From* [*C*] Furukawa T, Bassett AL, Furukawa N, et al. The ionic mechanism of reperfusion-induced early afterdepolarizations in feline left ventricular hypertrophy. J Clin Invest 1993;91:1521–31.)

of a normal or previously compromised circulation constitute a common mechanism of ischemia, angina pectoris, arrhythmias, and SCD. Coronary artery spasm or modulation of coronary collateral flow, predisposed to by local endothelial dysfunction, exposes the myocardium to the double hazard of transient ischemia and reperfusion (**Fig. 4**). Vascular susceptibility and humoral factors, notably those related to platelet activation and aggregation, are important mechanisms. Inflammatory responses in atherosclerotic plaques lead to lesion progression, including erosion, disruption, platelet activation, and thrombosis.

Acute ischemia causes the immediate onset of electrical, mechanical, and biochemical dysfunction of cardiac muscle. The His-Purkinje tissue is more resistant to acute ischemia than is working myocardium, and therefore the electrophysiologic consequences are less intense and more delayed in onset in specialized conduction tissue. In addition to the direct effect of ischemia on normal or previously abnormal tissue, reperfusion after

transient ischemia can cause lethal arrhythmias. Reperfusion of ischemic areas can occur by 3 mechanisms: (1) spontaneous thrombolysis, (2) recruitment of collateral vessels in response to local ischemia, and (3) relief of vasospasm (see **Fig. 4**A, B). Some mechanisms of life-threatening reperfusion-induced arrhythmias seem to result from the duration of ischemia. Experimental data, and some clinical observations,[19] suggest that there is a window of vulnerability beginning 5 to 10 minutes after the onset of ischemia and lasting up to 20 to 30 minutes.

Within the first minutes after experimental coronary ligation, there is a propensity to ventricular arrhythmias that abate after 30 minutes and reappear after several hours. The initial 30 minutes of arrhythmias is divided into 2 periods, the first of which lasts for approximately 10 minutes and is related to the acute ischemic burden. The next 20 to 30 minutes may be related either to reperfusion of ischemic areas or to the continuing evolution of nonuniform injury patterns in the affected myocardium. Multiple mechanisms of reperfusion arrhythmias have been observed experimentally, including slow conduction and reentry, enhanced normal automaticity in specialized conducting tissue, and afterdepolarizations and triggered activity. With regard to afterdepolarizations and triggered activity, reperfusion after 10 to 30 minutes of transient ischemia causes a transient prolongation of the time course of repolarization in the affected muscle (see **Fig. 4**C), a cellular equivalent of prolonged QT in the region.[22] This mechanism is associated with triggered activity.

At the level of the myocyte, the onset of ischemia is associated with efflux of K^+, influx of Ca^{2+}, acidosis, and reduction of transmembrane resting potentials, which are followed by a separate series of changes during reperfusion. Those of particular interest are the influx of Ca^{2+}, which may produce electrical instability and afterdepolarizations as triggering responses for Ca^{2+}-dependent arrhythmias. Other possible mechanisms studied experimentally include the formation of superoxide radicals in reperfusion arrhythmias and differential responses of endocardial and epicardial muscle activation times and refractory periods during ischemia or reperfusion. The adenosine triphosphate–dependent K^+ current, which is inactive during normal conditions, is activated during ischemia, resulting in efflux of K^+ ions from myocytes and marked shortening of the time course of repolarization, which leads to slow conduction and ultimately to inexcitability.[23] This response is more marked in epicardium than in endocardium, leading to a prominent dispersion of repolarization across the myocardium during transmural ischemia. At an intercellular level, ischemia alters the distribution of connexin 43, the primary gap junction protein between myocytes. This alteration results in uncoupling of myocytes, which is a factor that is arrhythmogenic because of altered patterns of excitation and regional changes in conduction velocity.[24]

Tissue that has healed after ischemic injury seems to be more susceptible to the destabilizing effects of acute ischemia, as is chronically hypertrophied muscle. Remodeling-induced local stretch, regional hypertrophy, or intrinsic cellular alteration may contribute to this vulnerability. Of more direct clinical relevance is K^+ depletion by diuretics because clinical hypokalemia may make ventricular myocardium more susceptible to potentially lethal arrhythmias, in part by its effect on repolarization (QT) duration. Other metabolic changes, including increase of cyclic adenosine monophosphate levels, accumulation of free fatty acids and their metabolites, formation of lysophosphoglycerides, and impaired myocardial glycolysis, are also suggested destabilizing influences.[24]

TRANSITION FROM MYOCARDIAL INSTABILITY TO LETHAL TACHYARRHYTHMIAS

A triggering event interacting with susceptible myocardium is a primary mechanism leading to the initiation of lethal arrhythmias (see **Figs. 2 and 3**). The triggering event for ventricular tachycardia (VT) or VF, or persisting risk for recurrence, can be electrophysiologic, ischemic, metabolic, or hemodynamic. For VF, the end point of these interactions is disorganization of patterns of myocardial activation into multiple uncoordinated reentrant pathways. Clinical, experimental, and pharmacologic data have suggested that triggering events in the absence of myocardial instability are less likely to initiate lethal arrhythmias.

ASYSTOLIC ARREST

The basic electrophysiologic mechanism in this form of arrest is failure of normal subordinate automatic activity to assume mechanical activation of the ventricular myocardium, caused by the absence of the electrical stimulus. Asystolic arrest is more common in severely diseased hearts and in patients with several end-stage disorders, both cardiac and noncardiac. These mechanisms may result, in part, from diffuse involvement of subendocardial Purkinje fibers in advanced heart disease.

PULSELESS ELECTRICAL ACTIVITY

PEA is separated into primary and secondary forms. No single unifying definition for PEA, mechanistically or clinically, is generally accepted. The common denominator is the presence of organized cardiac electrical activity in the absence of effective mechanical function.[25] The absence of rapid ROSC is important in that it excludes transient losses of cerebral blood flow, such as the various patterns of vasovagal reflex syncope, which have different clinical implications than the meaning attributed to true PEA. The secondary form of PEA results from an abrupt cessation of cardiac venous return, such as massive pulmonary embolism, acute malfunction of prosthetic valves, exsanguination, and cardiac tamponade from hemopericardium. The primary form is the more familiar; in this form none of these obvious mechanical factors is present, but ventricular muscle fails to produce an effective contraction despite continued electrical activity. It usually occurs as an end-stage event in advanced heart disease, but it can occur in patients with acute ischemic events or, more commonly, after electrical resuscitation from prolonged cardiac arrest. Although it is not thoroughly understood, it seems that diffuse disease, metabolic abnormalities, or global ischemia provides the pathophysiologic substrate. The proximate mechanism for failure of electromechanical coupling may be abnormal intracellular Ca^{2+} metabolism, intracellular acidosis, or perhaps depletion of ATP.

REFERENCES

1. Mozaffarian D, Benjamin EJ, Go AS, et al. American Heart Association Statistics Committee and Stroke Statistics Subcommittee: heart disease and stroke statistics–2016 update: a report from the American Heart Association. Circulation 2016;133:e38–360.
2. Myerburg RJ, Goldberger JJ. Sudden cardiac arrest risk assessment: population science and the individual risk mandate. JAMA Cardiol 2017;2(6):689–94.
3. Merchant RM, Yang L, Becker LB, et al, American Heart Association Get with the Guidelines–Resuscitation Investigators. Incidence of treated cardiac arrest in hospitalized patients in the United States. Crit Care Med 2011;39:2401–6.
4. Goldberger JJ, Buxton AE, Cain M, et al. Risk stratification for arrhythmic sudden cardiac death: identifying the roadblocks. Circulation 2011;123: 2423–30.
5. Fishman GI, Chugh SS, DiMarco JP, et al. Sudden cardiac death prediction and prevention. Report from a National Heart, Lung, and Blood Institute and Heart Rhythm Society workshop. Circulation 2010;122:2335–48.
6. Stecker EC, Reinier K, Marijon E, et al. Public health burden of sudden cardiac death in the United States. Circ Arrhythm Electrophysiol 2014;7:212–7.
7. Kim AS, Moffatt E, Ursell PC, et al. Sudden neurological death masquerading as out-of-hospital sudden cardiac death. Neurology 2016;87:1669–73.
8. Bagnall RD, Weintraub RG, Ingles J, et al. A prospective study of sudden cardiac death among children and young adults. N Engl J Med 2016;374:2441–52.
9. Myerburg RJ, Castellanos A. Cardiac arrest and sudden cardiac death. Chapter 39. In: Mann DL, Zipes DP, Libby P, et al, editors. Braunwald's heart disease: a textbook of cardiovascular medicine. 10th edition. Oxford (United Kingdom): Elsevier; 2015. p. 821–60.
10. Priori SG, Schwartz PJ, Napolitano C, et al. Risk stratification in the long-QT syndrome. N Engl J Med 2003;348:1866–74.
11. Youngquist ST, Kaji AH, Niemann JT. Beta-blocker use and the changing epidemiology of out-of-hospital cardiac arrest rhythms. Resuscitation 2008;76:376–80.
12. Junttila MJ, Hookana E, Kaikonnen K, et al. Temporal trends in the clinical and pathological characteristics of victims of sudden cardiac death in the absence of previously identified heart disease. Circ Arrhythm Electrophysiol 2016;9(6) [pii:e003723].
13. Hookana E, Junttila MJ, Puurunen V-P, et al. Causes of non-ischemic sudden cardiac death in the current era. Heart Rhythm 2011;8:1570–5.
14. Friedlander Y, Siscovick DS, Weinmann S, et al. Family history as a risk factor for primary cardiac arrest. Circulation 1998;97:155.
15. Jouven X, Desnos M, Guerot C, et al. Predicting sudden death in the population: the Paris Prospective Study I. Circulation 1978;99:1999.
16. Dekker LR, Bezzina CR, Henriques JP, et al. Familial sudden death is an important risk factor for primary ventricular fibrillation: a case-control study in acute myocardial infarction patients. Circulation 2006; 114:1140–5.
17. Kaikkonen KS, Kortelainen ML, Linna E, et al. Family history and the risk of sudden cardiac death as a manifestation of an acute coronary event. Circulation 2006;114:1462–7.
18. Myerburg RJ, Junttila MJ. Sudden cardiac death caused by coronary heart disease. Circulation 2012;125:1043.
19. Myerburg RJ, Kessler KM, Mallon SM, et al. Life-threatening ventricular arrhythmias in patients with silent myocardial ischemia due to coronary artery spasm. N Engl J Med 1992;326:1451–5.
20. Myerburg RJ. Sudden cardiac death: exploring the limits of our knowledge. J Cardiovasc Electrophysiol 2001;12:369.
21. Huikuri H, Castellanos A, Myerburg RJ. Sudden death due to cardiac arrhythmias. N Engl J Med 2001;345:1473.
22. Furukawa T, Bassett AL, Furukawa N, et al. The ionic mechanism of reperfusion-induced early afterdepolarizations in feline left ventricular hypertrophy. J Clin Invest 1993;91:1521–31.
23. Furukawa T, Kimura S, Furukawa N, et al. Role of cardiac ATP-regulated potassium channels in differential responses of endocardial and epicardial cells to ischemia. Circ Res 1991;68:1693–702.
24. Beardslee MA, Lerner L, Tadros PN, et al. Dephosphorylation and intracellular redistribution of ventricular connexin 43 during electrical uncoupling induced by ischemia. Circ Res 2000;87:656.
25. Myerburg RJ, Halperin H, Egan D, et al. Pulseless electrical activity – definition, causes, mechanisms, management, and research priorities for the next decade: report from a National Heart, Lung, and Blood Institute workshop. Circulation 2013;128: 2532.

Basic Electrophysiologic Mechanisms of Sudden Cardiac Death Caused by Acute Myocardial Ischemia and Infarction

CrossMark

Andrew L. Wit, PhD

KEYWORDS

- Ischemia • Action potentials • Gap junctions • Reentry

KEY POINTS

- Ischemia causes increased $[K^+]_o$ that depolarizes the resting potential.
- Ischemia causes reduction in phase 0 depolarization.
- Ischemia causes gap junction uncoupling.
- Slowing of conduction and conduction block lead to formation of reentrant circuits.
- Flow of injury currents cause arrhythmias.

INTRODUCTION

Sudden cardiac death has traditionally been defined as "the unexpected natural death from a cardiac cause within a short period, usually ≤1 hour from the onset of symptoms in a person without any prior conditions that would appear fatal."[1,2] A rapid death of this kind is often a result of cardiac arrhythmias, although a significant number of deaths are unwitnessed. Up to 80% of individuals who suffer sudden cardiac death have coronary artery disease.[1] Approximately 20% of patients who survive cardiac arrest develop transmural myocardial infarction. Transient myocardial ischemia caused by coronary vasospasm or unstable platelet thrombi also play a role in precipitating fatal arrhythmias.[1]

Myocardial ischemia, whether transient or long lasting, resulting in myocardial infarction causes changes in the electrical properties of myocardial cells. Experimental laboratory studies on animal models buttressed by clinical observations and studies during the past 50 years have established that all ventricular arrhythmias associated with myocardial ischemia and infarction do not have the same electrophysiologic mechanisms. Rather, arrhythmias can be subdivided into acute, subacute, and chronic phases according to their time of occurrence in relation to the ischemic event, for example, a coronary artery occlusion.[3,4] In the experimental laboratory, the time of onset of ischemia is controlled and, therefore, well-documented as compared with clinical arrhythmias where, sometimes, the time of onset of ischemia may be uncertain. Therefore, much of the information concerning these electrophysiologic mechanisms comes from experimental models of ischemic arrhythmias and sudden death.[3,4] In this brief review, some of the basic effects of ischemia on cardiac cells and how these effects lead to fatal ventricular arrhythmias, in particular ventricular fibrillation (VF), are described although the experimental models and methods of original data collection are not. Rather, the experimental results are presented in the form of a narrative that provides

Department of Pharmacology, College of Physicians and Surgeons of Columbia University, 630 West 168th Street, New York, NY 10032, USA
E-mail address: alw4@cumc.columbia.edu

Card Electrophysiol Clin 9 (2017) 525–536
http://dx.doi.org/10.1016/j.ccep.2017.07.004
1877-9182/17/© 2017 Elsevier Inc. All rights reserved.

a summary of current concepts of the mechanisms of sudden death in acute ischemia. For more complete reviews the reader is referred to references.[3–5]

THE ACUTE PHASE OF MYOCARDIAL ISCHEMIA AND INFARCTION

The term acute phase of myocardial ischemia refers to events occurring within the first 2 to 4 hours after the sudden reduction of blood flow through a coronary artery. In many individuals who develop VF outside the hospital, collapse occurs almost instantly (within 1 minute) after the onset of symptoms manifested as chest pain or dyspnea,[6,7] indicating that if the onset of symptoms can be equated with the onset of ischemia, ischemia need only to exist for a short time to induce arrhythmias. This proposed relationship between transient ischemia and arrhythmias has been corroborated by studies in patients with transient coronary artery spasm in whom ventricular arrhythmias, including VF, occur within minutes after the beginning of electrocardiographic signs of myocardial ischemia caused by the spasm.[8] Arrhythmias can result both from transient ischemia during ST segment changes and from reperfusion (after return of the ST segment to normal). When coronary artery occlusion is not transient but persists (because of, for example, occlusive thrombi or long-lasting spasm), ischemic cells become irreversibly damaged and myocardial infarction results. The incidence of ventricular arrhythmias during the acute phase of myocardial infarction is higher than for transient ischemic episodes, although it varies widely in different reports (for a review see reference[9]).

It is generally accepted that the occurrence of lethal arrhythmias is the result of the interplay between substrate, trigger, and modulating factors. The electrophysiologic changes brought about by acute ischemia directly on cardiac muscle cells creates the substrate. Arrhythmias in the setting of acute ischemia or infarction are more likely to become manifest in the presence of appropriate triggers, such as changes in autonomic nerve activity, heart rate, and so on. Modulating factors, such as the activity of the sympathetic nervous system, electrolyte disturbances (eg, low serum potassium levels),[10] or impaired left ventricular function may modify both the substrate and the trigger. The description that follows focuses on the substrate changes caused by acute ischemia.

Effects of Ischemia on Ventricular Muscle Substrate Electrophysiology

Myocardial ischemia that results from coronary artery occlusion has a profound effect on the electrophysiologic properties of cardiac cells resulting from a number of factors in the ischemic environment. Extracellular $[K^+]$ is initially elevated, along with hypoxia, a low pH, no substrates, high P_{CO_2}, and accumulation of substances such as lysophosphoglycerides and catecholamines. Each may have an influence on ion channels and the various combinations may exert effects that are not predictable from the action of each substance alone.[3–5]

Within a few minutes after coronary artery occlusion, the amplitude, upstroke velocity, and duration of ventricular muscle action potentials normally supplied by that artery, decrease along with the depolarization of the resting membrane potential (**Fig. 1**, lines 5–9 min of occlusion). After a reduction to resting membrane potentials from a normal value of approximately −80 mV, to around −60 to −65 mV, the cells become unresponsive (see **Fig. 1**, lines 11–13 min of occlusion).[11,12] The phase of unresponsiveness is transient: with maintained coronary occlusion, transmembrane potentials can again be recorded in previously unresponsive cells after about 15 to 30 minutes. The action potentials at that time are abnormal in that they have a short duration, a low amplitude, and a reduced upstroke velocity, yet they are able to propagate. After 40 to 60 minutes, these action potentials disappear and the cells in the center of the ischemic zone become inexcitable.

The changes in resting membrane potential and inward and outward currents during the action potential lead to alterations in conduction, refractoriness and impulse initiation, all of which contribute to the occurrence of ventricular arrhythmias. In addition to changes in these active membrane properties, passive electrical properties are changed as well, and these changes also influence propagation in ischemic myocardium and contribute to arrhythmogenesis (the mechanisms are described elsewhere in this article).

The dramatic changes in electrical activity are rapidly reversible within 20 to 30 minutes if occlusion is transient, owing to readmission of oxygen and nutrients and the washout of substances accumulated in the extracellular space. Rapid reversal of electrical changes cannot occur after prolonged periods of occlusion beyond 20 to 30 minutes.

Resting membrane potential

Cells in the ischemic region depolarize within minutes after coronary artery occlusion from normal values of around −80 mV to between −65 and −60 mV.[11–13] The decrease in resting potential is linked at least partly to alterations in distribution

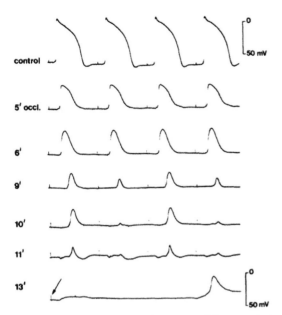

Fig. 1. Transmembrane action potentials recorded from the subepicardium of the left ventricle of an in situ pig heart before and after occlusion (occl.) of the proximal left anterior descending artery. Arrow after 13 minutes shows slight hyperpolarization. (*Reproduced from* Downar E, Janse MJ, Durrer D. The effect of acute coronary artery occlusion on subepicardial transmembrane potentials in the intact porcine heart. Circulation 1977;56:217–24.)

of K^+ across the cell membrane. Recall that the resting membrane potential is determined mainly by the K^+ equilibrium potential.[5] It is primarily caused by the selective permeability of the sarcolemma to K^+ that provide an outward membrane K^+ current flowing through I_{K1} channels down an electrochemical gradient (inside $[K^+]$ = approximately 145 mmol/L, outside $[K^+]$ = approximately 4 mmol/L). During these initial minutes, extracellular K^+ increase to as high as approximately 15 mmol/L in 2 phases. If reperfusion occurs within 15 minutes the first phase is reversible[14,15] and resting potential quickly returns to normal.[11]

Although the increase in extracellular K^+ in the first 10 minutes is substantial,[13,14] it represents only a relatively small decrease in intracellular K^+ concentration (from about 140 to 135 mmol/L) because the ions are transferred from an intracellular space that is 3 times larger than the extracellular space.[16] However, eventually there may also be a significant loss of intracellular K^+ that contributes to a decrease in the K^+ equilibrium potential and resting potential.

Much of the cause of the K^+ efflux is the lack of oxygen (hypoxia) that induces an increase in K^+ conductance (loss of rectifier properties of the time-independent I_{K1} current).[17] An increased conductance of adenosine triphosphate (ATP)-sensitive K^+ channels also might result from the effects of ATP depletion.[18] There is also a link between CO_2 accumulation and elevated $[K^+]_o$ early during ischemia, which might be mediated through changes in $[H^+]_i$. Elevated CO_2 can attenuate K^+ accumulation to maintain excitability in some regions.[19]

After 10 to 20 minutes, a second phase of increase in extracellular potassium begins, which is not reversed by reperfusion.[14,15] This phase is most likely due to disruption of the sarcolemma and irreversible cell damage.

Additional causes for depolarization beside extracellular K^+ accumulation might also occur concomitantly. There is a 3- to 5-fold increase in cytosolic Ca^{2+} between 10 and 20 minutes after the onset of ischemia that is reversible upon reperfusion, which may be involved.[20] After ischemic periods of longer than 10 to 15 minutes, an increase in intracellular calcium plays an important role in causing cellular uncoupling, which has important effects on conduction and arrhythmogenesis (described elsewhere in this article). Increased Ca^{2+} may also cause delayed afterdepolarizations and triggered action potentials in border zones.

A class of metabolites that accumulates in ischemic myocardium and that has been implicated as a cause of early electrical changes during ischemia, including the depolarization of the membrane potential, are the lysophosphoglycerides, among which lysophosphatidylcholine and lysophosphatidylethanolamine[21] cause membrane depolarization by reducing potassium conductance.[22] At higher concentrations, lysophosphoglycerides cause loss of membrane phospholipids, and eventually the membrane is disrupted. Massive calcium entry then leads to cell death.[23]

Phase 0 depolarization

As the resting potential becomes less negative, the velocity and amplitude of phase 0 depolarization decrease until action potentials no longer occur (see **Fig. 1**). A major cause is the inactivation of Na^+ channels at reduced resting potentials, although the direct depressant effect of hypoxia and low intracellular pH may also play a role and exaggerates many of the effects of elevated $[K^+]_o$.[24] A reduction in phase 0 is accompanied by a decrease in conduction velocity (described elsewhere in this article). Before ischemic cells become unresponsive, the amplitude and duration of the action potentials often alternate and sometimes 2:1 responses occur during normal sinus rhythm (see **Fig. 1** and 9 minutes). Conduction blocks during the small amplitude response are caused by activation of the small amount of remaining Na^+ current. In the larger action potentials, the upstroke is divided into 2 components. The fast Na^+ inward current, although depressed, is responsible for the first component of depolarization and carries the membrane potential to a level where the L-type Ca^{2+} current can be activated. The inward Ca^{2+} current is then thought to be responsible for the second phase of the upstroke and for the plateau phase.

The depressed upstrokes (decreased amplitude and velocity of phase 0 depolarization) of action potentials with partially depolarized membrane potentials in ischemic regions may be caused by either a reduced fast Na^+ current (depressed fast response) or by the slow inward L-type Ca^{2+} current (slow response).[25] The latter may occur when the level of the resting potential is reduced enough to inactivate most of the Na^+ current. A high local norepinephrine level caused by catecholamine released from sympathetic nerve endings after coronary occlusion[26] can increase L-type Ca^{2+} current so that it is sufficient to support conducting action potentials in the presence of elevated extracellular $[K^+]$. Even if the L-type Ca^{2+} inward current is not responsible for the entire action potential upstroke during ischemia, it may assume a greater role in causing phase 0 depolarization than in normal myocardial cells, as described.

Action potential duration and refractory period
The duration of the refractory period during the first 2 minutes after coronary artery occlusion increases concomitantly with the lengthening of the action potential.[11] Some of this change has been ascribed to the cooling that accompanies the decrease in coronary blood flow. Subsequently, the action potential duration shortens mainly because of a shortening of the plateau phase. A likely contributor to the action potential shortening during hypoxia is a decrease in the inward L-type calcium current caused by the depressant effect of hypoxia on L-type Ca^{2+} channels. An increase in K^+ conductance resulting from the effects of ATP depletion on ATP-sensitive K^+ channels also participates.[27,28] Other components of the ischemic environment, such as high K^+, and metabolic products may shorten action potential duration. Refractory periods of ischemic myocardium shorten along with the action potential duration, during the first few minutes after complete coronary artery occlusion. Subsequently, refractory periods prolong, even though the action potential duration is shortened.[29] In partially depolarized cells, recovery from inactivation of

both fast Na^+ and slow Ca^{2+} inward currents (the refractory period) is markedly delayed until many milliseconds after the completion of repolarization.

Passive properties
During the initial 15 minutes of ischemia, axial resistance through intracellular and intercellular pathways from cell to cell, reflecting mainly gap junction conductance, remains unchanged. Increased myocardial resistivity results from collapse of the vascular bed and osmotic cell swelling, reducing extracellular space and increasing extracellular resistance. A marked decrease in gap junction conductance at around 15 minutes[3–5] results from a combination of factors that are a consequence of decreased oxygen availability. Los of K^+ from cells and accumulation in extracellular space is associated with development of intracellular acidosis that closes gap junction channels.[3–5] The decrease in pH renders gap junctions more sensitive to the effects of increasing intracellular calcium.[5] Accumulation of lysophosphoglycerides, arachidonic acid, and other substances reduce gap junctional conductance. The presence of catecholamines may decrease conductance in the presence of calcium overload. Gap junction uncoupling is greater intramurally than in border zone regions, where some recovery of the severely depressed transmembrane potentials may occur.[30] Increased intercellular resistance resulting from decreased gap junction conductance is eventually accompanied by focal separation of intercalated disc membranes and a reduction in gap junction surface density.[31] This occurrence is related to reduction of connexin (Cx)43 quantity accompanied by appearance of Cx43 on lateral sarcolemmal membranes (lateralization),[32] where it is not normally located. Lateralized Cx43 likely represents protein, that is not functional junctions, and is part of the process of the removal of gap junctions from intercalated disks triggered by decreased intracellular pH. Changes in phosphorylation of Cx43 impacts both functional and structural remodeling. Reduced phosphorylation at some sites on the Cx43 molecule contributes to decreased Cx43 protein and lateralization (S325, S328, and S330), and a decrease in gap junction conductance (S364/365, S297, and S306). In contrast, S368 becomes phosphorylated through the activation of protein kinase C, also decreasing conductance.[33]

Effects of ischemia on Purkinje cell substrate electrophysiology
The specialized ventricular conducting system sends Purkinje ramifications throughout the left

ventricle. These Purkinje cells form a layer overlying ventricular muscle that is adjacent to the ventricular cavity. Purkinje fibers located immediately beneath the endocardium probably receive adequate amounts of oxygen and substrate via diffusion from the cavitary blood to maintain normal electrophysiologic properties for a while after they are deprived of their coronary arterial supply.[34] Purkinje fibers are also more resistant to hypoxia than muscle fibers.[35] Purkinje fibers that are embedded more deeply within the subendocardial muscle are more dependent on coronary artery blood supply and, therefore, are more affected by coronary occlusion. However, the Purkinje fibers adjacent to the ventricular cavity might still be influenced by substances leaking out from the subjacent ischemic muscle cells. For example, lysophosphoglycerides have been shown to induce triggered activity in Purkinje fibers exposed to high K^+ and acidosis[36] (discussed elsewhere in this article). Purkinje fibers that survive the acute phase of ischemia and infarction eventually undergo electrophysiologic changes and cause subacute arrhythmias many hours later.[3,4]

Arrhythmogenic consequences of changes in ventricular muscle and Purkinje cell electrophysiology Alterations in conduction and refractoriness related to the changes in action potentials that occur in ventricular muscle cells deprived of coronary blood flow, described in the previous sections, lead to the occurrence of reentrant circuits in the ischemic region. In particular, slowing of conduction and conduction block are prerequisite conditions for reentry to occur.

After several minutes of coronary occlusion, slowing of conduction is especially prominent in ischemic subepicardium related to the decrease in blood flow, whereas activation of subendocardial layers is relatively unaffected[37,38] because of the diffusion of oxygen and nutrients from the ventricular chamber. Conduction velocity decreases in concert with a decrease in action potential amplitude and an increase in extracellular resistance. Large delays in epicardial activation are caused by irregular conduction from endocardium to epicardium at reduced speed around multiple sites of intramural conduction block. After 10 to 30 minutes of coronary occlusion, activation delay in the subepicardium diminishes.[39,40] The improvement of conduction is related to the appearance of transmembrane potentials in previously unresponsive cells.[41] This is possibly related to the release of norepinephrine from sympathetic nerve endings as described, which increases resting potential by stimulating the Na^+/K^+ pump

and increasing L-Type Ca^{2+} current even in the presence of hypoxia.

As described, the decrease in the resting potential inactivates Na^+ channels, reducing the inward Na^+ current (I_{Na}) during phase 0 of the action potential. As a consequence, conduction velocity can slow by about two-thirds. The safety factor for conduction also decreases in parallel until conduction blocks when the safety factor falls below 1.[42] Much slower conduction, as slow as 1.00 to 0.05 cm/s, sometimes occurs in ischemic myocardium. Action potentials with phase 0 depolarization owing to I_{CaL} can conduct this slowly. In cells with resting potentials less than −60 mV that completely inactivates I_{Na}, the normally weak I_{CaL} may give rise to phase 0 of conducting action potentials (the slow response) under the influence of catecholamines.[25,42]

After more prolonged ischemia (about 15 minutes in some experimental studies), intracellular resistance increases markedly from cellular uncoupling, and conduction velocity decreases more steeply than action potential amplitude. Rapid cellular uncoupling causes conduction to become even slower and discontinuous, and eventually leads to complete conduction block. As coupling (conductance) decreases, conduction velocity can decline to a very low value of less than 0.5 cm/s before block occurs. At these very low conductance values, I_{CaL} assumes an important role in conduction by providing additional inward source current to that provided by I_{Na}, to depolarize the sink. The minimum conduction velocity that can be attained before block occurs is much slower than that associated with a reduction of I_{Na} alone. At the same time, there is a transient increase in the safety factor, meaning that, despite the very slow conduction, there is less of a possibility of conduction block until conduction becomes very slow (block occurs when the safety factor reaches 1). This property is different than the continuous decline in safety factor with reduction of I_{Na}.[42]

In addition, inhomogeneities in conduction and refractoriness, within the ischemic zone, largely caused by differences in extracellular K^+ are crucial in setting the stage for reentrant arrhythmias. Although ischemic cells are sharply demarcated from nonischemic cells at the border of the region deprived of its blood supply, this boundary is irregular, with interdigitating peninsulae of ischemic and nonischemic tissue, which form the lateral ischemic border zone.[43] One of the reasons for this inhomogeneity at the border is that K^+ diffuses from the ischemic zone toward the normal zone. The diffusion alters membrane potential in a relatively broad area interposed between the center of the ischemic zone and the normally perfused area, affecting conduction and refractoriness within this area. In regions toward the border, $[K^+]_o$ is not as increased as much (approximately 13 mmol) and can support very slow conduction, and refractory periods may not be prolonged as much as in the central ischemic region, or they may even be shorter, resulting in significant inhomogeneities. In the presence of hypoxia, small differences in extracellular K^+ concentrations produce marked changes in the recovery kinetics of phase 0 depolarization.[44]

The changes described are responsible for the rate-dependent properties of conduction velocity in the ischemic region. Because of the strong time dependence of recovery of excitability, the interval between successive depolarizations markedly influences amplitude and upstroke velocity of the action potentials. As this time interval (cycle length) decreases, phase 0 decreases, conduction slows, and eventually conduction block occurs. This effect may be a trigger for initiation of arrhythmias by an increase in heart rate.

Mechanisms of arrhythmias during acute ischemia

During the first 30 minutes after experimental, complete coronary artery occlusion, ventricular arrhythmias (ventricular premature depolarizations, ventricular tachycardia, and VF) occur in 2 distinct phases. The first phase, called phase 1a or immediate ventricular arrhythmias, usually occurs between 2 and 10 minutes after occlusion, the second phase called phase 1b ventricular arrhythmias occurs from approximately 12 to 30 minutes after occlusion.[3,4] Whether or not similar 2 phases of arrhythmias occurs in patients after coronary artery occlusion is unknown.

Phase 1a arrhythmias occur when there is a high degree of conduction slowing manifested as delayed activation in subepicardial muscle of the ischemic region resulting in reentry.[41,45] **Fig. 2** shows the pattern of reentrant excitation in subepicardium (indicated by the arrows) after coronary occlusion in a pig heart. A large single circus movement occurred during the initial ventricular tachycardia (beats 27–35 shown in **Fig. 2**). The reentrant impulse revolves around regions of myocardium that are inexcitable because of the resting membrane depolarization and gap junction uncoupling as described. However, because changes in electrophysiology are inhomogeneous, cells in the pathway around this region of block are still excitable. Tachycardia degenerates into fibrillation when a single reentrant wave front splits into multiple independent wavelets traveling around multiple islets of functional block in the ischemic

region shown in **Fig. 3**. This pattern may be more likely to occur toward the lateral border or even in bordering nonischemic but slightly depressed myocardium where refractory periods are shorter than in the center of the ischemic region, resulting in smaller circuits and more rapid activity.[46] Intramural reentry may occur as well, causing tachycardia that eventually degenerates into VF.[45,47] In summary, the reentrant circuits occurring in ventricular muscle that cause VT and VF are functional, supported by the heterogeneous changes in cellular electrophysiology as described.

Microreentry or reflection might also occur in segments of the Purkinje network that are located more deeply within the ischemic myocardium and subjected to high extracellular K^+ concentrations.[48] The surviving Purkinje network that is not severely depressed may also provide a rapid conducting pathway from these small circuits to the rest of the ventricles, leading to fibrillatory conduction and VF.

Rapid activity emanating from the ischemic border zone causes fibrillation globally. The dynamics of electrical activity undergo rapid change after the onset of VF characterized by a transient phase of increased periodicity and organization followed by a rapid decrease in organization.[49] Changes are likely linked to development of global ischemia. The increase in the organization of VF and stabilization of reentrant sources sometimes occurring in the epicardium may result from more rapid accumulation of $[K^+]_o$, which can stabilize rotor reentry.[50] After ischemia becomes prolonged during VF, focal activity arising from subendocardial Purkinje fibers also contributes to VF maintenance.[51] Focal activity might result from abnormal automaticity or triggered activity.

Nonreentrant mechanisms of impulse formation also occur that cause premature ventricular depolarizations that initiate reentry, the triggering component of arrhythmogenesis. These premature depolarizations arise toward the lateral border, blocking in regions within the ischemic area with longer refractory periods and conducting in regions that are less depressed with shorter refractory periods, to initiate the functional reentry that causes VT and eventually VF (see **Figs. 2** and **3**). The exact mechanism underlying the nonreentrant ectopic activity is unknown. Triggered activity, either induced by early or delayed afterdepolarizations is a possibility. The occurrence of early afterdepolarizations in ischemic myocardium is unlikely because increased K^+ concentrations suppresses this mechanism. However, they may still occur in Purkinje fibers in the subendocardium adjacent to ischemic myocardium (endocardial border zone) that are exposed to lysophosphoglycerides leaking

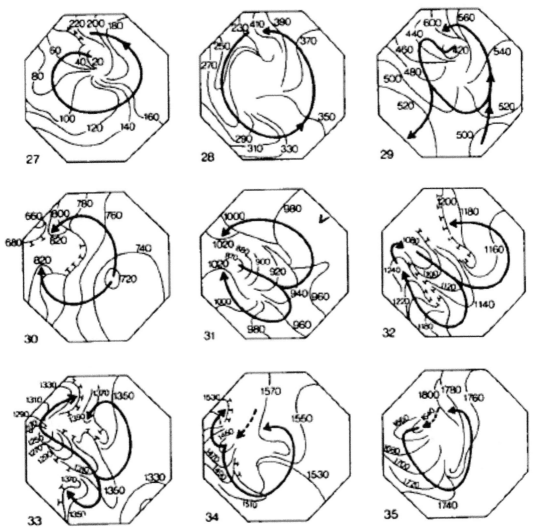

Fig. 2. Patterns of excitation of the area covered by the electrode from beat 27 to 35 ($t = 0$ is chosen arbitrarily). Note that, basically, 1 circus movement of fairly large dimensions is responsible for the continuation of the tachycardia, although both dimension and position of the reentrant circuit change from beat to beat. (*Reproduced from Janse MJ, Van Capelle FJL, Morsink H, et al. Flow of "injury" current and patterns of excitation during early ventricular arrhythmias in acute regional myocardial ischemia in isolated porcine and canine hearts. Evidence for two different arrhythmogenic mechanisms. Circ Res 1980;47:151–65.*)

out of the ischemic myocardium, as well as to protons but to lower concentrations of K^+, because they are bathed in ventricular cavity blood. Delayed afterdepolarizations are also unlikely to occur in severely ischemic myocardium because the Ca^{2+} release and reuptake that underlies their occurrence is inhibited by ischemia,[52] but also might arise from subendocardial Purkinje fibers in the vicinity of ischemic muscle. Here, Po_2 and extracellular K^+ are only moderately changed because of the exposure to oxygenated blood of the ventricular cavity. Ca^{2+} release and reuptake by sarcoplasmic reticulum might still occur to cause delayed afterdepolarizations.[53] Stretch caused by

loss of contractility and systolic bulging of ischemic myocardium could be additional factors that induce repetitive activity owing to triggered activity. In addition, the relatively large membrane resistance of Purkinje fibers makes them more likely to develop spontaneous automaticity as well as triggered activity.[54]

The flow of current across the boundary between ischemic and normal myocardium also contributes to the genesis of ectopic activity. Such current flow is generated by the differences in membrane potential between closely adjacent regions either during diastole or during the action potential; the differences in membrane potential

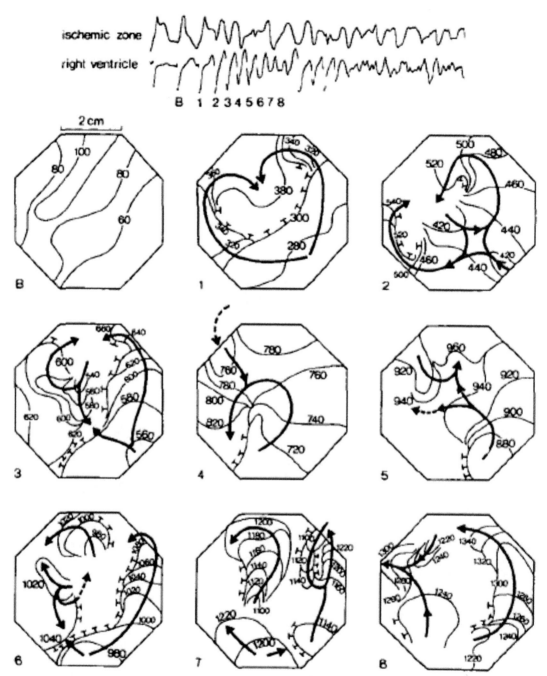

Fig. 3. Same experiment as in **Fig. 2** and 30 seconds later. A ventricular premature beat with the same coupling interval as the one that initiated a run of tachycardia in **Fig. 2** now initiates ventricular fibrillation. Note reentry between first and second ectopic beats. Note fragmentation of wave fronts in beats, 6, 7, and 8 and microcircus movement in beat 7. (*Reproduced from* Janse MJ, Van Capelle FJL, Morsink H, et al. Flow of "injury" current and patterns of excitation during early ventricular arrhythmias in acute regional myocardial ischemia in isolated porcine and canine hearts. Evidence for two different arrhythmogenic mechanisms. Circ Res 1980;47:151–65.)

being caused by injury to the ischemic region. As described, ischemic cells have lower membrane potentials and a different time course of repolarization than normal cells. Depression of the T-Q segment in direct current extracellular electrograms recorded from the ischemic tissue indicate injury current flowing during diastole.[12] It is predicted from a theoretic analysis that, in diastole, when the intracellular compartments of partially depolarized ischemic cells are positive to the intracellular compartments of normal cells, intracellular current flows from ischemic toward normal cells. This current flowing between the ischemic cells with delayed activity and the normal cells, which have repolarized or are repolarizing, through an inexcitable segment of depolarized cells interposed between the two, reexcites the normal cells to cause premature depolarizations.[45] The normal cells may be ventricular muscle at the lateral margins of the ischemic region or Purkinje cells in the subendocardial border zone. This current can also initiate early or delayed after depolarizations or accelerate automatic firing.

After 15 to 20 minutes of ischemia, some of the depressed action potentials in the ischemic region are restored; resting membrane potential increases, action potential amplitude increases, and action potentials occur in regions that were previously inexcitable. These changes accompany the occurrence of phase 1b arrhythmias. Ischemia causes an increased release of noradrenaline only after 15 to 20 minutes.[55,56] Thus, accumulation of catecholamines in the extracellular space of the ischemic region may play a role in the genesis of phase 1b arrhythmias. Catecholamines hyperpolarize resting membrane potential either by increasing Na^+/K^+ pump activity[57] or K^+ conductance,[58] and these effects may be the cause of hyperpolarization of the ischemic cells. Catecholamines also restore conduction in muscle fibers partly depolarized by high extracellular K^+ to membrane potentials less than about -60 mV.[25] The effect is a result of an increase in inward L-type calcium current and the induction of slow response action potentials.

In addition to the arrhythmia-promoting changes in ventricular muscle action potentials coincident with the phase 1b arrhythmias, as described, a marked decrease in gap junction conductance at around 15 minutes[30] is implicated in this second phase of arrhythmias. Both the occurrence of action potentials with depressed phase 0 depolarization and the uncoupling of gap junctions can lead to a reentrant mechanism. However, ischemia-induced depression of action potentials, gap junction coupling, and conduction in border zones of surviving myocardium subjected to less intense ischemia than dying intramural regions may not be sufficient to provide a reentrant substrate. A novel hypothesis proposes that the combination of slow conduction, block, and reentry may still occur in border zones because of the electrotonic current sink through gap junctional connections with the large mass of the highly ischemic region with depressed membrane potentials.[30] Injury currents flowing between normal and ischemic myocardium at ischemic borders as tissue resistance increases because of partial gap junction uncoupling can trigger premature beats by either reexcitation of cells or increasing diastolic depolarization. Injury current and propagation wane when complete uncoupling occurs.

Reperfusion arrhythmias

VF may occur within seconds after restoration of blood flow to myocardium made ischemic by a period of coronary occlusion (reperfusion). At least a 3-minute ischemic period during occlusion is necessary before reperfusion arrhythmias occur in experimental animals.[59,60] The incidence of reperfusion-induced VF increases when occlusion periods are lengthened to about 30 minutes,[61] after which arrhythmias decrease because of the onset of irreversible injury.[60] Reperfusion after a 30-minute occlusion in dog hearts results in 2 distinct periods of arrhythmias.[62] Immediately after reperfusion, VF is the dominant arrhythmia. If no fibrillation occurs immediately upon reperfusion, a delayed period of arrhythmias may occur 2 to 7 minutes later, characterized by ventricular premature depolarizations and ventricular tachycardia but usually not fibrillation. It is not known if these are characteristics of reperfusion arrhythmias in humans.

During relatively brief periods of ischemia of 20 minutes or less, there is marked depression of ventricular muscle transmembrane action potentials, and even inexcitability as described. Sudden reperfusion results in a very rapid restoration of action potentials to the ischemic myocardium,[11,62,63] although the return of electrical activity is not equally rapid for all cells.[11] These restored action potentials have reduced upstroke velocities and low amplitudes, and the duration and amplitude often alternate between high amplitude and long duration and low amplitude and short duration, similar to changes that occur during acute occlusion. Within 1 minute of reperfusion, the action potential duration is markedly shortened. This shortening may be due to the fact that substances that accumulated in the extracellular space of the ischemic compartment such as K^+, lactate, and other metabolites transiently influence the electrophysiologic characteristics of normal cells close to the ischemic zone as they are washed out of the ischemic compartment.[64] In contrast, action potential shortening of previously ischemic cells during reperfusion is accompanied by a rapid return of extracellular K^+ concentration to normal values.

During the first minutes of reperfusion, there is a marked inhomogeneity in the action potentials within the ischemic area and at the border leading to the formation of reentrant circuits similar to those described that occur during acute ischemia. The origin of the initial ectopic impulses that induce fibrillation is close to the border and these impulses usually are not caused by reentry.[65] Some of these initiating impulses might be a result of enhanced abnormal automaticity or triggered activity in Purkinje cells that remain partially depolarized after blood flow is restored.[66] After readmission of oxygen, washout of metabolites, and normalization of pH, there is a rapid decrease in intracellular Na^+ activity associated with hyperpolarization. This change is most likely owing to stimulation of Na^+/K^+ pump activity and of the Na^+/Ca^+ exchanger.[67] The increase of intracellular Ca^{2+} (also probably occurring from calcium release from the sarcoplasmatic reticulum) could then activate a nonselective cation channel, leading to an inward current and cause the membrane depolarization that enables abnormal automaticity to occur.[67] Reperfusion is also likely to result in Ca^{2+} overload[68,69] owing to spontaneous release of calcium from the sarcoplasmatic reticulum that might cause delayed or early afterdepolarizations.[70,71]

An increase in automaticity in the surviving Purkinje system is evident during the delayed reperfusion arrhythmias.[62] Accelerated idioventricular rhythm, an arrhythmia that may be caused by automaticity, often occurs after thrombolytic procedures designed to disrupt a coronary occlusion in patients, and in such patients ischemia must have been present for some time.

REFERENCES

1. Zipes DP, Wellens HJJ. Sudden cardiac death. Circulation 1998;98:2334–51.
2. Myerburg RJ, Castellanos A. Cardiac arrest and sudden death. In: Braunwald E, editor. Heart disease: a textbook of cardiovascular medicine. Philadelphia: WB Saunders; 1997. p. 742–79.
3. Janse MJ, Wit AL. Electrophysiological mechanisms of ventricular arrhythmias resulting from myocardial ischemia and infarction. Physiol Rev 1989;69:1049–169.
4. Wit AL, Janse MJ. The ventricular arrhythmias of ischemia and infarction. Electrophysiological mechanisms. Mount Kisco (NY): Futura; 1993.
5. Carmeliet E. Cardiac ionic currents and acute ischemia: from channels to arrhythmias. Physiol Rev 1999;79:917–87.
6. Liberthson RR, Nagel EL, Hirschman JC, et al. Pathophysiologic observations in prehospital ventricular fibrillation and sudden cardiac death. Circulation 1974;49:790–8.
7. Liberthson RR, Nagel EL, Ruskin JN. Pathophysiology, clinical course, and management of prehospital ventricular fibrillation and sudden cardiac death. In: Adgey AAJ, editor. Acute phase of ischemic heart disease and myocardial infarction. The Hague (Netherlands): Martinus Nijhoff; 1982. p. 165–82.
8. Maseri AS, Severi S, Marzullo P. Role of coronary arterial spasm in sudden coronary ischemic death. In: Greenberg HM, Dwyer Jr EM, editors. Sudden Coronary Death. Ann NY Acad Sci 1982;382:204–16.
9. Bigger JT Jr, Dresdale RJ, Heissenbuttel RH, et al. Ventricular arrhythmias in ischemic heart disease: mechanism, prevalence, significance, and management. Prog Cardiovasc Dis 1977;19:255–300.
10. Nordrehaug JE, von der Lippe G. Hypokalaemia and ventricular fibrillation in acute myocardial infarction. Br Heart J 1983;50:525–9.
11. Downar E, Janse MJ, Durrer D. The effect of acute coronary artery occlusion on subepicardial transmembrane potentials in the intact porcine heart. Circulation 1977;56:217–24.
12. Kleber AG, Janse MJ, Van Capelle FJL, et al. Mechanism and time course of S-T and T-Q segment changes during acute regional myocardial ischemia in the pig heart determined by extracellular and intracellular recordings. Circ Res 1978;42:603–13.
13. Kleber AG. Resting membrane potential, extracellular potassium activity, and intracellular sodium activity during acute global ischemia in isolated perfused Guinea pig hearts. Circ Res 1983;52:442–50.
14. Hill JL, Gettes LS. Effects of acute coronary artery occlusion on local myocardial extracellular K+ activity in swine. Circulation 1980;61:768–78.
15. Hirche HJ, Franz C, Bos L, et al. Myocardial extracellular K+ and H+ increase and noradrenaline release as possible cause of early arrhythmias following acute coronary artery occlusion in pigs. J Mol Cell Cardiol 1980;12:579–93.
16. Polimeni PI. Extracellular space and ionic distribution in rat ventricle. Am J Physiol 1974;227:676–83.
17. Weiss JN, Lamp ST, Shine KI. Cellular K+ loss and anion efflux during myocardial ischemia and metabolic inhibition. Am J Physiol 1989;256:H1165–75.
18. Noma A, Shibasaki T. Membrane current through adenosine-triphosphate-regulated potassium channels in Guinea-pig ventricular cells. J Physiol 1985;363:463–80.
19. Cascio WE, Yan GX, Kleber AG. Early changes in extracellular potassium in ischemic rabbit myocardium. The role of carbon dioxide accumulation and diffusion. Circ Res 1992;70:409–22.
20. Clusin WT, Buchbinder M, Ellis AK, et al. Reduction of ischemic depolarization by the calcium blocker diltiazem. Correlation with improvement of ventricular conduction and early arrhythmias in the dog. Circ Res 1984;54:10–20.

21. Sobel BE, Corr PB, Robison AK, et al. Accumulation of lysophosphoglycerides with arrhythmogenic properties in ischemic myocardium. J Clin Invest 1978;62:546–53.

22. Clarkson CW, Ten Eick RE. On the mechanism of lysophosphatidylcholine- induced depolarization of cat ventricular myocardium. Circ Res 1983;52:543–56.

23. Corr PB, Sobel BE. Amphiphilic lipid metabolism and ventricular arrhythmias. In: Parratt JR, editor. Early arrhythmias resulting from myocardial ischaemia. New York: Oxford University Press; 1982. p. 199–218.

24. Cascio WE, Johnson TA, Gettes LS. Electrophysiological changes in ischemic myocardium: I. Influence of ionic, metabolic and energetic changes. J Cardiovasc Electrophysiol 1995;6:1039–62.

25. Cranefield PF. The conduction of the cardiac impulse. The slow response and cardiac arrhythmias. Mount Kisco (NY): Futura Publishing Co.; 1975.

26. Carlsson L. Mechanisms of local noradrenaline release in acute myocardial ischemia. Acta Physiol Scand 1987;129(Suppl. 559):7–85.

27. Noma A. ATP-regulated K+ channels in cardiac muscle. Nature 1983;305:147–8.

28. Isenberg G, Vereecke J, Heyden G, et al. The shortening of the action potential by DNP in Guinea-pig ventricular myocytes is mediated by an increase of a time-independent K conductance. Pflugers Arch 1983;397:251–9.

29. Lazzara R, El-Sherif N, Hope RR, et al. Ventricular arrhythmias and electrophysiological consequences of myocardial ischemia and infarction. Circ Res 1978;42:740–9.

30. De Groot JR, Wilms-Schopman FJG, Opthof T, et al. Late ventricular arrhythmias during acute regional ischemia in the isolated blood perfused pig heart. Role of electrical cellular coupling. Cardiovasc Res 2001;50:362–72.

31. Peters NS, Wit AL. Myocardial architecture and ventricular arrhythmogenesis. Circulation 1998;97:1746–54.

32. Kieken F, Mutsaers N, Dolmatova E, et al. Structural and molecular mechanisms of gap junction remodeling in epicardial border zone myocytes following myocardial infarction. Circ Res 2009;104:1103–12.

33. Wit AL, Peters NS. The role of gap junctions in the arrhythmias of ischemia and infarction. Heart Rhythm 2012;9:308–11.

34. Dangman KH, Wang HH, Wit AL. Effects of intracoronary potassium chloride on electrograms of canine Purkinje fibers in six-hour - to four-week-old myocardial infarcts. An indication of time-dependent changes in collateral blood flow. Circ Res 1979;44:392–405.

35. Bagdonas AA, Stuckey JH, Piera J, et al. Effects of ischemia and hypoxia on the specialized conducting system of the canine heart. Am Heart J 1961;61:206–18.

36. Pogwizd SM, Onufer JR, Kramer JB, et al. Induction of delayed afterdepolarizations and triggered activity in canine Purkinje fibers by lysophosphoglycerides. Circ Res 1986;59:416–26.

37. Ruffy R, Lovelace DE, Mueller TM, et al. Relationship between changes in left ventricular bipolar electrograms and regional myocardial blood flow during acute coronary artery occlusion in the dog. Circ Res 1979;45:764–70.

38. Honjo H, Hirai M, Osaka T, et al. Effects of acute ischemia on the endocardial activation sequence of canine left ventricle. Environ Med 1986;30:83–8.

39. Kaplinsky E, Ogawa S, Balke CW, et al. Two periods of early ventricular arrhythmia in the canine acute myocardial infarction model. Circulation 1979;60:397–403.

40. Scherlag BJ, El-Sherif N, Hope RR, et al. Characterization and localization of ventricular arrhythmias resulting from myocardial ischemia and infarction. Circ Res 1974;35:372–83.

41. Janse MJ, Kleber AG. Electrophysiological changes and ventricular arrhythmias in the early phase of regional myocardial ischemia. Circ Res 1981;49:1069–81.

42. Shaw RM, Rudy Y. Ionic mechanisms of propagation in cardiac tissue. Roles of the sodium and L-type calcium currents during reduced excitability and decreased gap junction coupling. Circ Res 1997;81:727–41.

43. Janse MJ, Cinca J, Morina H, et al. The "border zone" in myocardial ischemia. An electrophysiological, metabolic and histochemical correlation in the pig heart. Circ Res 1979;44:576–88.

44. Wilde AAM, Kleber AG. The combined effects of hypoxia, high K+, and acidosis on the intracellular sodium activity and resting potential in Guinea pig papillary muscle. Circ Res 1986;58:249–56.

45. Janse MJ, Van Capelle FJL, Morsink H, et al. Flow of "injury" current and patterns of excitation during early ventricular arrhythmias in acute regional myocardial ischemia in isolated porcine and canine hearts. Evidence for two different arrhythmogenic mechanisms. Circ Res 1980;47:151–65.

46. Zaitsev AV, Sarmast F, Kolli A, et al. Wavebreak formation during ventricular fibrillation in the isolated regionally ischemic pig heart. Circ Res 2003;92:546–53.

47. Janse MJ, van Capelle FJL. Ectopic activity in the early phase of regional myocardial ischemia. In: Bouman LN, Jongsma HJ, editors. Cardiac rate and rhythm. physiological, morphological and developmental aspects. The Hague (Netherlands): Martinus Nijhoff Publishers; 1982. p. 297–320.

48. Wit AL, Cranefield PF, Hoffman BF. Slow conduction and reentry in the ventricular conducting system. II.

Single and sustained circus movement in networks of canine and bovine Purkinje fibers. Circ Res 1972;30:11–22.

49. Huang J, Rogers JM, Killingsworth CR, et al. Evolution of activation patterns during long-duration ventricular fibrillation in dogs. Am J Physiol Heart Circ Physiol 2004;286:H1193–200.

50. Zaitsev AV. Mechanisms of ischemic ventricular fibrillation: who's the killer. In: Zipes DP, Jalife J, editors. Cardiac electrophysiology: from cell too bedside. Philadelphia: Saunders; 2004.

51. Tabereaux PB, Walcott GP, Rogers JM, et al. Activation patterns of Purkinje fibers during long-duration ventricular fibrillation in an isolated canine heart model. Circulation 2007;116:1113–9.

52. Overend CL, Eisner DA, O'Neil SC. Altered cardiac sarcoplasmic reticulum function of intact myocytes of rat ventricle during metabolic inhibition. Circ Res 2001;88:181–7.

53. Tsujii E, Tanaka H, Oyamada M, et al. In situ visualization of the intracellular Ca2+ dynamics at the border of the acute myocardial infarct. Mol Cell Biochem 2003;248:135–9.

54. Huelsing DG, Spitzer KW, Pollard AE. Spontaneous activity induced in rabbit Purkinje myocytes during coupling to a depolarized model cell. Cardiovasc Res 2003;59:620–7.

55. Forfar JC, Riemersma RA, Oliver MF. a-adrenoceptor control of norepinephrine release from acutely ischaemic myocardium: effects of blood flow, arrhythmias, and regional conduction delay. J Cardiovasc Pharmacol 1983;5:752–9.

56. Riemersma RA. Myocardial catecholamine release in acute myocardial ischaemia; Relationship to cardiac arrhythmias. In: Parratt JR, editor. Early arrhythmias resulting from myocardial ischaemia. New York: Oxford University Press; 1982. p. 125–38.

57. Desilets M, Baumgarten CM. Isoproterenol directly stimulates the Na+-K+ pump in isolated cardiac myocytes. Am J Physiol 1986;251:H218–25.

58. Boyden PA, Cranefield PF, Gadsby DC. Noradrenaline hyperpolarizes cells of the canine coronary sinus by increasing their permeability to potassium ions. J Physiol 1983;339:185–206.

59. Balke CW, Kaplinsky E, Michelson EL, et al. Reperfusion ventricular tachyarrhythmias: correlation with antecedent coronary artery occlusion tachyarrhythmias and duration of myocardial ischemia. Am Heart J 1981;101:449–56.

60. Manning AS, Hearse DJ. Reperfusion-induced arrhythmias: mechanisms and prevention. J Mol Cell Cardiol 1984;16:497–518.

61. Corbalan R, Verrier RL, Lown B. Differing mechanisms for ventricular vulnerability during coronary artery occlusion and release. Am Heart J 1976;92:223–30.

62. Kaplinsky ES, Ogawa B, Michelson EL, et al. Instantaneous and delayed ventricular arrhythmias after reperfusion of acutely ischemic myocardium: evidence for multiple mechanisms. Circulation 1981;63:333–40.

63. Murdock DK, Loeb JM, Euler DE, et al. Electrophysiology of coronary reperfusion. A mechanism for reperfusion arrhythmias. Circulation 1980;61:175–82.

64. Nakata T, Hearse DJ, Curtis MJ. Are reperfusion-induced arrhythmias caused by disinhibition of an arrhythmogenic component of ischemia? J Mol Cell Cardiol 1990;22:843–58.

65. Pogwizd SM, Corr PB. Electrophysiologic mechanisms underlying arrhythmias due to reperfusion of ischemic myocardium. Circulation 1987;76:404–26.

66. Ferrier GR, Moffat MP, Lukas A. Possible mechanisms of ventricular arrhythmias elicited by ischemia followed by reperfusion. Studies on isolated canine ventricular tissues. Circ Res 1985;56:184–94.

67. Strauss HC, Yee R, Hill JA Jr, et al. Mechanisms of reperfusion arrhythmias. In: Rosen MR, Palti Y, editors. Lethal arrhythmias resulting from myocardial ischemia and infarction. Boston: Kluwer Academic Publishers; 1989. p. 55–73.

68. Smith GL, Allen DG. Effects of metabolic blockade on intracellular calcium concentration in isolated ferret ventricular muscle. Circ Res 1988;62:1223–36.

69. Stern MD, Weisman HF, Renlund DG, et al. Laser backscatter studies of intracellular Ca2+ oscillations in isolated hearts. Am J Physiol 1989;257:H665–73.

70. Priori SG, Mantica M, Napolitano C, et al. Early afterdepolarizations induced in vivo by reperfusion of ischemic myocardium. A possible mechanism for reperfusion arrhythmias. Circulation 1990;81:1911–20.

71. Goldberg S, Greenspon AJ, Urban PL, et al. Reperfusion arrhythmia: a marker of restoration of antegrade flow during intracoronary thrombolysis for acute myocardial infarction. Am Heart J 1983;105:26–32.

Channelopathies as Causes of Sudden Cardiac Death

Peter J. Schwartz, MD[a],*, Michael J. Ackerman, MD, PhD[b,c,d],
Arthur A.M. Wilde, MD, PhD[e,f]

KEYWORDS

- Brugada syndrome • Catecholaminergic polymorphic ventricular tachycardia • Genetic testing
- Ion channels • Long QT syndrome • Ryanodine receptor • Left cardiac sympathetic denervation

KEY POINTS

- All patients with channelopathies should undergo genetic screening because the identification of the disease-causing mutation allows diagnosis or exclusion of the disease in the entire family.
- For patients with long QT syndrome and catecholaminergic polymorphic ventricular tachycardia, left cardiac sympathetic denervation should be considered before the implantable cardiovert-defibrillator (ICD) for quality of life.
- Risk stratification for asymptomatic patients with the Brugada syndrome remains ill-defined and, even with a spontaneous type 1 pattern, the low risk suggests careful judgment before implanting an ICD.

LONG QT SYNDROME

There is little doubt that congenital long QT syndrome (LQTS) is the best known and best understood of the channelopathies. Partly, because its first description goes back already 60 years, when Professor Anton Jervell recognized the unique clinical entity present in a Norwegian family and described it so carefully[1] to facilitate the initial studies of the syndrome[2] and of the specific variant with congenital deafness that, appropriately, bears his name.[3] Partly, because the genetic discoveries of 1995 and 1996[4–6] have brought a

Disclosure Statement: P.J. Schwartz has no conflict of interest to disclose. M.J. Ackerman is a consultant for Boston Scientific, Gilead Sciences, Invitae, Medtronic, MyoKardia, and St. Jude Medical. M.J. Ackerman and Mayo Clinic have received sales based royalties from Transgenomic (FAMILION-LQTS and FAMILION-CPVT tests). M.J. Ackerman and Mayo Clinic have a license agreement with AliveCor. However, none of these companies have been involved in this study in any way. A.A.M. Wilde is member of the Scientific Advisory Board of LilaNova. Both the IRCCS Istituto Auxologico Italiano and the Heart Center, Academic Medical Center, University of Amsterdam, are members of the European Reference Network for rare, low prevalence and complex diseases of the heart – ERN GUARD-Heart.
[a] Center for Cardiac Arrhythmias of Genetic Origin, IRCCS Istituto Auxologico Italiano, c/o Centro Diagnostico e di Ricerca S. Carlo, Via Pier Lombardo, 22, Milan 20135, Italy; [b] Department of Cardiovascular Diseases, Division of Heart Rhythm Services, Windland Smith Rice Sudden Death Genomics Laboratory, Mayo Clinic, Guggenheim 501, Rochester, MN 55905, USA; [c] Department of Pediatrics, Division of Pediatric Cardiology, Windland Smith Rice Sudden Death Genomics Laboratory, Mayo Clinic, Guggenheim 501, Rochester, MN 55905, USA; [d] Department of Molecular Pharmacology and Experimental Therapeutics, Windland Smith Rice Sudden Death Genomics Laboratory, Mayo Clinic, Guggenheim 501, Rochester, MN 55905, USA; [e] Heart Center, Academic Medical Center, University of Amsterdam, PO-Box 22700, 1100DE, Amsterdam, The Netherlands; [f] Princess Al-Jawhara Al-Brahim Centre of Excellence in Research of Hereditary Disorders, Jeddah, Saudi Arabia
* Corresponding author.
E-mail addresses: peter.schwartz@unipv.it; p.schwartz@auxologico.it

true revolution to the entire field of channelopathies and because of the impact on management of the genotype–phenotype correlation, which is indeed best understood for LQTS.[7]

Clinical Manifestations and Diagnosis

The most common presentation of LQTS is that of a syncope triggered by an abrupt emotional or physical stress. A sequence of syncopal episodes culminating in cardiac arrest and/or sudden death is typical for symptomatic patients left untreated. However, the clinical picture is often much more complex and sudden death as a sentinel event has been found to occur in 13% of the affected subjects[8]; this observation has contributed to the current concept that most patients should be treated once the diagnosis has been established. Furthermore, a variety of potential triggers for the arrhythmic events have been identified—ranging from swimming to acoustic stimuli to disrupted sleep—and has been recognized to associate with specific disease genes.[9] This in turn is guiding what now has become a rather advanced gene-specific management.[10]

The diagnosis of LQTS is straightforward in typical cases, but can be complex especially when the patient is asymptomatic and the QT interval is only modestly prolonged. The diagnosis of LQTS should not be made on the basis of a single parameter, with the reasonable exception of a QTc of well over 500 ms—in the absence of an acquired explanation such as, for example, a QT-prolonging drug or hypokalemia.[11] Experts usually do not take long to recognize LQTS, but for cardiologists with limited experience with the disease, the use of a diagnostic score can be very valuable to enhance the probability of a correct diagnosis.

The "Schwartz score" (**Table 1**) includes a series of clinical elements and is useful for assessing the probability that the proband is affected by LQTS. A diagnostic score of 3.5 or greater implies a high probability of LQTS, and mandates additional investigations.[12] It is important to realize that "high probability" is not equivalent to an established diagnosis. When in doubt, repeated clinical visits help, and especially the use of 12-lead 24-hour Holter monitor is helpful because it allows the unmasking of often transient but important morphologic changes in the T wave, which facilitate the diagnosis. Indeed, the diagnosis of LQTS represents a good example of "pattern recognition" and this explains why the clinical experience is so valuable. The exercise stress test is useful mostly to assess the degree of QT adaptation to heart rate increase and the changes occurring in the recovery period, regarding both T wave morphology and QT lengthening.[12,13] When the clinical suspicion is sound, genetic testing becomes mandatory, not only for diagnostic purposes but for a more targeted management.

Role of Genetics

Since 1995, at least 16 LQTS disease-causing genes have been identified.[7] Currently, in experienced laboratories, a disease-causing mutation is identified in 75% of clinically definite cases. This implies that, when the clinical diagnosis is certain, a negative genetic test should not modify confidence in the diagnosis; conversely, when the clinical suspicion is weak, a negative genotype contributes to make the diagnosis even less likely. The 3 canonical genes (KCNQ1, KCNH2, SCN5A, causing respectively LQT1, LQT2, and LQT3) contribute to the majority of diagnosed cases.

Once the genotype of the proband is identified, 2 things should follow. One is cascade screening of all first- and second-degree family members, because this is likely to reveal that approximately 50% of them is mutation positive.[14] The second is gene-specific management.

Cascade screening should not be viewed as an option, because not to perform it is tantamount to willingly ignore whether other family members are affected and thereby at risk for life-threatening arrhythmias, and it could carry medicolegal implications.[15] Gene-specific management, as proposed in 2005,[16] has become a reality, and is discussed in the subsequent section on therapy. An additional issue, of growing interest and importance, is that of the "modifier genes," that is, of those genetic variants able to modify—in either direction—the arrhythmic risk created by the disease-causing mutations.[17] These findings may impact both risk stratification and management.

Therapy

There is not much that is new in therapy for LQTS compared with what has been repeatedly said in the last few years.[10] For all LQTS patients, there is a universal recommendation for avoidance, whenever possible, of medications with known QT-prolonging potential (www.crediblemeds.org). The cornerstones of therapy remain β-blockers, left cardiac sympathetic denervation (LCSD), and the implantable cardioverter-defibrillator (ICD). Only a few points will be made herein, because the available literature offers all the necessary details.

β-blockers

Propranolol and nadolol are the 2 β-blockers to be used. There is evidence that metoprolol and atenolol are associated with a significant risk of

Table 1
The 1993-2011 LQTS diagnostic criteria

			Points
Electrocardiographic findings[a]			
A	QTc[b]	≥480 ms	3
		460–479 ms	2
		450–459 ms (male)	1
B	QTc[b] fourth minute of recovery from exercise stress test ≥480 ms		1
C	Torsade de pointes[c]		2
D	T wave alternans		1
E	Notched T wave in 3 leads		1
F	Low heart rate for age[d]		0.5
Clinical history			
A	Syncope[c]	With stress	2
		Without stress	1
B	Congenital deafness		0.5
Family history			
A	Family members with definite LQTS[e]		1
B	Unexplained sudden cardiac death below age 30 among immediate family members[e]		0.5

Abbreviation: LQTS, long QT syndrome.

Score: ≤1 point, low probability of LQTS; 1.5–3.0 points, intermediate probability of LQTS; ≥3.5 points, high probability.

[a] In the absence of medications or disorders known to affect these electrocardiographic features.

[b] QTc calculated by Bazett's formula where QTc = QT/√RR.

[c] Mutually exclusive.

[d] Resting heart rate below the second percentile for age.

[e] The same family member cannot be counted in A and B.

(*From* Schwartz PJ, Crotti L. QTc behavior during exercise and genetic testing for the long-QT syndrome. Circulation 2011;124:2182; with permission.)

recurrences[18] and should be avoided in LQTS. Once the diagnosis of LQTS is made, therapy should begin because the risk of death as a first event is unacceptably high at 13%, particularly if the resting QTc exceeds 500 ms.[8] The only 2 reasonable exceptions are (1) the LQT1 men who when diagnosed are already over age 20 to 25 and completely asymptomatic while off therapy and (2) the so-called genotype positive/phenotype negative (concealed LQTS) subjects who have a QTc either within normal limits or just borderline with a possible doubt for LQT2. The concept that β-blockers would not be useful for LQT3 patients has been proven wrong,[19,20] and there should be no hesitation in using β-blockers also in this group of patients.

Left cardiac sympathetic denervation
The rationale for LCSD is clear and solid,[21] because of its high efficacy in LQTS.[22,23] It is always worth reminding the 2 key mechanisms of the protection afforded by LCSD: (1) the major reduction in the localized release of norepinephrine at ventricular level (which would increase the heterogeneity of repolarization thus enhancing the probability of reentry); and (2) the increase in the ventricular fibrillation (VF) threshold, which makes it more difficult for a heart to fibrillate.[21] There are several specific conditions in which there should be no hesitation in proceeding with LCSD: in the presence of specific contraindications to β-blockers, whenever an episode of syncope occurs despite β-blockers or when despite events on therapy there are signs of high cardiac electrical instability (eg, episodes of T wave alternans), whenever there are electrical storms in patients with an ICD, and in still asymptomatic patients with a QTc of 550 ms or greater.

Implantable cardioverter defibrillator
The ICD represents an important tool for management, but should be used when necessary and not just because a patient has had an episode of syncope. Before recommending an ICD in a patient who had not had a cardiac arrest, the cardiologist should consider the greater than 30% of major adverse effects that occur within 5 years from the ICD implant.[24] This dramatic price to be paid, especially in children and adolescents, should lead to more caution to avoid unnecessary

implants. The difference in the rate of ICD implants between LQTS specialty centers and general cardiac electrophysiology centers is staggering.[10] The cases when an ICD is recommended, or should be seriously considered, have been described in detail.[24] The subcutaneous ICD, of potential interest in the young, may not be ideal in LQTS because of the lack of pacing ability.

Gene-specific management

The progress in the understanding of the correlation between genotype and phenotype, with specific reference to the triggers for cardiac events[9] (**Fig. 1**), has guided an approach that allows modulation management according to the disease-causing gene and, partially, even to the disease-causing mutation.

LQT1 patients, because their mutations impair the I_{Ks} current, which accelerates repolarization whenever the RR interval shortens, are exquisitely sensitive to rapid changes in heart rate. This is obviously true for increases in heart rate, but also for sudden decreases resulting in long pauses.[25,26] This issue raises concerns for conditions associated with significant physical stress, such as competitive sports. However, a low event rate has been observed among athletes with LQTS, even LQT1, who have elected to remain in competitive sports.[27] One specific condition, potentially dangerous for LQT1 patients, is swimming and we recommend that this activity be performed in the presence of an adult able to swim. Conversely, as mentioned, there is strong evidence that male patients with LQT1 who remained asymptomatic without ever being treated until age 25 or more are extremely unlikely to become symptomatic; accordingly, and especially if their QTc is less than 500 ms, it may be reasonable to not initiate therapy.

The LQT2 patients are sensitive to hypokalemia and to sudden noise. Their potassium level should be monitored, also because some of these patients tend to lose potassium and in these cases appropriate countermeasures should be taken. In any case, a potassium-rich diet should be recommended. It is very important to try (although it is not always possible) to minimize the occurrence of sudden noises, especially while at rest. Accordingly, we recommend avoiding telephones and alarm clocks in the bedroom and that parents, when waking up their children, do it gently and without yelling. LQT2 women are also at higher risk in the post partum period and when their sleep is disrupted. Accordingly, we recommend that, in the first 4 to 6 months after delivery, the nighttime feeding of the infants be taken care of by their partners to protect their sleep, unless the infant is being breastfed.

The LQT3 patients are at higher risk while resting, and cardiac events not infrequently occur during sleep. This phenomenon does not necessarily imply that these events occur while sympathetic activity is low, because the phases of REM sleep are characterized by burst of both vagal and sympathetic activity. Because death would follow a relatively slow decrease in blood pressure, owing the horizontal position, this would not be an instantaneous event, but would allow time for progressive cerebral hypoxia leading to gasping noises. These can be heard by whoever sleeps in the same room and has resulted in many patients saved by bed partners. Accordingly, we recommend that, whenever possible, LQT3 patients sleep with an adult or that—in the case of children—there is an intercom connected to the parents' bedroom.

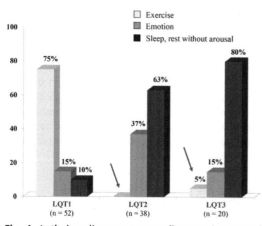

Fig. 1. Lethal cardiac events according to triggers and genotype. Numbers in parenthesis are triggers, not patients. The arrows point to the rare occurrence of lethal events during exercise among LQT2 and LQT3 patients. (*Modified from* Schwartz PJ, Priori SG, Spazzolini C, et al. Genotype-phenotype correlation in the long-QT syndrome: gene-specific triggers for life-threatening arrhythmias. Circulation 2001;103:92; with permission.)

CATECHOLAMINERGIC POLYMORPHIC VENTRICULAR TACHYCARDIA

Catecholaminergic polymorphic ventricular tachycardia (CPVT) is a potentially heritable arrhythmia syndrome that classically manifests with exercise-induced syncope, seizures or sudden cardiac death (SCD). A first large cohort of CPVT patients was described in 1995.[28] These 21 patients were displaying a unique and uniform pattern of stress-induced, bidirectional ventricular tachycardia (VT) in the absence of structural heart disease.[28] CPVT predominantly presents before puberty, although older ages have been reported.

In fact, once thought to manifest only during child-hood, more recent studies have suggested that the age of first presentation can vary from during infancy to 40 years of age. CPVT closely mimics some of the LQT1 clinical features, such as adren-ergically triggered cardiac events (syncope, sei-zures, SCD) in the setting of a structurally normal heart. For example, akin to LQT1, swimming is a potentially lethal arrhythmia-precipitating trigger in CPVT, because both have been shown to under-lie several cases of unexplained drowning or near drowning in a seemingly healthy swimmer.[29] However, in contrast with LQT1, patients with CPVT always have a normal resting 12-lead elec-trocardiogram (ECG) without QT prolongation. The current estimated prevalence of CPVT is approximately 1 in 10,000. However, because CPVT can only be detected electrocardiographi-cally by a stress test ECG or 24-hour Holter moni-toring, the true prevalence may be higher. The underlying causes of cardiac events in CPVT are cardiac arrhythmias of bidirectional or polymorphic VT that can either self-terminate or progress to life-threatening VF. Although exercise-associated bidi-rectional VT is essentially pathognomonic for CPVT, it is very uncommon.[30] Instead, an index of suspicion for CPVT should be raised when a pa-tient presents with an exercise-associated symp-tom of concern and when the stress test yields normal sinus rhythm at rest but onset of premature ventricular contractions (PVCs) in isolation with onset around 110 to 130 beats/min. The isolated PVCs then progress to PVCs in bigeminy and into more complex arrhythmias as the heart rate increases.

Perturbations in key components of intracellular calcium-induced calcium release from the sarco-plasmic reticulum underlie the pathogenic basis for approximately two-thirds of CPVT. Mutations in the RYR2-encoded cardiac ryanodine recep-tor/calcium release channel represent the most common genetic subtype of CPVT (CPVT1), ac-counting for 60% of robust CPVT cases.[31,32] Although an oversimplification, conceptually gain-of-function mutations in RyR2 produce "leaky" calcium release channels that cause increased intracellular calcium levels during dias-tole, particularly during sympathetic stimulation. This increased diastolic calcium can precipitate calcium overload, delayed afterdepolarizations, and ventricular arrhythmias. As a corollary, the pharmacologic mimicker of the CPVT-associated bidirectional VT is digoxin toxicity.

Most unrelated CPVT families have their own unique, private RYR2 mutation and about 5% of unrelated mutation-positive patients host multiple putative pathogenic mutations. Although there are not any specific mutation hot spots in the large gene RYR2, there are 3 regional hot spots or do-mains where CPVT-causing mutations cluster. Before next-generation sequencing technologies emerged, this observation lent itself to targeted genetic testing of RYR2 (~61 exons, approxi-mately two-thirds of the complete gene) rather than a complete scan of RYR2's 105 exons, which is one of the largest genes in the human genome.[32] In fact, two-thirds of all CPVT1-associated muta-tions in RYR2 are confined to fewer than 20 of its 105 translated exons.

More than 90% of RYR2 mutations discovered to date represent missense mutations; however, perhaps as much as 5% of unrelated CPVT pa-tients host large gene rearrangements consistent with large whole exon deletions. Interpretation of the genetic test is complicated by the rate of back-ground noise variants in the normal population of 3%, yielding a favorable signal-to-noise ratio of approximately 20:1 (ie, a 5% chance of being a false positive).[33] Importantly, however, this signal-to-noise ratio requires the case to be a robust CPVT case. As the veracity of the CPVT diagnosis weakens, the probability that an identi-fied variant within RYR2 is a pathogenic mutation decreases. In addition to CPVT1, mutations in KCNJ2-encoded inwardly rectifying potassium channel (KCNJ2), a phenocopy of LQTS type 7 (LQT7) or Andersen-Tawil syndrome, and CALM1-encoded calmodulin 1 (CALM1) have been described. Although mutations in these genes are associated with an autosomal dominant inheritance pattern, a less common form of autosomal-recessive CPVT stemming from homo-zygous or compound heterozygous mutations in CASQ2-encoded calsequestrin have been described.[34,35]

Clinical Manifestation and Diagnosis

Typically, the sentinel event for a patient with CPVT is a self-limiting, exercise-induced faint or a faint followed by a generalized seizure with sub-sequent recovery. However, a sentinel event of SCD in an undiagnosed and untreated patient is probably highest for CPVT compared with either LQTS or the Brugada syndrome. Overall, the pos-sibility of CPVT should be suspected in patients (i) experiencing syncope or generalized seizure dur-ing exercise or emotion, (ii) with SCD triggered by acute emotional stress or exercise, (iii) with a family history of SCD during acute emotional stress or exercise, (iv) with a stress test that yields increasing ventricular ectopy and ectopy complexity during exercise that normalizes in the recovery phase, and (v) VF in setting of acute stress, all in the absence of structural cardiac abnormalities.[36] Clinically, a presentation of exercise-induced syncope and a QTc of less than 460 ms should always prompt first consideration of CPVT rather than the so-called electrocardiographically concealed LQTS.

The diagnostic workup for a patient with suspected CPVT should include complete personal and extensive family history of disease, resting ECG, 24-hour Holter monitor (to determine the number of arrhythmias over time and at different heart rates), echocardiogram and/or cardiac MRI (to confirm a structurally normal heart), and a consult with genetic counselor. Additionally, a loop recorder could be implanted to track a patient's arrhythmia burden over time, although this monitoring is not used very commonly in most CPVT centers. Given that the CPVT phenotype is adrenergically driven, the most critical diagnostic test is the exercise stress test. As an aside, many young out-of-hospital cardiac arrest survivors are dismissed from the hospital with an ICD after an extensive workup that often fails to include a stress test. Given the growing concerns that an ICD could be part of a CPVT patient's problem rather than their therapeutic solution, it is vital that CPVT be ruled out with a normal stress test in out-of-hospital cardiac arrest survivors who are younger than 40 years of age.

During the treadmill or cycle stress test (alternatively chemical stress test with isoproterenol), isolated PVCs commence around 110 to 130 beats/min and progress to bigeminal PVCs as the heart rate and workload increase (**Fig. 2**). Then, ventricular couplets emerge. In the correct story, these stress test finds are sufficient to compel a preliminary diagnosis of CPVT and pursue CPVT genetic testing. Occasionally, bidirectional couplets will follow and rarely, the ventricular arrhythmias will ensue with nonsustained VT.

To reemphasize, although pathognomonic for CPVT, the emergence of exercise-associated bidirectional VT is not a sensitive finding. At the highest workload, the ectopy often ceases. If it persisted until the patient's maximum heart rate was achieved, the ventricular ectopy characteristically stops immediately in the recovery phase rather than continuing until the heart rate decreases below the original ectopy onset heart rate.[30,37]

If an SCD is the sentinel event, first-degree relatives should undergo extensive clinical evaluation (including exercise testing) and subsequent genetic testing should be performed in a living relative who shows a diagnostic profile consistent with an identifiable channelopathy. If not, postmortem genetic testing (aka, molecular autopsy) should be performed on the decedent.[38] More than 30% of patients with CPVT have a positive family history of premature SCD. This number increases to approximately 60% of families hosting CPVT1-associated *RyR2* mutations. Moreover, approximately 15% of autopsy negative sudden unexplained deaths in the young and some cases of sudden infant death syndrome have been attributed to CPVT.[39,40] In 1 study, nearly one-third of patients diagnosed as possible/atypical LQTS (QTc <480 ms) cases with exertion-induced syncope were instead *RYR2* mutation positive and subsequently diagnosed with CPVT.[32]

Risk Stratification

Risk stratifiers for CPVT include male gender, the occurrence of aborted cardiac arrest before diagnosis, and early diagnosis.[41] Most important, although a cardiac arrest before diagnosis is associated with a higher risk of future events, this is not the case for a history of syncope. After diagnosis, the persistence of ectopy (ventricular couplets or nonsustained VT) on exercise testing, despite medical treatment, has been associated with a worse outcome.[41] Additionally, mutations located in the C-terminus of *RyR2* carry a higher risk.[42]

Therapy

The treatment options and recommendation for CPVT are summarized in **Table 2** per international guidelines[36]; however, these recommendations were written before the full evidence of the efficacy of LCSD in CPVT had been published. First, unlike LQTS and Brugada syndrome, where there are QT-prolonging drugs to avoid or Brugada syndrome–aggravating drugs to avoid, no particular drugs are contraindicated in patients with CPVT, except perhaps epinephrine/isoproterenol in the case of resuscitation. In contrast with Brugada syndrome, where there was never evidence regarding proarrhythmic potential in athletes, or in LQTS, where there is growing observational evidence that a well-treated athlete may remain an athlete, CPVT is the cardiac channelopathy where there is greatest concern about exercise-triggered events, including SCD in patients wishing to remain an athlete. As such, in accordance with the 2013 expert opinion guideline,[36] disqualification from competitive sports is advised. However, even for CPVT, preliminary evidence is emerging to suggest that a well-treated athlete may be able to safely remain an athlete.[43] With this information and with an increasing embrace of shared decision making regarding return-to-play considerations, the 2015 American Heart Association/

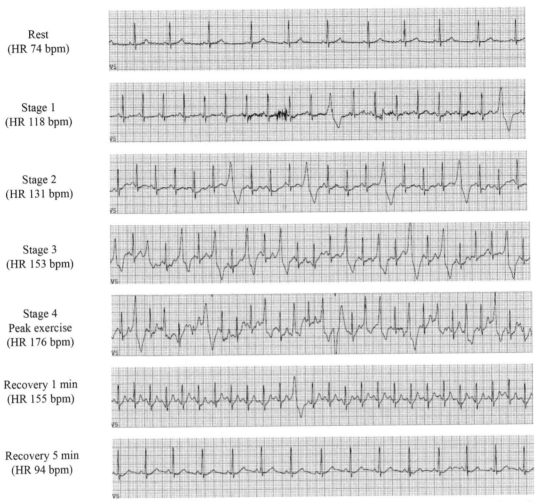

Rest
(HR 74 bpm)

Stage 1
(HR 118 bpm)

Stage 2
(HR 131 bpm)

Stage 3
(HR 153 bpm)

Stage 4
Peak exercise
(HR 176 bpm)

Recovery 1 min
(HR 155 bpm)

Recovery 5 min
(HR 94 bpm)

Fig. 2. Exercise test in a genotype-positive patient with catecholaminergic polymorphic ventricular tachycardia showing normal sinus rhythm at rest with increasing ectopy with exercise. Patient demonstrated single premature ventricular contractions (PVCs) starting at a heart rate (HR) of 118 bpm (stage 1) increasing in frequency to PVCs in bigeminy with couplets and a bidirectional couplet at peak exercise (stage 4). Ectopy disappears during the recovery phase.

American College of Cardiology scientific statement advised that athletes with CPVT who desired to remain an athlete should be evaluated, risk stratified, treated, and counseled by an expert in CPVT to ensure that a well-informed decision could be made.[44] The legislation concerning the possibility for a patient affected by a channelopathy to practice competitive sports varies between countries. In Italy, for example, a sport physician is not allowed by a state law to provide an LQTS or CPVT patient with the certificate necessary to practice sports.

β-Blockers (preferably nadolol, 1–2 mg/kg divided 2 times per day until age 10, and once a day thereafter) are the first line of pharmacotherapy in CPVT by inhibition of adrenergic activity, heart rate reduction (or blunting during exercise, emotion) or possibly direct effect on calcium release form sarcoplasmic reticulum.[36] β-Blockers have a proven efficacy of approximately 60%, and are dosed by uptitration until a significant reduction of exercise-induced arrhythmias is achieved on repeated treadmill exercise tests. For patients who still experience breakthrough cardiac events or fail to show a reduction of ectopy on exercise testing, combination drug therapy with the addition of flecainide can further reduce ectopy burden.[45,46] Although individualization of therapy is appropriate for CPVT, flecainide monotherapy is not yet supported by enough evidence, although early observations are encouraging.[47]

If syncope recurs despite pharmacotherapy or if the patient is not tolerating their medications, the

Table 2
Treatment options for CPVT

Therapy	Expert Guideline Recommendation
Lifestyle changes (disqualification from competitive sports and avoidance of strenuous exercise, stressful situations)	Recommended for all patients (class I, 2013 HRS/EHRA). But, if shared decision making is being considered, an athlete with CPVT who desires to remain an athlete should be evaluated, risk stratified, treated, and counseled by a cardiologist with expertise in CPVT (class I, 2015 AHA/ACC).
β-Blockers (nadolol, propranolol, or carvedilol)	Recommended for all symptomatic patients (class I).
	Can be useful in asymptomatic, mutation-positive patients (class IIa).
Flecainide	Can be useful as an addition to β-blockers in patients with recurrent syncope or polymorphic/bidirectional VT while on β-blockers (class IIa).
ICD	Recommended in patients with a previous cardiac arrest, or recurrent syncope of polymorphic/bidirectional VT despite optimal medical treatment and/or LCSD (class I).
LCSD	May be considered in patients with recurrent syncope or polymorphic/bidirectional VT while on β-blockers, or contraindicated for ICD (Class IIb by 2013 guidelines, class IIa by current evidence).

Abbreviations: AHA/ACC, American Heart Association/American College of Cardiology; CPVT, catecholaminergic polymorphic ventricular tachycardia; HRS/EHRA, Heart Rhythm Society/European Heart Rhythm Association; ICD, implantable cardioverter-defibrillator; LCSD, left cardiac sympathetic denervation; VT, ventricular tachycardia.

most recent data suggest that LCSD should be considered before an ICD.[23,48–50] Although still a class IIb recommendation by 2013 guidelines,[36] subsequent studies have demonstrated a significant reduction in arrhythmia burden after LCSD in patients with CPVT. In fact, a recent large, multicenter study has shown that LCSD has a potent, antifibrillatory effect in patients with CPVT, especially when the denervation surgery is performed correctly, suggesting a growing and possible alternative role for this procedure over ICD implantation.[50]

However, according to the 2013 guidelines, an ICD is recommended (class I recommendation) in CPVT patients who have experienced either (i) a cardiac arrest, (ii) recurrent syncope/seizures while on drug therapy, or (iii) persistent nonsustained VT on stress testing, despite optimal medical treatment.[36] However, unlike symptomatic Brugada syndrome where ICD monotherapy is indicated universally, an ICD should never be used alone in a patient with CPVT. In fact, over the past decade, the ICD has gone from being one of the first therapies in CPVT (secondary to

the recognition that there may be a 25% chance of CPVT-triggered recurrence on β-blocker therapy) to being one of the last therapies in CPVT and never the only therapy. This practice change has occurred because of the increased risk in CPVT for a so-called electrical storm (VF–shock–VF–shock cycles), where ultimately there is a failure to restore the cardiac rhythm.[51] In fact, there are now tragic examples where the inciting shock was an inappropriate shock secondary to sinus tachycardia or atrial fibrillation, which then "woke up" the proverbial CPVT beast and an electrical storm and subsequent death followed. In other words, the ICD itself was the direct cause of death for the CPVT patient rather than the intended life-saving solution. When an ICD is being used in a patient's treatment program, we always recommend dual therapy (β-blocker and flecainide, β-blocker and LCSD, or LCSD and flecainide) and sometimes triple therapy (β-blocker, flecainide, and LCSD) as part of the patient's anti–electrical storm strategy. The growing use of LCSD, in CPVT as well as in LQTS, also reflects its favorable impact on quality of life.[52,53]

BRUGADA SYNDROME

Brugada syndrome is one of the inherited arrhythmia syndromes that, in recent years, has obtained a lot of attention. Many aspects of the disease are heavily discussed and that includes whether it is a pure electrical disease or it represents part of a spectrum (ie, its pathophysiological [and genetic] basis), and which (asymptomatic) patient is at risk.[54,55] The diagnosis is fortunately agreed upon[36] and that is a type 1 pattern of ST elevation ($\geq$2 mm) in the right precordial leads (either placed at the normal fourth intercostal space or in a higher intercostal space). The disease associates with an arrhythmic risk based on VF that usually starts with short-coupled ectopy from the right ventricular outflow tract area.

As stated, the diagnosis is an electrophysiological entity and does not, in contrast with LQTS, include genetic information. In fact, the genetics seems to be complex, with a suggested involvement of more than 20 genes. In recent studies, however, the concept that Brugada syndrome is an oligogenetic disease has gained interest. In a genome-wide association study performed on more than 300 cases of Brugada syndrome, 3 genomic areas, including the SCN5A, SCN10A, and Hey2 loci, were linked to the disease.[56] The phenotype was more prevalent in individuals with a greater number of risk alleles.[56] Other next-generation sequencing efforts have indicated that rare variants in all, except SCN5A, putative Brugada syndrome susceptibility genes are found in equal numbers in controls as well.[57] Importantly, if the patient has a type 1 Brugada ECG pattern and a prolonged PR interval, the rate of SCN5A positivity is about 40%. In contrast, if the PR interval is normal, the SCN5A yield is less than 10%.[58,59] SCN5A mutations with a higher degree of loss-of-function are associated with a more severe disease (wider conduction intervals) than mutation with less disruptive effect on the function of the cardiac sodium channel.[60] However, in all these studies, probably do to a relatively small number of symptomatic patients, no effect could be demonstrated in symptoms/outcome. Hence, at present genetic testing is not useful for determining future risk. Of importance, the presence of a causal SCN5A variant(s), although not leading to active treatment, should result in lifestyle adjustments (ie, avoidance of drugs, and avoidance of fever and high-dose alcohol intake).

Clinical Manifestation and Diagnosis

SCD owing to VF is the most severe clinical symptom in Brugada syndrome and, not rarely, this is the first manifestation. Patients can also present with syncope but the vast majority of patients with Brugada syndrome are asymptomatic for life. The mean age of VF episodes is around 41 years old and men have a 5.5-fold greater risk of SCD as compared with women.[55] However, arrhythmic events may occur from infancy to old age.[55] Most frequently, arrhythmic events are observed at rest or while asleep, most frequently from midnight to 6 AM.[61] Vagal tone might play a role in arrhythmic events.[55] Fever is a very important factor for ECG changes and successive VF.[62] Children were reported to manifest coved-type ST elevation during fever quite frequently, indeed.[63]

Supraventricular arrhythmias are also frequently observed in patients with the Brugada syndrome, including atrial fibrillation.[55] Interestingly, almost 30% of patients with atrioventricular nodal reentry respond with the development of a type 1 Brugada ECG pattern to ajmaline.[64] Rarely, monomorphic VT is observed.[55] Bradycardia, sick sinus node syndrome, and atrioventricular conduction disturbances are frequently reported in patients with the Brugada syndrome with SCN5A mutations.[65,66]

The diagnostic criteria for the Brugada syndrome have been changed several times since its initial description. Central in all consensus documents is a type 1 Brugada ECG pattern ($\geq$2 mm ST elevation in a right precordial lead). In the first consensus document,[67] only the standard placement (fourth intercostal space) of electrodes was accepted, but based on studies demonstrating the diagnostic value of the ECG recordings in the upper precordial leads[68] or the manifestation of coved type ST-segment elevation in inferolateral leads in Brugada syndrome.[69] The criteria changed and accepted a type 1 Brugada ECG pattern in alternative lead positions as well. The clinical criteria, initially requested for the diagnosis in the first consensus document, in the latest consensus document have become part of the scoring system and are only relevant in the setting of a drug-induced type 1 ECG.[55] The ECG may vary from day to day and is under the influence of several factors, including vagal tone, testosterone levels, and body temperature.[55] Confounding factors, including acute myocardial ischemia, myocarditis, electrolyte disorders, arrhythmogenic right ventricular dysplasia, pulmonary embolism, or mechanical compression of the right ventricular outflow tract, need to be excluded before the definite diagnosis of the Brugada syndrome can be made.[55,67]

Risk Stratification

There is little doubt that symptomatic patients with the Brugada syndrome, that is, with a past history of VT/VF or syncope of suspected cardiac origin, are at risk for future arrhythmic events.[55,62,67,70] The risk varies from 7.7% to 10.2% in resuscitated patients to 0.6% to 1.9% in patients with a history of syncope.[55] Unfortunately, for asymptomatic patients with the Brugada syndrome, the risk for (near) lethal events is poorly defined. A recent review summarized the literature through 2014[70] and emphasizes that, on most parameters, there is disagreement as to their prognostic value. An exception is the presence of a spontaneous type 1 Brugada ECG pattern that in all studies is associated with an increased risk. The annual risk for (near) lethal arrhythmias associated with a spontaneous type 1 Brugada ECG pattern is estimated to be around 0.5% to 0.8%.[55,62,70] In mid life, this risk may accumulate over years but at advanced age patients with a spontaneous type 1 Brugada ECG pattern seem to be at a lower risk.[71] More recent studies emphasize a role for a pronounced S-wave in lead I.[72] Finally, a large metaanalysis on the role of electrophysiological testing concludes that induction with a mild protocol, that is, 1 or 2 extra systoles, may bear some prognostic value in asymptomatic individuals.[73]

Therapy

Given the recurrent risk on lethal arrhythmias, an ICD is the first line therapy in symptomatic patients with the Brugada syndrome with a past history of VT/VF or syncope suggestive of malignant arrhythmia origin.[55] Considering the relatively low annual rate of arrhythmic events in asymptomatic patients (see above), an ICD indication in asymptomatic patients needs careful consideration. However, alternative treatment options are not readily available. Quinidine has been advocated to be effective, also in the long term.[74]

Specific lifestyle adjustments are pertinent in all Brugada syndrome patients. A number of drugs are to be avoided. Most of these drugs, among which are psychotropic drugs and anesthetics, block the cardiac sodium channel. The list is, however, much longer and can be found on the website www.brugadadrugs.org.[75] Fever is another important trigger for symptoms and the general advice is to lower body temperature as soon as possible with antipyretic drugs or to come to the nearest hospital for monitoring. Alcohol intake has been associated with events and a large quantity is better avoided.

For patients with electrical storms, isoproterenol is effective in suppressing VF.[55] For patients with a history of appropriate VF-terminating ICD shocks, long-term chronic oral medication with quinidine, denopamine, cilostazol, and bepridil (available only in Japan) are effective in VF suppression.[55] In more recent years, exciting invasive ablation options have come to the surface. Ablation of the epicardial surface of the right ventricular outflow track was shown to be effective for VF suppression and the disappearance of type 1 ECG in a first series of 8 of 9 patients with the Brugada syndrome (at 2 years follow-up)[76] and this technique (right ventricular outflow tract epicardial ablation) now seems so promising that a randomized trial comparing epicardial ablation with conservative treatment has been called for.[77] This development is relevant because an epicardial ablation is a more difficult procedure compared with endocardial approach and does not go without risk.[78] Clearly, the latter also implies that it is much too early to perform epicardial ablation in asymptomatic patients. Endocardial ablation of initiating extra systoles has also been reported to be successful in single cases.[79]

ACKNOWLEDGMENTS

The authors are grateful to Pinuccia De Tomasi, BS, for expert editorial support.

REFERENCES

1. Jervell A, Lange-Nielsen F. Congenital deaf-mutism, functional heart disease with prolongation of the Q-T interval, and sudden death. Am Heart J 1957;54: 59–68.
2. Schwartz PJ, Periti M, Malliani A. The long Q-T syndrome. Am Heart J 1975;89:378–90.
3. Schwartz PJ, Spazzolini C, Crotti L, et al. The Jervell and Lange-Nielsen Syndrome. Natural history, molecular basis, and clinical outcome. Circulation 2006;113:783–90.
4. Wang Q, Shen J, Splawski I, et al. SCN5A mutations associated with an inherited cardiac arrhythmia, long QT syndrome. Cell 1995;80:805–11.
5. Curran ME, Splawski I, Timothy KW, et al. A molecular basis for cardiac arrhythmia: HERG mutations cause long QT syndrome. Cell 1995;80:795–803.
6. Wang Q, Curran ME, Splawski I, et al. Positional cloning of a novel potassium channel gene: KvLQT1 mutations cause cardiac arrhythmias. Nat Genet 1996;12:17–23.
7. Schwartz PJ, Ackerman MJ, George AL Jr, et al. Impact of genetics on the clinical management of channelopathies. J Am Coll Cardiol 2013;62:169–80.
8. Priori SG, Schwartz PJ, Napolitano C, et al. Risk stratification in the long-QT syndrome. N Engl J Med 2003;348:1866–74.
9. Schwartz PJ, Priori SG, Spazzolini C, et al. Genotype-phenotype correlation in the long-QT

syndrome: gene-specific triggers for life-threatening arrhythmias. Circulation 2001;103:89–95.

10. Schwartz PJ, Ackerman MJ. The long QT syndrome: a transatlantic clinical approach to diagnosis and therapy. Eur Heart J 2013;34:3109–16.

11. Schwartz PJ, Woosley RL. Predicting the unpredictable: drug-induced QT prolongation and Torsades de Pointes. J Am Coll Cardiol 2016;67:1639–50.

12. Schwartz PJ, Crotti L, Insolia R. Arrhythmogenic disorders of genetic origin: long QT syndrome: from genetics to management. Circ Arrhythm Electrophysiol 2012;5:868–77.

13. Schwartz PJ, Crotti L. QTc behavior during exercise and genetic testing for the long-QT syndrome. Circulation 2011;124:2181–4.

14. Hofman N, Tan HL, Alders M, et al. Active cascade screening in primary inherited arrhythmia syndromes: does it lead to prophylactic treatment? J Am Coll Cardiol 2010;55:2570–6.

15. Schwartz PJ. Efficacy of left cardiac sympathetic denervation has an unforeseen side effect: medicolegal complications. Heart Rhythm 2010;7:1330–2.

16. Schwartz PJ. Management of the long QT syndrome. Nat Clin Pract Cardiovasc Med 2005;2:346–51.

17. Schwartz PJ. Sudden cardiac death, founder populations and mushrooms. What is the link with gold mines and modifier genes? Heart Rhythm 2011;8: 548–50.

18. Chockalingam P, Crotti L, Girardengo G, et al. Not all beta-blockers are equal in the management of long QT syndrome types 1 and 2: higher recurrence of events under metoprolol. J Am Coll Cardiol 2012; 60:2092–9.

19. Schwartz PJ, Spazzolini C, Crotti L. All LQT3 patients need an ICD. True or false? Heart Rhythm 2009;6:113–20.

20. Wilde AAM, Moss AJ, Kaufman ES, et al. Clinical aspects of type 3 long QT syndrome. An international multicenter study. Circulation 2016;134:872–82.

21. Schwartz PJ. Cardiac sympathetic denervation to prevent life-threatening arrhythmias. Nat Rev Cardiol 2014;11:346–53.

22. Schwartz PJ, Priori SG, Cerrone M, et al. Left cardiac sympathetic denervation in the management of high-risk patients affected by the long QT syndrome. Circulation 2004;109:1826–33.

23. Collura CA, Johnson JN, Moir C, et al. Left cardiac sympathetic denervation for the treatment of long QT syndrome and catecholaminergic polymorphic ventricular tachycardia using video-assisted thoracic surgery. Heart Rhythm 2009;6:752–9.

24. Schwartz PJ, Spazzolini C, Priori SG, et al. Who are the long-QT syndrome patients who receive an implantable cardioverter defibrillator and what happens to them? Data from the European long-QT syndrome implantable cardioverter-defibrillator (LQTS ICD) Registry. Circulation 2010;122:1272–82.

25. Schwartz PJ, Vanoli E, Crotti L, et al. Neural control of heart rate is an arrhythmia risk modifier in long QT syndrome. J Am Coll Cardiol 2008;51:920–9.

26. Crotti L, Spazzolini C, Porretta AP, et al. Vagal reflexes following an exercise stress test: a simple clinical tool for gene-specific risk stratification in the long QT syndrome. J Am Coll Cardiol 2012;60: 2515–24.

27. Johnson JN, Ackerman MJ. Competitive sports participation in athletes with congenital long QT syndrome. JAMA 2012;308:764–5.

28. Leenhardt A, Lucet V, Denjoy I, et al. Catecholaminergic polymorphic ventricular tachycardia in children. A 7-year follow-up of 21 patients. Circulation 1995;91:1512–9.

29. Choi G, Kopplin LJ, Tester DJ, et al. Spectrum and frequency of cardiac channel defects in swimming-triggered arrhythmia syndromes. Circulation 2004; 110:2119–24.

30. Horner JM, Ackerman MJ. Ventricular ectopy during treadmill exercise stress testing in the evaluation of long QT syndrome. Heart Rhythm 2008;5:1690–4.

31. Priori SG, Napolitano C, Tiso N, et al. Mutations in the cardiac ryanodine receptor gene (hRyR2) underlie catecholaminergic polymorphic ventricular tachycardia. Circulation 2001;103:196–200.

32. Medeiros-Domingo A, Bhuiyan ZA, Tester DJ, et al. The RYR2-encoded ryanodine receptor/calcium release channel in patients diagnosed previously with either catecholaminergic polymorphic ventricular tachycardia or genotype negative, exercise-induced long QT syndrome: a comprehensive open reading frame mutational analysis. J Am Coll Cardiol 2009;54:2065–74.

33. Ackerman MJ, Priori SG, Willems S, et al. HRS/EHRA expert consensus statement on the state of genetic testing for the channelopathies and cardiomyopathies. Heart Rhythm 2011;8:1308–39.

34. Lahat H, Eldar M, Levy-Nissenbaum E, et al. Autosomal recessive catecholamine- or exercise-induced polymorphic ventricular tachycardia: clinical features and assignment of the disease gene to chromosome 1p13-21. Circulation 2001;103: 2822–7.

35. Lahat H, Pras E, Olender T, et al. A missense mutation in a highly conserved region of CASQ2 is associated with autosomal recessive catecholamine-induced polymorphic ventricular tachycardia in Bedouin families from Israel. Am J Hum Genet 2001;69:1378–84.

36. Priori SG, Wilde AA, Horie M, et al. HRS/EHRA/APHRS expert consensus statement on the diagnosis and management of patients with inherited primary arrhythmia syndromes: document endorsed by HRS, EHRA, and APHRS in May 2013 and by ACCF, AHA, PACES, and AEPC in June 2013. Heart Rhythm 2013;10:1932–63.

37. Priori SG, Blomström-Lundqvist C, Mazzanti A, et al. 2015 ESC guidelines for the management of patients with ventricular arrhythmias and the prevention of sudden cardiac death: the Task Force for the Management of Patients with Ventricular Arrhythmias and the Prevention of Sudden Cardiac Death of the European Society of Cardiology (ESC). Endorsed by: Association for European Paediatric and Congenital Cardiology (AEPC). Eur Heart J 2015;36:2793–867.

38. Tester DJ, Spoon DB, Valdivia HH, et al. Targeted mutational analysis of the RyR2-encoded cardiac ryanodine receptor in sudden unexplained death: a molecular autopsy of 49 medical examiner/coroner's cases. Mayo Clin Proc 2004;79:1380–4.

39. Tester DJ, Ackerman MJ. The role of molecular autopsy in unexplained sudden cardiac death. Curr Opin Cardiol 2006;21:166–72.

40. Tester DJ, Dura M, Carturan E, et al. A mechanism for sudden infant death syndrome (SIDS): stress-induced leak via ryanodine receptors. Heart Rhythm 2007;4:733–9.

41. Hayashi M, Denjoy I, Extramiana F, et al. Incidence and risk factors of arrhythmic events in catecholaminergic polymorphic ventricular tachycardia. Circulation 2009;119:2426–34.

42. van der Werf C, Nederend I, Hofman N, et al. Familial evaluation in catecholaminergic polymorphic ventricular tachycardia: disease penetrance and expression in cardiac ryanodine receptor mutation-carrying relatives. Circ Arrhythm Electrophysiol 2012;5:748–56.

43. Ostby SA, Bos JM, Owen HJ, et al. Competitive sports participation in patients with catecholaminergic polymorphic ventricular tachycardia. A single center's early experience. J Am Coll Cardiol 2016; 2:253–62.

44. Ackerman MJ, Zipes DP, Kovacs RJ, et al, American Heart Association Electrocardiography and Arrhythmias Committee of Council on Clinical Cardiology, Council on Cardiovascular Disease in Young, Council on Cardiovascular and Stroke Nursing, Council on Functional Genomics and Translational Biology, and American College of Cardiology. Eligibility and disqualification recommendations for competitive athletes with cardiovascular abnormalities: task force 10: the cardiac channelopathies: a scientific statement from the American Heart Association and American College of Cardiology. Circulation 2015;132(22):e326–9.

45. Watanabe H, Chopra N, Laver D, et al. Flecainide prevents catecholaminergic polymorphic ventricular tachycardia in mice and humans. Nat Med 2009;15: 380–3.

46. van der Werf C, Kannankeril PJ, Sacher F, et al. Flecainide therapy reduces exercise-induced ventricular arrhythmias in patients with catecholaminergic polymorphic ventricular tachycardia. J Am Coll Cardiol 2011;57:2244–54.

47. Padfield GJ, AlAhmari L, Lieve KV, et al. Flecainide monotherapy is an option for selected patients with catecholaminergic polymorphic ventricular tachycardia intolerant of β-blockade. Heart Rhythm 2016;13:609–13.

48. Wilde AA, Bhuiyan ZA, Crotti L, et al. Left cardiac sympathetic denervation for catecholaminergic polymorphic ventricular tachycardia. N Engl J Med 2008;358:2024–9.

49. Coleman MA, Bos JM, Johnson JN, et al. Videoscopic left cardiac sympathetic denervation for patients with recurrent ventricular fibrillation/malignant ventricular arrhythmia syndromes besides congenital long QT syndrome. Circ Arrhythm Electrophysiol 2012;5:782–8.

50. De Ferrari GM, Dusi V, Spazzolini C, et al. Clinical management of catecholaminergic polymorphic ventricular tachycardia: the role of left cardiac sympathetic denervation. Circulation 2015;131:2185–93.

51. Roses-Noguer F, Jarman JW, Clague JR, et al. Outcomes of defibrillator therapy in catecholaminergic polymorphic ventricular tachycardia. Heart Rhythm 2014;11:58–66.

52. Antiel RM, Bos JM, Joyce DD, et al. Quality of life after videoscopic left cardiac sympathetic denervation in patients with potentially life-threatening cardiac channelopathies/cardiomyopathies. Heart Rhythm 2016;13:62–9.

53. Schwartz PJ. When the risk is sudden death, does quality of life matter? Heart Rhythm 2016;13:70–1.

54. Mizusawa Y, Wilde AAM. Brugada syndrome. Circ Arrhythm Electrophysiol 2012;5:606–16.

55. Antzelevitch C, Yan GX, Ackerman MJ, et al. J-Wave syndromes, expert consensus conference report: emerging concepts and gaps in knowledge. Heart Rhythm 2016;13:e295–324.

56. Bezzina CR, Barc J, Mizusawa Y, et al. Common variants at SCN5A/SCN10A and HEY2 are associated with Brugada syndrome, a rare disease with high risk of sudden cardiac death. Nat Genet 2013;45: 1044–9.

57. LeScouarnec S, Karakachoff M, Gourraud JB, et al. Testing the burden of rare variation in arrhythmia-susceptibility genes provides new insights into molecular diagnosis for Brugada syndrome. Hum Mol Genet 2015;24:2757–63.

58. Kapplinger JD, Tester DJ, Alders M, et al. An international compendium of mutations in the SCN5A-encoded cardiac sodium channel in patients referred for Brugada syndrome genetic testing. Heart Rhythm 2010;7:33–46.

59. Crotti L, Marcou CA, Tester DJ, et al. Spectrum and prevalence of mutations involving BrS1-through BrS12-susceptibility genes in a cohort

of unrelated patients referred for Brugada Syndrome genetic testing. J Am Coll Cardiol 2012; 60:1410–8.

60. Meregalli PG, Tan HL, Probst V, et al. Type of SCN5A mutation determines clinical severity and degree of conduction slowing in loss-of-function sodium channelopathies. Heart Rhythm 2009;6:341–8.

61. Takigawa M, Noda T, Shimizu W, et al. Seasonal and circadian distributions of ventricular fibrillation in patients with Brugada syndrome. Heart Rhythm 2008; 5:1523–7.

62. Mizusawa Y, Morita H, Adler A, et al. The prognostic significance of fever-induced Brugada Syndrome. Heart Rhythm 2016;13:1515–20.

63. Probst V, Denjoy I, Meregalli PG, et al. Clinical aspects and prognosis of Brugada syndrome in children. Circulation 2007;115:2042–8.

64. Hasdemir C, Payzin S, Kocabas U, et al. High prevalence of concealed Brugada syndrome in patients with atrioventricular nodal reentrant tachycardia. Heart Rhythm 2015;12:1584–94.

65. Smits JP, Koopmann TT, Wilders R, et al. A mutation in the human cardiac sodium channel (E161K) contributes to sick sinus syndrome, conduction disease and Brugada syndrome in two families. J Mol Cell Cardiol 2005;38:969–81.

66. Rodríguez-Mañero M, Sacher F, Asmundis C, et al. Monomorphic ventricular tachycardia in patients with Brugada syndrome: a multicenter retrospective study. Heart Rhythm 2016;13:669–82.

67. Wilde AA, Antzelevitch C, Borggrefe M, et al. Proposed diagnostic criteria for the Brugada syndrome: consensus report. Circulation 2002;106:2514–9.

68. Shimizu W, Matsuo K, Takagi M, et al. Body surface distribution and response to drugs of ST segment elevation in Brugada syndrome: clinical implication of eighty-seven-lead body surface potential mapping and its application to twelve-lead electrocardiograms. J Cardiovasc Electrophysiol 2000;11: 396–404.

69. Sarkozy A, Chierchia GB, Paparella G, et al. Inferior and lateral electrocardiographic repolarization abnormalities in Brugada syndrome. Circ Arrhythm Electrophysiol 2009;2:154–61.

70. Adler A, Rosso R, Chorin E, et al. Risk stratification in Brugada syndrome: clinical characteristics, electrocardiographic parameters, and auxiliary testing. Heart Rhythm 2015;13:299–310.

71. Kitamura T, Fukamizu S, Kawamura I, et al. Clinical characteristics and long-term prognosis of senior patients with Brugada syndrome. J Am Coll Cardiol, in press.

72. Caló L, Giustetto C, Martino A, et al. A new ECG marker of sudden death in Brugada Syndrome. The S-wave in lead I. J Am Coll Cardiol 2016;67: 1427–40.

73. Sroubek J, Probst V, Mazzanti A, et al. Programmed ventricular stimulation for risk stratification in the Brugada syndrome. A pooled analysis. Circulation 2016;133:622–30.

74. Viskin S, Wilde AA, Tan HL, et al. Empiric quinidine therapy for asymptomatic Brugada syndrome: time for a prospective registry. Heart Rhythm 2009;6: 401–4.

75. Postema PG, Wolpert C, Amin AS, et al. Drugs and Brugada syndrome patients: review of the literature, recommendations, and an up-to-date website (www.brugadadrugs.org). Heart Rhythm 2009;6: 1335–41.

76. Nademanee K, Veerakul G, Chandanamattha P, et al. Prevention of ventricular fibrillation episodes in Brugada syndrome by catheter ablation over the anterior right ventricular outflow tract epicardium. Circulation 2011;123:1270–9.

77. Wilde AAM, Nademanee K. Epicardial substrate ablation in Brugada syndrome. Time for a randomized trial! Circ Arrhythm Electrophysiol 2015;8: 1306–8.

78. Sacher F, Roberts-Thomson K, Maury P, et al. Epicardial ventricular tachycardia ablation a multicenter safety study. J Am Coll Cardiol 2010;55: 2366–72.

79. Shah AJ, Hocini M, Lamaison D, et al. Regional substrate ablation abolishes Brugada Syndrome. J Cardiovasc Electrophysiol 2011;22:1290–1.

Public Access Defibrillation

Is This Making Any Difference? Controversial Issues in Resuscitation from Cardiac Arrest

Myron L. Weisfeldt, MD[a],*, Ross A. Pollack, BS[b]

KEYWORDS

- Defibrillation • Cardiopulmonary resuscitation • Bystander AED • Automated external defibrillator
- Epinephrine

KEY POINTS

- Public access defibrillation is particularly valuable in witnessed cardiac arrests that occur in public locations. There has been considerable growth in bystander and police use of automated external defibrillators (AEDs) over the past 15 years for this subset of all cardiac arrests.
- Although defibrillators are used by bystanders or police in only a very small (but growing) percentage of all cardiac arrests, use among patients with cardiac arrest who survive, and survive with normal or near-normal neurologic function, is substantial.
- There is great promise for increasing the use of bystander defibrillators as communication technology links the patients with shockable arrests to volunteers committed to bringing AED's and applying the device to the patient.
- There are several important strategies that could increase the availability and use of AEDs, such as optimizing their location within public buildings and reducing their size and weight.
- Although the value of early shock in increasing survival from shockable cardiac arrest is well established, there continues to be considerable controversy and little definite evidence as to the value of using epinephrine, antiarrhythmic drugs, hypothermia, or mechanical chest compression devices in resuscitation from cardiac arrest.

INTRODUCTION

In 2002, Weisfeldt and Becker[1] proposed a 3-element model for the best strategy for resuscitation from cardiac arrest. Because this model has to some extent passed the test of time, the model frames this discussion (**Box 1**). Phase I of the model (the first 3–4 minutes after collapse) states that, if the cause of cardiac arrest is shockable rhythm and a defibrillator is available, the patient should be defibrillated first. Also, occasionally, correction of bradycardia or asystole may occur by pacing or repeated chest blows during phase 1.

Phase II is between 4 and 10 minutes after arrest. After 4 minutes, it is important to provide chest compressions to create artificial circulation that provides myocardial blood flow. After 4 minutes, defibrillation without prior circulation frequently leads to irreversible myocardial changes, often called stone heart. Phase III, after

The investigators have no conflicts of interest.

a Department of Medicine, Johns Hopkins University School of Medicine, 1812 Ashland Avenue Suite 110, Baltimore, MD 21205, USA; b Johns Hopkins University School of Medicine, 733 North Broadway, Baltimore, MD 21205, USA

* Corresponding author.

E-mail address: mlw5@jhmi.edu

Box 1
The 3-phase model of cardiac resuscitation

I. Electrical: 0 to 4 minutes

II. Circulatory: 4 to 10 minutes

III. Metabolic: greater than 10 minutes

Time intervals are from the onset of arrest. During the electrical phase, immediate electrical correction is advised. During the circulatory phase cardiopulmonary resuscitation (chest compressions) are advised before electrical correction. In the metabolic phase, the hope is to identify lifesaving interventions.

   Data from Weisfeldt ML, Becker L. Resuscitation after cardiac arrest: a 3-phase time-sensitive model [Commentary]. JAMA 2002;288(23):3035–8.

---

10 minutes of untreated arrest, is likely to be fatal. Very rarely does a patient with no chest compression or defibrillation survive. It is hoped that at some point an effective metabolic intervention will be identified that might allow survival without severe neurologic injury. No intervention is currently established to provide such benefit in humans. It was hoped that hypothermia might be such an intervention but there is no clear proof of benefit at this time.

LAUNCHING OF BYSTANDER USE OF AUTOMATIC DEFIBRILLATORS: PUBLIC ACCESS DEFIBRILLATION

In the early 1990s, the American Heart Association in a task force report[2] recommended to industry that simple-to-use, reliable, and inexpensive defibrillators be developed for use by lay bystanders. Automatic detection of ventricular tachycardia or fibrillation was essential. Once it was clear that such devices were going to become available, the American Heart Association led an effort with others to publicize, promote, and seek regulatory approval of defibrillation by any willing and adequately trained individual, whether a health care professional or not. Two consensus meetings featuring survivors of defibrillation arrest and attended by health care professionals, representatives of government (including the US Food and Drug Administration [FDA]), and the press were held in Washington, DC, and the results published.[3,4] Public interest was enhanced by the press and automated external defibrillators (AEDs) were approved for use, but not by non–health care professionals. The American Heart Association successfully pursued the inclusion of defibrillation under each state's so-called Good Samaritan statutes. Favorable results from the use of

defibrillators by security guards in Las Vegas casinos[5] and aboard American Airlines flights[6] showed both safety and efficacy in the hands of lay individuals with a duty to respond. Proof of benefit in the hands of lay volunteers awaited the FDA allowing the use of AEDs by lay responders and the randomized National Heart Lung and Blood Institute Public Access Defibrillation (PAD) study published in 2004.[7] In that study, 1000 community site volunteers were trained to perform cardiopulmonary resuscitation (CPR) and call 911. At 500 randomly chosen sites, volunteers were also trained in the use of AEDs and the sites were equipped with AEDs. The number of survivors increased from 15 to 30 in control versus AED sites ($P<.03$). Following this publication, sales of AEDs increased exponentially.

EQUIPPING OF POLICE VEHICLES AND TRAINING OF POLICE IN THE USE OF AUTOMATED EXTERNAL DEFIBRILLATORS

Long before the advent of easy-to-use automatic AEDs for public use, Roger White led a successful effort in Rochester, Minnesota, to improve survival from cardiac arrest in that community. Dr White trained police in defibrillation and CPR and summoned both the nearest emergency medical services (EMS) vehicle and the nearest police vehicle to every call that was likely to be related to a patient with cardiac arrest. The results of this effort were reported in serial publications documenting improved survival after successful police defibrillation when the police arrived before EMS.[8]

   Following this successful effort, Koster and associates progressively implemented a similar police effort, again with impressive results of improving survival from shockable out-of-hospital arrests from 29.1% to 41.4%.[9] The limited studies analyzing police AED defibrillation in major US cities have had mixed results. The Rochester experience pertains to small to middle-sized communities, whereas the extent of use by police in larger, more densely populated communities may be more variable.

COMMUNITY-BASED STUDIES OF USE AND OUTCOME

Several prospective registries of patients with cardiac arrest have documented improved survival and little evidence of harm from implementing bystander AED use in out-of-hospital cardiac arrests. The Resuscitation Outcomes Consortium (ROC) implemented an extensive prospective registry called EPISTRY (Epidemiology and Registry) under the leadership of Laurie Morrison in 2005, functioning as the backbone for prospective randomized trials.[10] The initial experience with bystanders applying an AED was published in 2010.[11] In 7 major cities or regions (Toronto, Ottawa, and Vancouver in Canada; and Seattle/King County, Portland, Oregon, San Diego, Dallas, Milwaukee and Pittsburgh) 259 patients had an AED applied by a bystander, with 149 of these patients shocked by the bystander (**Fig. 1**). Survival was 36% in those shocked and 23% in those applied whether there was a shock or not. These survival rates compared favorably with the 16% survival for those patients first shocked by EMS after bystander CPR and were nearly identical if arrest was observed and shocked by EMS (32%). There was no evidence of harm by applying an AED and clearly better survival than waiting for the first shock for EMS to arrive.

Patients shocked by an AED were only 149 out of 10,663 cardiac arrests. However, those shocked by a bystander AED were more than 11% of those with CPR and then shocked by EMS (149 out of 1293). Extrapolating these results to the entire population of the United States and Canada suggested that 500 patients per year survived because of a bystander applying and using an AED to treat a shockable rhythm. Similar overall results from similar periods of time have been reported by other substantial networks (CARES [Cardiac Arrest Registry to Enhance Survival])[12] and a regional system in North Carolina.[13]

CONCENTRATION OF SHOCKABLE CARDIAC ARRESTS IN PUBLIC LOCATIONS

Using the same ROC database, the overall incidence of shockable out-of-hospital cardiac arrest

was only 25%, whereas 30 years ago 75% were shockable.[14] For patients with an AED applied by a bystander, 149 out of 259 (58%) patients were shocked. Exploring this high rate of shock,[15] the ROC investigators found that arrests witnessed in public locations with an AED applied were 80% shockable and, of all 1003 witnessed arrests in public, 60% were shockable. Of 3451 witnessed arrests in the home, only 35% were shockable (**Fig. 2**). The ROC investigators rationalized that people who arrest in public are active individuals likely with mild or unknown cardiac disease and they had classic primary ventricular tachycardia (VT)/ventricular fibrillation (VF) shockable arrests, whereas patients who had arrests at home, even if witnessed, likely had chronic heart disease on medication and were more likely to have a non-VT/VF arrest. These data also point to the great value of PAD programs that concentrate attention on public locations. A single major study of arrest in the home failed to show any benefit of AEDs and training of spouses or friends.[16] Thus, rapid defibrillation saves lives, AEDs are particularly useful in public location arrests, and asystole and pulseless electrical activity are common in arrests occurring at home or in nursing homes.

CONTEMPORARY USE OF AUTOMATED EXTERNAL DEFIBRILLATORS IN CARDIAC ARRESTS WITNESSED IN PUBLIC LOCATIONS

In unpublished data from ROC (Pollack R, 2017) from between 2011 and 2015 there was an increase in shock by a bystander in shockable observed public out-of-hospital cardiac arrests (SOP-OHCAs) from ~10% to ~20%. Details of

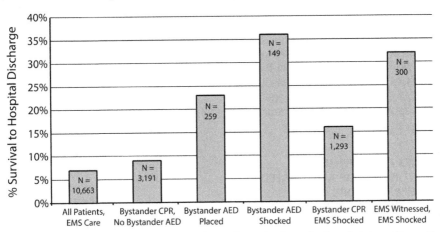

Fig. 1. Overall and subgroup survival to hospital discharge from the Resuscitation Outcomes Consortium, 2005 to 2007. Of note is the survival of 259 patients with an AED applied whether or not a shock was delivered and the survival of 149 patients in whom a shock was delivered. The latter compares favorably with survival of those receiving bystander CPR and waiting for EMS to arrive for a shock to be delivered. (*Data from* Weisfeldt ML, Sitlani CM, Ornato JP, et al. Survival after application of automatic external defibrillators before arrival of the emergency medical system: evaluation in the resuscitation outcomes consortium population of 21 million. J Am Coll Cardiol 2010;55(16):1713–20.)

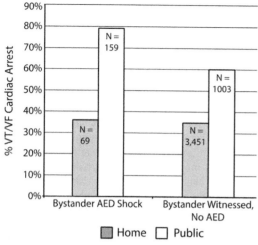

Fig. 2. High frequency of shockable cardiac arrests occurring in public versus home and particularly if an AED is applied by a bystander. From Resuscitation Outcomes Consortium (2005–2007). VF, ventricular fibrillation; VT, ventricular tachycardia. (*Data from* Weisfeldt ML, Everson-Stewart S, Sitlani C, et al. Ventricular tachyarrhythmias after cardiac arrest in public versus at home. N Engl J Med 2011;364(4):313–21.)

this increase will be available but the data strongly suggest a growing public commitment to the purchase of AEDs, training in the use of AEDs, and public willingness to use AEDs in witnessed public arrests.

The original study[11] estimated 500 lives per year saved by extrapolating to the population of the United States and Canada. Doing the same extrapolation based on the more recent data, ~1200 patients per year are being saved by AED use in public locations in the United States and Canada. Assuming that, through communication technology and more AEDs and training, 70% to 90% bystander shock for SOP-OHCA can be achieved, this will increase survival from the current of 8.3% of all cardiac arrests in the United States to 11.3%. Such a prediction suggest that about 10,000 people per year in the United States will be saved by bystanders using AEDs.

OPPORTUNITIES FOR FURTHER IMPROVEMENT IN USE OF AUTOMATED EXTERNAL DEFIBRILLATORS IN ALL CARDIAC ARRESTS OCCURRING IN PUBLIC LOCATIONS

Several studies have shown that the location of AED installations and their availability during hours when out-of-hospital cardiac arrest occur are far from ideal.[17,18] This situation could be improved without great financial investment by enactment of municipal ordinances similar to those for fire

extinguishers in public buildings. Given the data discussed earlier, every building with more than 300 people 8 hours a day needs to have an AED in full public view near the entrance of the building, most likely near the security desk. Signage needs to be prominent, as in airports. Security desk individuals should be trained in AED use and have a security backup if a call comes to the security desk looking for an AED for an arrest.

In a different direction, efforts such as Pulse-Point[19] using GPS (global positioning system) technology and dispatcher mapping and instructions to link the arrest location, the AED location, and a willing rescuer are currently being implemented in forward-looking US cities and regions. Others are experimenting with cell phone acquisition of an electrocardiogram (ECG) to identify shockable arrests in individual persons in similar models. For example, in persons at higher risk who do not have implanted or wearable defibrillators, inventors are working toward simple pulse or ECG wearable monitoring systems emitting a loud noise in the event of a positive detection, allowing the person to turn off the alarm. If not turned off, the information is transmitted directly to the EMS dispatcher with the location of the arrest. In addition, AEDs, like other technology, are becoming smaller (**Fig. 3**) and thus more likely to be inserted in a brief case, car glove compartment, or large purse.

CIRCULATORY PHASE OF CARDIAC RESUSCITATION IN RELATION TO SHOCK AND USE OF AUTOMATED EXTERNAL DEFIBRILLATORS

The impressive simple experiments of Niemann and colleagues,[20] repeated subsequently by others in pigs, have stood the test of time. They placed anesthetized dogs into VF and after

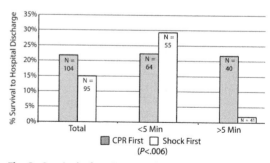

Fig. 3. Survival of patients in shockable cardiac arrest randomized to immediate defibrillation or 3 minutes of CPR before defibrillation (*left*) and subgroups of EMS response time of greater than (*right*) or less than (*center*) 5 minutes. For those with longer EMS response times, 3 minutes of CPR was associated with improved survival.

7.5 minutes randomized the dogs to immediate defibrillation without CPR or 3 minutes of CPR with epinephrine and then defibrillation. Survival was greater in the CPR group, although VF continued for 3 minutes longer. Others have studied nonsurvival hearts with a shock without CPR and found myocardial contracture, or what has been called stone heart, as the result. Thus, for experimental large animals, circulation via chest compression is essential in improving survival after some minutes of untreated VF. The most similar data in humans are those from Wik and colleagues[21] (**Fig. 4**), who randomized patients to immediate defibrillation or 3 minutes of CPR before defibrillation. They arbitrarily divided the patients with EMS response times of less than or more than 5 minutes and showed improved survival with 3 minutes of CPR in those with greater than 5-minute EMS response time. Results were insignificantly better with immediate shock if the EMS response time was less than 5 minutes. These results seem to confirm the animal data. Thus, in the 3-element model (see **Box 1**), after 4 minutes it is essential to provide a period of circulation before defibrillation. With use of an AED, this suggest that, in a patient with uncertain onset time, 3 minutes of CPR before shock from an AED is advised but also there is likely to be no value in the delay if the arrest is witnessed and the AED is ready to shock in less than 4 minutes.

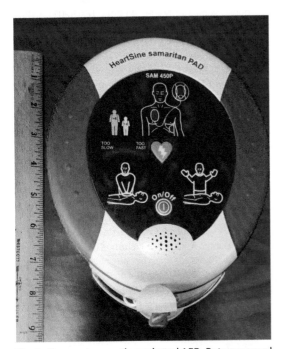

Fig. 4. Compact, recently marketed AED. Put your novel on your phone and carry an AED in your purse or briefcase! (*Courtesy of* HeartSmart.com; with permission.)

CONTROVERSIAL AND NONCONTROVERSIAL ASPECTS OF CARDIOPULMONARY RESUSCITATION

Among the recent advances in clinical resuscitation is the acceptance of hands-only CPR as a lifesaving procedure for use by lay rescuers before EMS arrival.[22,23] In true primary cardiac arrest there is little question that there is sufficient oxygen available in the lung for many minutes and that more bystanders will administer CPR with chest compression–only CPR. With drowning, acute airway obstruction and severe pulmonary disease or congestion ventilation is essential. Studies in animals also suggest that excessive ventilation is harmful during resuscitation,[24] perhaps by blocking passive venous return or interrupting coronary blood flow as arterial pressure decreases during the interruption of compression.

ROC investigators clustered randomized patients to 1 minute of CPR versus 3 minutes of CPR and found no difference overall in outcome, but when the study was reanalyzed separating the resuscitation effort into good and poor performing quality of CPR, good quality of CPR was associated with better outcome for 3 minutes versus 1 minute of CPR.[25,26] In a second cluster randomized study, EMS resuscitation ventilation as the American Heart Association recommends was marginally superior to continuous compression with ventilation without chest compression interruption.[27]

Controversies that are under active investigation currently include the use of all drugs and/or metabolic interventions as applied in the third phase of CPR. A major randomized trial comparing targeted temperature management of 36°C versus 32°C to 34°C after hospital admission while unconscious showed no benefit for the colder temperature. Also, field administration of large volumes of cold saline seem to be of no value.[28,29] In most EMS systems, epinephrine is administered well into failed resuscitative efforts, with administration occurring 8 to 20 minutes after EMS arrival. This finding is unlike the administration of epinephrine at the onset of CPR in most VF animal models. Epidemiologic data from several settings suggest short-term survival benefit of epinephrine and long-term detriment to survival.[30,31] Placebo-controlled studies of epinephrine are progressing and early administration of epinephrine by some effective means is an idea that is receiving attention in experimental laboratories. A complex study of amiodarone, lidocaine, and placebo in refractory VF/VT suggested some benefit for both active agents but was short of a definitive positive result.[32] Mechanical aids to chest compression are useful during transport. In randomized trials against manual CPR, mechanical devices have not proved to be superior.[33,34]

SUMMARY

Immediate defibrillation in patients with sudden-onset VF is lifesaving. Bystander use of AEDs has improved survival by about 2-fold in shockable arrests relative to survival if the shock awaits EMS arrival. Efforts to expand and focus bystanders on attaining an AED and bring both the AED and the bystander to the patient with an arrest are many and progressing well. Placement of AEDs uniformly and adequate signage, as well as modern communication technology, could do much to increase effective AED use and patient survival. Despite the introduction of modern CPR near 60 years ago, clinicians do not know the place of drugs or any metabolic interventions following or during resuscitation.

For patients who can be shocked in 4 minutes after collapse, shock first. For patients with no AED or defibrillator available, administer hands-only CPR until an AED or EMS arrive. For arrests caused by pulmonary problems such as drowning, airway obstruction, or pulmonary congestion, ventilation is essential as part of CPR.

REFERENCES

1. Weisfeldt ML, Becker L. Resuscitation after cardiac arrest: a 3-phase time-sensitive model [Commentary]. JAMA 2002;288(23):3035–8.
2. Cobb LA, Eliastam M, Kerber RE, et al. AHA Task Force report: the future of cardiopulmonary resuscitation. Circulation 1992;85(6):2346–55.
3. Weisfeldt ML, Kerber RE, McGoldrick RP, et al. American Heart Association report on the Public Access Defibrillation Conference December 8-10, 1994. Circulation 1995;92:2740–7.
4. Nichol G, Hallstrom AP, Kerber R, et al. American Heart Association report on the second public access defibrillation conference, April 17-19, 1997, special report. Circulation 1998;97:1309–14.
5. Valenzuela TD, Roe DJ, Nichol G, et al. Outcomes of rapid defibrillation by security officers after cardiac arrest in casinos. N Engl J Med 2000;343(17):1206–9.
6. Page RL, Joglar JA, Kowal RC, et al. Use of automated external defibrillators by a U.S. airline. N Engl J Med 2000;343(17):1210–6.
7. Hallstrom AP, Ornato JP, Weisfeldt M, et al. Public-access defibrillation and survival after out-of-hospital cardiac arrest. N Engl J Med 2004;351(7):637–46.
8. Agarwal DA, Hess EP, Atkinson EJ, et al. Ventricular fibrillation in Rochester, Minnesota: experience over 18 years. Resuscitation 2009;80(11):1253–8.
9. Blom MT, Beesems SG, Homma PC, et al. Improved survival after out-of-hospital cardiac arrest and use of automated external defibrillators. Circulation 2014;130(21):1868–75.
10. Morrison LJ, Nichol G, Rea TD, et al. Rationale, development and implementation of the Resuscitation Outcomes Consortium Epistry-Cardiac Arrest. Resuscitation 2008;78(2):161–9.
11. Weisfeldt ML, Sitlani CM, Ornato JP, et al. Survival after application of automatic external defibrillators before arrival of the emergency medical system: evaluation in the resuscitation outcomes consortium population of 21 million. J Am Coll Cardiol 2010;55(16):1713–20.
12. Abrams HC, McNally B, Ong M, et al. A composite model of survival from out-of-hospital cardiac arrest using the Cardiac Arrest Registry to Enhance Survival (CARES). Resuscitation 2013;84:1093–8.
13. Malta Hansen C, Kragholm K, Pearson DA, et al. Association of bystander and first- responder intervention with survival after out-of-hospital cardiac arrest in North Carolina, 2010-2013. JAMA 2015;314(3):255–64.
14. Becker L, Gold LS, Eisenberg M, et al. Ventricular fibrillation in King County, Washington: a 30-year perspective. Resuscitation 2008;79(1):22–7.
15. Weisfeldt ML, Everson-Stewart S, Sitlani C, et al. Ventricular tachyarrhythmias after cardiac arrest in public versus at home. N Engl J Med 2011;364(4):313–21.
16. Bardy GH, Lee KL, Mark DB, et al. Home use of automated external defibrillators for sudden cardiac arrest. N Engl J Med 2008;358(17):1793–804.
17. Hansen CM, Wissenberg M, Weeke P, et al. Automated external defibrillators inaccessible to more than half of nearby cardiac arrests in public locations during evening, nighttime, and weekends. Circulation 2013;128(20):2224–31.
18. Chrisinger BW, Grossestreuer AV, Laguna MC, et al. Characteristics of automated external defibrillator coverage in Philadelphia, PA, based on land use and estimated risk. Resuscitation 2016;109:9–15.
19. Brooks SC, Simmons G, Worthington H, et al. The PulsePoint Respond mobile device application to crowdsource basic life support for patients with out-of-hospital cardiac arrest: challenges for optimal implementation. Resuscitation 2016;98:20–6.
20. Niemann JT, Cairns CB, Sharma J, et al. Treatment of prolonged ventricular fibrillation. Immediate countershock versus high-dose epinephrine and CPR preceding countershock. Circulation 1992;85(1):281–7.
21. Wik L, Hansen TB, Fylling F, et al. Delaying defibrillation to give basic cardiopulmonary resuscitation

to patients with out-of-hospital ventricular fibrillation: a randomized trial. JAMA 2003;289(11):1389–95.

22. Ewy GA, Sanders AB, Kern KB. Compression-only cardiopulmonary resuscitation improves survival. Am J Med 2011;124(5):383–5.

23. Bobrow BJ, Clark LL, Ewy GA, et al. Minimally interrupted cardiac resuscitation by emergency medical services for out-of-hospital cardiac arrest. JAMA 2008;299(10):1158–65.

24. Yannopoulos D, Aufderheide TP, Gabriella A, et al. Clinical and hemodynamic comparison of 15:2 and 30:2 compression-to-ventilation ratios for cardiopulmonary resuscitation. Crit Care Med 2006;34(5):1444–9.

25. Stiell IG, Nichol G, Leroux BG, et al. Early versus later rhythm analysis in patients with out-of-hospital cardiac arrest. N Engl J Med 2011;365:787–97.

26. Rea T, Prince D, Morrison L, et al. Association between survival and early versus late rhythm analysis in out-of-hospital cardiac arrest: do agency level factors influence outcome? Ann Emerg Med 2014;64:1–8.

27. Graham N, Leroux B, Wang H, et al. Trial of continuous or interrupted chest compressions during CPR. N Engl J Med 2015;373:2203–14.

28. Nielsen N, Wetterslev J, Cronberg T, et al. Targeted temperature management at 33°C versus 36°C after cardiac arrest. N Engl J Med 2013;369(23):2197–206.

29. Kim F, Nichol G, Maynard C, et al. Effect of prehospital induction of mild hypothermia on survival and neurological status among adults with cardiac arrest: a randomized clinical trial. JAMA 2014;311(1):45–52.

30. Olasveengen TM, Sunde K, Brunborg C, et al. Intravenous drug administration during out-of-hospital cardiac arrest: a randomized trial. JAMA 2009;302(20):2222–9.

31. Hagihara A, Hasegawa M, Abe T, et al. Prehospital epinephrine use and survival among patients with out-of-hospital cardiac arrest. JAMA 2012;307(11):1161–8.

32. Kudenchuk PJ, Brown AP, Daya M, et al. Amiodarone, lidocaine or placebo in out of hospital cardiac arrest. N Engl J Med 2016;374:1711–22.

33. Hallstrom A, Rea TD, Sayre MR, et al. Manual chest compression vs use of an automated chest compression device during resuscitation following out-of-hospital cardiac arrest: a randomized trial. JAMA 2006;295(22):2620–8.

34. Wik L, Olsen JA, Persse D, et al. Manual vs. integrated automatic load-distributing band CPR with equal survival after out of hospital cardiac arrest. The randomized CIRC trial. Resuscitation 2014;85:741–7.

Sudden Cardiac Death During Sports Activities in the General Population

Kumar Narayanan, MD[a,b], Wulfran Bougouin, MD, PhD[a,c],
Ardalan Sharifzadehgan, MD, MPH[a,c,d,e],
Victor Waldmann, MD, MPH[a,c,d,e],
Nicole Karam, MD, PhD[a,c,d,e], Eloi Marijon, MD, PhD[a,c,d,e,*],
Xavier Jouven, MD, PhD[a,c,d,e]

KEYWORDS

• Sports • Athlete • Prevention • General population • Sudden cardiac arrest

KEY POINTS

- Although sports-related sudden cardiac death (SCD) is often a devastating event in a young individual, exercise is beneficial and has a role in the prevention and therapy of cardiac disease.
- The goal for health care providers should be not to discourage sports participation.
- However there should be concerted efforts to enhance prevention and management of sports-related SCD, which seems to be a particularly suitable model for specific therapies.
- Targeted prevention through tailored and individualized preparticipation screening as well as education of participants and other stakeholders in sporting events could be of particular benefit.

Participating athletes in competitive sport events as well as sports participants in general are usually healthy and are perceived to be fit. It is also accepted that regular sports activity is beneficial in reducing long-term overall as well as cardiovascular mortality, including sudden cardiac death (SCD).[1–7] However, the occasional instance of SCD during a sporting event in full public glare serves as a grim reminder of the small but definite arrhythmic risk of extreme exercise. This paradox of exercise has been described for more than 30 years,[2–4] wherein, although regular physical activity has proven benefits for cardiovascular health, vigorous exercise could increase the short-term risk of dying suddenly (during or shortly after exercise).

Therefore, fairly extensive attention has focused on physical exertion as a potential trigger for SCD. To add to the complexity, the risk of sports-related SCD decreases with regular exercise training.[7,8] Notwithstanding these facts, the occurrence of such unexpected and tragic events among athletes, who epitomize health and well-being, invariably begs the question as to whether they cannot be prevented or better managed. The ability to screen athletes to prevent such events has been the subject of considerable scientific attention and controversy.[9–11] The devastating and traumatic consequences of sports-related SCD, therefore, mandate a thorough understanding of this phenomenon across the general population.[12,13]

[a] Paris Cardiovascular Research Center–INSERM U970 (PARCC), Paris, France; [b] Cardiology Department, Maxcure Hospitals, Hitec City, Hyderabad 500081, India; [c] Paris Sudden Death Expertise Center (SDEC), European Georges Pompidou Hospital, 56 rue Leblanc, Paris 75987, France; [d] Paris Descartes University, Rue de l'Ecole de Médecine, Paris 75006, France; [e] Cardiology Department, European Georges Pompidou Hospital, 20, Rue Leblanc, Paris 75015, France
* Corresponding author. Hôpital Européen Georges Pompidou, Département de Cardiologie, Unité de Rythmologie, 20-40 Rue Leblanc, 75908 Paris Cedex 15, France
E-mail address: eloi_marijon@yahoo.fr

In this review, we summarize the current knowledge in this field, to provide an overview of the connection between sports and SCD, and to place into perspective the current thoughts on screening and other measures to improve outcomes.

SPORTS ACTIVITY: CONCLUSIVELY BENEFICIAL FOR LONG-TERM SUDDEN CARDIAC DEATH RISK

The cardiovascular advantages of physical activity are well-established, and the excessive attention often focused on sports-related SCD should not overshadow the broad issue that regular exercise has irrefutable benefits.[14] Several studies have demonstrated a strong and consistent reduction of risk through regular physical activity with regard to cardiovascular mortality,[5] atrial fibrillation,[15] and coronary artery disease,[16] with the last mentioned being described more than 35 years ago.[17] Considering that coronary artery disease is one of the major underlying causes of SCD (especially during sports activity in subjects over 30 years of age[18,19]), regular physical activity could, through reduction of coronary artery

disease, lead to a decreased SCD risk. Concordant with this, studies have clearly established that regular physical activity is associated with a lower long-term risk of SCD.[7,20–24] Therefore, there is scientific consensus that a certain amount of physical activity is strongly recommended to reduce overall mortality,[25] including SCD.

In contrast, for sports-related SCD, an analogy of "drug overdosage"[26] has been used, considering that sports (exercise) is in fact an effective "drug" for SCD risk reduction. This analogy suggests that the association between sports and mortality may follow a U-curve[27]; moderate sports would confer a lower overall mortality, whereas strenuous sports activity would be associated with a similar mortality as a nonexercising population owing to a counterbalancing effect of short-term SCD risk (**Fig. 1**). However, this concept remains controversial: for instance, recent data from healthy elite athletes (French participants in the Tour de France) reported a significantly lower mortality when compared with the general population.[28] Such results need careful interpretation, considering the potential selection bias in a population of elite athletes.[29]

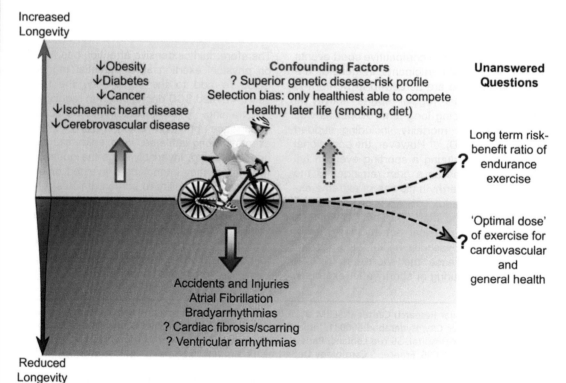

Fig. 1. Potential effects of endurance sport on longevity. (*From* Zaidi A, Sharma S. Reduced mortality in former Tour de France participants: the benefits from intensive exercise or a select genetic tour de force? Eur Heart J 2013;34(40):3106–8.)

SUDDEN DEATH IN THE YOUNG COMPETITIVE ATHLETE: THE APPARENT PART OF THE ICEBERG

A young competitive athlete is traditionally defined as any person 10 to 35 years old who participates in an organized sports program (team or individual sport) that requires regular competition and training.[11,19,30–32] SCD occurring among young competitive athletes has always attracted major media attention, with emblematic examples in footballers[33] or, more recently, cyclists.[34] To date, the large majority of data on sports-related SCD have focused on the burden among young competitive athletes and the extent to which intensive physical activity may be actually harmful. The focus on healthy young athletes is highly understandable given the substantial social and emotional impact of sudden and unexpected deaths in this population.

However, there are some noteworthy facts in this regard. Sudden death in competitive athletes is a very low-frequency event.[35,36] Furthermore, several studies published on this subject included not only sudden deaths owing to cardiovascular causes, but also trauma[9] or even suicide.[37] Other studies included SCD occurring in circumstances unassociated with sport.[9] Overall, although an accurate estimation of the incidence of sports-related SCD among young competitive athletes is challenging, it is estimated to be fewer than 10 per million per year in a recent metaanalysis.[36] In contrast, considering the burden of sports participation in the general population, focusing on competitive athletes alone could lead to a rather biased perspective on sports-related SCD.

SUDDEN CARDIAC DEATH AMONG RECREATIONAL SPORTS PARTICIPANTS: THE MAJORITY OF SPORTS-RELATED SUDDEN CARDIAC DEATH

Sports-related SCD accounts for a small but significant proportion of all SCD, with recent studies consistently reporting around 5% of overall SCD occurring during sporting activity.[38,39] Because the incidence of SCD is around 300,000 cases per year in Europe[40,41] and North America,[42,43] it may be estimated that sports-related SCD likely accounts for 15,000 cases annually in North America and in Europe. This estimation underlines the important magnitude of this entity. Literature on sports-related SCD, during recreational sports activities in the community, remains relatively sparse. The emphasis on young competitive athletes as opposed to recreational sports participants is discordant with the relative magnitudes of the respective problems, which was recently highlighted by a population-based registry.[30] Overall, among all sports-related SCD, only 6% occurred in young competitive athletes, as compared with 94% among recreational sports participants (**Fig. 2**).[30] This is intuitive given the large pool of recreational sports participants as compared with competitive athletes. Thus, there is a crucial need to focus attention on this large at-risk population of subjects.

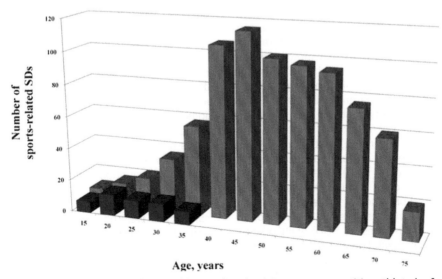

Fig. 2. Distribution by age of sports-related sudden cardiac death in young competitive athlete (*red*) and general population (*blue*). SD, sudden death. (*From* Marijon E, Tafflet M, Celermajer DS, et al. Sports-related sudden death in the general population. Circulation 2011;124(6):672–81.)

SPORTS-RELATED SUDDEN CARDIAC DEATH PRESENTS WITH HIGHLY HOMOGENOUS CHARACTERISTICS

Results from 3 large population-based registries recently published have elucidated the fairly uniform characteristics of sports-related SCD.[30,38,39] This form of SCD usually afflicts middle-aged patients, with a striking male predominance (>90% of cases), even after consideration of differences in participation rate according to sex. This predominance is notably higher than observed in non–sports-related SCD.[44–46] Several hypotheses can be advanced as an explanation for this.[47,48] First, this difference can be related to sex differences in the extent and type of sports participation (eg, beyond the lower participation rate of women in sports, a lower duration or intensity of physical activity). Second, an intrinsic physiologic difference related to sex is possible, considering the sex-specific prevalence of coronary heart disease. Moreover, sex differences can also involve differences in arrhythmogenic substrate, trigger, or autonomic modulators. As an example, vagal activation has been shown to be more common in women than in men during abrupt coronary occlusion[49] and may have beneficial antiarrhythmic effects. Sex-based differences with regard to nutritional factors and adherence to healthy lifestyles may be implicated as well. Finally, the contribution of other medical conditions (comorbidities) and treatments received may also have played a role in this observed difference.

In terms of medical history, a significant fraction of patients had previous heart disease[30,38] and, interestingly, several patients presented with symptoms (chest pain, dyspnea) during the week before the event[38] (similar to non–sports-related SCD[50]). In fact, up to one-third of sports-related SCD patients reported warning symptoms in the days before the event,[38] which were usually neglected. Attention to this could potentially create room for subacute prevention, with better identification of high-risk patients and education for self-assessment of risk.

Regarding circumstances, most sports-related SCD occurred in public places,[51] and a large majority of cases (around 90%) were witnessed by bystanders, with often multiple witnesses. This almost-universal presence of a bystander permits precise phenotyping of sports-related SCD (often difficult with other cases of SCD), with precise information on presentation and delays (including from collapse to cardiopulmonary resuscitation [CPR]). Rates of bystander CPR were substantially higher than those described in the non-sports setting, from 30% to 80%, and an initial shockable rhythm was found in 50% to 80% of cases (as compared with 3- to 4-fold lower in a nonsports setting[46,52]). However, rates of automated external defibrillator (AED) use were disappointingly low, especially in France (<1% of cases[30] vs 36% in the Netherlands[39,53,54]). This consistent phenotype has provided a reliable model to study determinants of survival in this population, and to identify areas for improvement.

Owing to these characteristics, survival is notably higher in sports-related SCD, ranging from 16% to 45% in multiple international reports,[30,39] compared with less than 10% for overall SCD.[40,46] In fact, several studies have reported even higher survival rates, for example, up to 85% in US high school subjects.[55] The opportunities to intervene early in this form of SCD suggest that these figures can be improved on.

HOW TO TACKLE SPORTS-RELATED SUDDEN CARDIAC DEATH?

Strategies to reduce the burden of sports-related SCD can be considered under 2 approaches, namely, primary prevention (through preparticipation screening and population education) and improved management of the SCD event (to increase survival rate). These approaches should ideally complement each other to achieve best results.

Primary prevention of sports-related SCD relies on the preparticipation screening of sports participants, as well as education of participants and other stakeholders in sporting events. Considering that most of these events are owing to cardiovascular diseases, there is an ongoing controversy regarding the way of delivering preparticipation screening and early identification of asymptomatic structural or electrical abnormalities in this population, with postulated benefits[11] but uncertainty regarding cost effectiveness.[56] A seemingly attractive and logical way for prevention would be to screen patients for asymptomatic cardiac lesions before sports participation. Toward this end, an understanding of the usual underlying causes of sports-related SCD is crucial. In a retrospective analysis of 1500 forensic autopsies, Tabib and colleagues[18] reported different etiologic patterns according to the age of occurrence of the sports-related SCD event. Under 30 years of age, the main causes were heritable diseases, such as hypertrophic cardiomyopathy and arrhythmogenic right ventricular cardiomyopathy. Over 30 years of age, atherosclerotic coronary disease strongly prevailed. Guidelines regarding cardiovascular evaluation before sports activity[57] suggest that to assess sport-related SCD risk among aged sport participants, the main issues to consider are medical history, level of physical activity, and previous exercise training. To further enhance screening, especially among young competitive athletes, strategies based on systematic performance of 12-lead electrocardiograph have been proposed.[11,58,59,60] Although this measure has had some promising results, there is significant ongoing controversy on such an approach with regard to cost effectiveness, false-positive rates, and the potential psychological impact on a young target population.[56,61] Notwithstanding these issues, considering the potential benefits, current guidelines advocate preparticipation electrocardiographic screening.[62] Although even governmental legislation has been considered, for instance, with regard to sports participation, this debate has been often emotionally fraught and a difficult dilemma for clinicians. A universal and undifferentiated strategy of screening is probably not an effective approach. However, identification of select subgroups that might benefit from such screening remains problematic. One would need to start with certain broad areas of focus, such as among middle-aged men, where, considering the greater risk, effective ways to enhance preparticipation screening need to be actively sought. Considering the recent data that previous warning

symptoms were present in several instances of sports-related SCD,[38] systematic assessment of such symptoms, and education of participants to identify them and take appropriate action, seems to be necessary.[63] This could indeed be an easy and cost-effective intervention to identify patients at increased risk.

SCD occurring during sports activity offers a particularly suitable setting to achieve a favorable outcome that needs to be capitalized on. Compared with other SCD, survival is relatively high after sports-related SCD, which can reach even up to 80% with immediate use of AEDs. However, one needs to bear in mind that this overall picture often masks major regional disparities in survival across regions, varying, for instance, from less than 10% to almost 50% (**Fig. 3**) in France.[64] This heterogeneity in survival rates is similar to results from studies performed in overall SCD.[65] However, in contrast with all SCD occurring in general population, sports-related SCD almost universally presents with homogenous characteristics (almost constantly witnessed, similar delays to intervention, similar rates of shockable rhythm).[64] Therefore, the specific setting of sports-related SCD offers a unique opportunity to better analyze the key determinants of survival in SCD (**Fig. 4**). Interestingly, bystander CPR seems to be one of

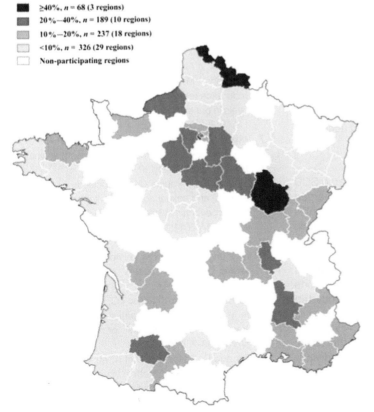

≥40%, n = 68 (3 regions)
20%–40%, n = 189 (10 regions)
10%–20%, n = 237 (18 regions)
<10%, n = 326 (29 regions)
Non-participating regions

Fig. 3. Survival rates after sport-related sudden cardiac death across districts in France. (*From* Marijon E, Bougouin W, Celermajer DS, et al. Major regional disparities in outcomes after sudden cardiac arrest during sports. Eur Heart J 2013;34(47):3632–40.)

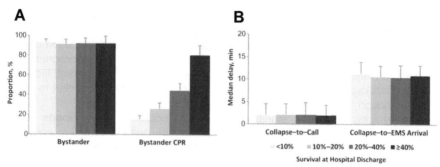

Fig. 4. Factors associated with rates of survival at hospital discharge after sport-related sudden cardiac death. (*A*) Progressive increase in rates of survival at hospital discharge with increasing bystander CPR but not by bystander presence alone. (*B*) No significant difference in the Collapse-to-Call and Collapse-to-EMS Arrival times across survival strata. CPR, cardiopulmonary resuscitation; EMS, emergency medical services. (*From* Marijon E, Bougouin W, Celermajer DS, et al. Major regional disparities in outcomes after sudden cardiac arrest during sports. Eur Heart J 2013;34(47):3632–40.)

the main prognostic factors, a result highly consistent in recent reports.[40] Finally, sports-related SCD could be considered as a "quasiexperimental" situation to demonstrate the potential benefit of a particular intervention in a relatively controlled environment, as previously described for implementation of public access defibrillation (in sports facilities[66–68]) or extracorporeal life support for selected cases.[69] The widespread deployment of AEDs in sport facilities, for example, may be a major tool available to enhance survival in sports-related SCD.[66,67] To this end, recent guidelines advocated that AEDs should be widely distributed throughout the arena or on mobile emergency responders to achieve the goal of first defibrillation within 5 minutes of a witnessed collapse.[67] Thus, although survival in sports-related SCD is better than for all SCD, room for improvement clearly remains in the form of public education, improved bystander CPR rates, and greater AED access.

SUMMARY

Although the specific entity of sports-related SCD is often a devastating and emotionally charged event in a young individual, exercise in general is clearly beneficial and has a role in the prevention and therapy of cardiac disease, and even in long-term prevention of sports-related SCD. Therefore, the goal for health care providers should certainly not be to discourage sports participation. However, there should be concerted efforts to enhance prevention and management of sports-related SCD, which seems to be a particularly suitable model for specific therapies. Targeted prevention through tailored and individualized preparticipation screening and an enhanced focus on middle-aged men during recreational sports could be of particular benefit.

REFERENCES

1. Sharma S, Merghani A, Mont L. Exercise and the heart: the good, the bad, and the ugly. Eur Heart J 2015;36(23):1445–53.
2. Siscovick DS, Weiss NS, Fletcher RH, et al. The incidence of primary cardiac arrest during vigorous exercise. N Engl J Med 1984;311(14):874–7.
3. Albert CM, Mittleman MA, Chae CU, et al. Triggering of sudden death from cardiac causes by vigorous exertion. N Engl J Med 2000;343(19):1355–61.
4. Maron BJ. The paradox of exercise. N Engl J Med 2000;343(19):1409–11.
5. Lee D-C, Pate RR, Lavie CJ, et al. Leisure-time running reduces all-cause and cardiovascular mortality risk. J Am Coll Cardiol 2014;64(5):472–81.
6. Conraads VM, Beckers P, Vaes J, et al. Combined endurance/resistance training reduces NT-proBNP levels in patients with chronic heart failure. Eur Heart J 2004;25(20):1797–805.
7. Whang W, Manson JE, Hu FB, et al. Physical exertion, exercise, and sudden cardiac death in women. JAMA 2006;295(12):1399–403.
8. Dahabreh IJ, Paulus JK. Association of episodic physical and sexual activity with triggering of acute cardiac events: systematic review and meta-analysis. JAMA 2011;305(12):1225–33.
9. Maron BJ, Doerer JJ, Haas TS, et al. Sudden deaths in young competitive athletes: analysis of 1866 deaths in the United States, 1980-2006. Circulation 2009;119(8):1085–92.
10. Maron BJ, Shirani J, Poliac LC, et al. Sudden death in young competitive athletes. Clinical, demographic, and pathological profiles. JAMA 1996; 276(3):199–204.
11. Corrado D, Basso C, Pavei A, et al. Trends in sudden cardiovascular death in young competitive athletes after implementation of a preparticipation screening program. JAMA 2006;296(13):1593–601.

12. Waldmann V, Bougouin W, Karam N, et al. Sudden cardiac death: a better understanting for a better prevention. Ann Cardiol Angeiol (Paris) 2017;66(4):230–8.

13. Jouven X, Bougouin W, Karam N, et al. Epidemiology of sudden cardiac death: data from the paris sudden death expertise center registry. Rev Prat 2015;65(7):916–8.

14. Arena R, Guazzi M, Lianov L, et al. Healthy lifestyle interventions to combat noncommunicable disease-a novel nonhierarchical connectivity model for key stakeholders: a policy statement from the American Heart Association, European Society of Cardiology, European Association for Cardiovascular Prevention and Rehabilitation, and American College of Preventive Medicine. Eur Heart J 2015;36(31):2097–109.

15. Morseth B, Graff-Iversen S, Jacobsen BK, et al. Physical activity, resting heart rate, and atrial fibrillation: the Tromsø Study. Eur Heart J 2016;37(29):2307–13.

16. Tanasescu M, Leitzmann MF, Rimm EB, et al. Exercise type and intensity in relation to coronary heart disease in men. JAMA 2002;288(16):1994–2000.

17. Morris JN, Everitt MG, Pollard R, et al. Vigorous exercise in leisure-time: protection against coronary heart disease. Lancet 1980;2(8206):1207–10.

18. Tabib A, Miras A, Taniere P, et al. Undetected cardiac lesions cause unexpected sudden cardiac death during occasional sport activity. A report of 80 cases. Eur Heart J 1999;20(12):900–3.

19. Marijon E, Bougouin W, Jouven X. Sports-related sudden death: lessons from the french registry. Rev Prat 2015;65(7):919–23.

20. Lemaitre RN, Siscovick DS, Raghunathan TE, et al. Leisure-time physical activity and the risk of primary cardiac arrest. Arch Intern Med 1999;159(7):686–90.

21. Chiuve SE, Fung TT, Rexrode KM, et al. Adherence to a low-risk, healthy lifestyle and risk of sudden cardiac death among women. JAMA 2011;306(1):62–9.

22. Deo R, Vittinghoff E, Lin F, et al. Risk factor and prediction modeling for sudden cardiac death in women with coronary artery disease. Arch Intern Med 2011;171(19):1703–9.

23. Deo R, Albert CM. Epidemiology and genetics of sudden cardiac death. Circulation 2012;125(4):620–37.

24. Wannamethee G, Shaper AG, Macfarlane PW, et al. Risk factors for sudden cardiac death in middle-aged British men. Circulation 1995;91(6):1749–56.

25. Wen CP, Wai JPM, Tsai MK, et al. Minimum amount of physical activity for reduced mortality and extended life expectancy: a prospective cohort study. Lancet 2011;378(9798):1244–53.

26. O'Keefe JH, Lavie CJ. Run for your life … at a comfortable speed and not too far. Heart 2013;99(8):516–9.

27. Schnohr P, O'Keefe JH, Marott JL, et al. Dose of jogging and long-term mortality: the Copenhagen city heart study. J Am Coll Cardiol 2015;65(5):411–9.

28. Marijon E, Tafflet M, Antero-Jacquemin J, et al. Mortality of French participants in the Tour de France (1947-2012). Eur Heart J 2013;34(40):3145–50.

29. Zaidi A, Sharma S. Reduced mortality in former Tour de France participants: the benefits from intensive exercise or a select genetic tour de force? Eur Heart J 2013;34(40):3106–8.

30. Marijon E, Tafflet M, Celermajer DS, et al. Sports-related sudden death in the general population. Circulation 2011;124(6):672–81.

31. Pelliccia A, Di Paolo FM, Corrado D, et al. Evidence for efficacy of the Italian national pre-participation screening programme for identification of hypertrophic cardiomyopathy in competitive athletes. Eur Heart J 2006;27(18):2196–200.

32. Corrado D, Basso C, Rizzoli G, et al. Does sports activity enhance the risk of sudden death in adolescents and young adults? J Am Coll Cardiol 2003;42(11):1959–63.

33. Dvorak J. A lion never dies: pro memoria of Marc-Vivien Foé. Br J Sports Med 2009;43(9):628.

34. Daan Myngheer: cycling mourns second Belgian death [Internet]. BBC Sport. Available at: http://www.bbc.com/sport/cycling/35914893. Accessed April 1, 2016.

35. Kim JH, Malhotra R, Chiampas G, et al. Cardiac arrest during long-distance running races. N Engl J Med 2012;366(2):130–40.

36. Gerardin B, Collet J-P, Mustafic H, et al. Registry on acute cardiovascular events during endurance running races: the prospective RACE Paris registry. Eur Heart J 2016;37(32):2531–41.

37. Harmon KG, Asif IM, Klossner D, et al. Incidence of sudden cardiac death in National Collegiate Athletic Association athletes. Circulation 2011;123(15):1594–600.

38. Marijon E, Uy-Evanado A, Reinier K, et al. Sudden cardiac arrest during sports activity in middle age. Circulation 2015;131(16):1384–91.

39. Berdowski J, de Beus MF, Blom M, et al. Exercise-related out-of-hospital cardiac arrest in the general population: incidence and prognosis. Eur Heart J 2013;34(47):3616–23.

40. Hasselqvist-Ax I, Riva G, Herlitz J, et al. Early cardiopulmonary resuscitation in out-of-hospital cardiac arrest. N Engl J Med 2015;372(24):2307–15.

41. Berdowski J, Berg RA, Tijssen JGP, et al. Global incidences of out-of-hospital cardiac arrest and survival rates: systematic review of 67 prospective studies. Resuscitation 2010;81(11):1479–87.

42. Kudenchuk PJ, Brown SP, Daya M, et al. Amiodarone, lidocaine, or placebo in out-of-hospital cardiac arrest. N Engl J Med 2016;374(18):1711–22.

43. Mozaffarian D, Benjamin EJ, Go AS, et al. Heart disease and stroke statistics–2015 update: a report from the American Heart Association. Circulation 2015;131(4):e29–322.

44. Adrie C, Cariou A, Mourvillier B, et al. Predicting survival with good neurological recovery at hospital admission after successful resuscitation of out-of-hospital cardiac arrest: the OHCA score. Eur Heart J 2006;27(23):2840–5.

45. Gräsner J-T, Meybohm P, Lefering R, et al. ROSC after cardiac arrest–the RACA score to predict outcome after out-of-hospital cardiac arrest. Eur Heart J 2011;32(13):1649–56.

46. Bougouin W, Lamhaut L, Marijon E, et al. Characteristics and prognosis of sudden cardiac death in Greater Paris: population-based approach from the Paris Sudden Death Expertise Center (Paris-SDEC). Intensive Care Med 2014;40(6):846–54.

47. Marijon E, Bougouin W, Celermajer DS, et al. Characteristics and outcomes of sudden cardiac arrest during sports in women. Circ Arrhythm Electrophysiol 2013;6(6):1185–91.

48. Marijon E, Bougouin W, Périer M-C, et al. Incidence of sports-related sudden death in France by specific sports and sex. JAMA 2013;310(6):642–3.

49. Airaksinen KE, Ikäheimo MJ, Linnaluoto M, et al. Gender difference in autonomic and hemodynamic reactions to abrupt coronary occlusion. J Am Coll Cardiol 1998;31(2):301–6.

50. Marijon E, Uy-Evanado A, Dumas F, et al. Warning symptoms are associated with survival from sudden cardiac arrest. Ann Intern Med 2016;164(1): 23–9.

51. Marijon E, Bougouin W, Karam N, et al. Survival from sports-related sudden cardiac arrest: in sports facilities versus outside of sports facilities. Am Heart J 2015;170(2):339–45.e1.

52. Rea TD, Eisenberg MS, Becker LJ, et al. Temporal trends in sudden cardiac arrest: a 25-year emergency medical services perspective. Circulation 2003;107(22):2780–5.

53. Karam N, Pechmajou L, Marijon E, et al. How often does athlete sudden cardiac death occur outside the context of exertion? J Am Coll Cardio 2016; 68(19):2125–6.

54. Karam N, Narayanan K, Bougouin W, et al. Major regional differences in Automated External Defibrillator placement and Basic Life Support training in France: further needs for coordinated implementation. Resuscitation 2017;118:49–54.

55. Drezner JA, Toresdahl BG, Rao AL, et al. Outcomes from sudden cardiac arrest in US high schools: a 2-year prospective study from the National Registry for AED Use in Sports. Br J Sports Med 2013;47(18): 1179–83.

56. Halkin A, Steinvil A, Rosso R, et al. Preventing sudden death of athletes with electrocardiographic screening: what is the absolute benefit and how much will it cost? J Am Coll Cardiol 2012;60(22): 2271–6.

57. Borjesson M, Urhausen A, Kouidi E, et al. Cardiovascular evaluation of middle-aged/senior individuals engaged in leisure-time sport activities: position stand from the sections of exercise physiology and sports cardiology of the European Association of Cardiovascular Prevention and Rehabilitation. Eur J Cardiovasc Prev Rehabil 2011;18(3):446–58.

58. Corrado D, Pelliccia A, Bjørnstad HH, et al. Cardiovascular pre-participation screening of young competitive athletes for prevention of sudden death: proposal for a common European protocol. Consensus statement of the Study Group of Sport Cardiology of the Working Group of Cardiac Rehabilitation and Exercise Physiology and the Working Group of Myocardial and Pericardial Diseases of the European Society of Cardiology. Eur Heart J 2005;26(5):516–24.

59. Sharma S, Drezner JA, Baggish A, et al. International recommendations for electrocardiographic interpretation in athletes. J Am Coll Cardiol 2017; 69(8):1057–75.

60. Mont L, Pelliccia A, Sharma S, et al. Pre-participation cardiovascular evaluation for athletic participants to prevent sudden death: Position paper from the EHRA and the EACPR, branches of the ESC. Endorsed by APHRS, HRS, and SOLAECE. Eur J Prev Cardiol 2017;24(1):41–69.

61. Wheeler MT, Heidenreich PA, Froelicher VF, et al. Cost-effectiveness of preparticipation screening for prevention of sudden cardiac death in young athletes. Ann Intern Med 2010;152(5):276–86.

62. Corrado D, Schmied C, Basso C, et al. Risk of sports: do we need a pre-participation screening for competitive and leisure athletes? Eur Heart J 2011;32(8):934–44.

63. Karam N, Marijon E, Jouven X. Opening a new front in the fight against sudden cardiac death: is it time for near-term prevention? Int J Cardiol 2017;237: 10–2.

64. Marijon E, Bougouin W, Celermajer DS, et al. Major regional disparities in outcomes after sudden cardiac arrest during sports. Eur Heart J 2013;34(47): 3632–40.

65. Girotra S, van Diepen S, Nallamothu BK, et al. Regional variation in out-of-hospital cardiac arrest survival in the United States. Circulation 2016; 133(22):2159–68.

66. Borjesson M, Dugmore D, Mellwig K-P, et al. Time for action regarding cardiovascular emergency care at sports arenas: a lesson from the Arena study. Eur Heart J 2010;31(12):1438–41.

67. Borjesson M, Serratosa L, Carre F, et al. Consensus document regarding cardiovascular safety at sports

arenas: position stand from the European Association of Cardiovascular Prevention and Rehabilitation (EACPR), section of Sports Cardiology. Eur Heart J 2011;32(17):2119–24.

68. Page RL, Husain S, White LY, et al. Cardiac arrest at exercise facilities: implications for placement of automated external defibrillators. J Am Coll Cardiol 2013;62(22):2102–9.

69. Lebreton G, Pozzi M, Luyt C-E, et al. Out-of-hospital extra-corporeal life support implantation during refractory cardiac arrest in a half-marathon runner. Resuscitation 2011;82(9):1239–42.

Sudden Cardiac Death in Children and Adolescents

Elizabeth D. Sherwin, MD[a,b,*], Charles I. Berul, MD[a,b]

KEYWORDS

- Pediatric • Arrhythmia • Sudden cardiac death • Sudden arrhythmic death syndrome
- Cardiomyopathy • Genetics

KEY POINTS

- Sudden cardiac death (SCD) is rare in childhood; the true incidence is not well understood.
- SCD etiologies in the young include anatomic and functional heart disease, primary arrhythmia syndromes, and other rare conditions.
- Sudden death can be the first symptom in a young person, although warning signs may be present: unexplained syncope or seizure, exertional chest pain or dyspnea, and a family history of early sudden death.
- Diagnosing disorders predisposing to pediatric SCD can be challenging; a strong index of suspicion and referral to experienced specialists are critical.
- Cascade screening of first-degree relatives is indicated after unexplained sudden death in individuals younger than 50 years or when a heritable cardiac condition is identified or suspected.

INTRODUCTION

"Sudden cardiac death has left no age untouched. Sparing neither saint nor sinner, it has burdened man with a sense of uncertainty and fragility."[1] Children, although commonly pictures of health, may be susceptible to sudden cardiac death (SCD). The definition is similar as for adults: sudden unexplained death in an otherwise healthy person within 1 hour of symptom onset, or unwitnessed death within 24 hours after seeing that person alive and well. In pediatrics, etiologies and challenges in SCD sometimes differ from adults.

SCD can be differentiated in the pediatric population based on age (**Table 1**), with variable etiologies. The younger the child, the less likely a cause of death will be identified with standard investigations.[2] When no etiology is found after comprehensive evaluation, including autopsy, toxicology, and histology, unexplained SCD is termed sudden arrhythmic death syndrome (SADS) or sudden unexplained death syndrome (SUDS).

Infant death during the first year of life is a distinct category that includes prenatal factors, congenital malformations, chromosomal abnormalities, premature births, and maternal, social, and environmental factors. An estimated 10% of sudden infant death syndrome (SIDS) is presumed due to an arrhythmia, predominantly congenital long QT syndrome (LQTS). The infant often carries a spontaneous, malignant mutation, typically without antecedent symptoms or known family history.

SCD is tragic for a family and community; there is high awareness of these uncommon but highly publicized events. A cardiac cause may be identified through a thorough postmortem evaluation.

Conflicts of Interest: None.
[a] Division of Cardiology, Children's National Health System, 111 Michigan Avenue Northwest, Washington, DC 20010, USA; [b] Department of Pediatrics, George Washington University School of Medicine, 2300 Eye Street NW, Washington, DC 20037, USA
* Corresponding author. Division of Cardiology, Children's National Health System, 111 Michigan Avenue Northwest, Washington, DC 20010.
E-mail address: edsherwin@childrensnational.org

Card Electrophysiol Clin 9 (2017) 569–579
http://dx.doi.org/10.1016/j.ccep.2017.07.008

Table 1
Pediatric sudden death terminology varies by age

SUID	Sudden unexplained infant death	Death in a child <1 y without obvious cause before investigation • Includes SIDS, accidental suffocation, strangulation in bed • Also called SUDI (sudden unexplained death in infancy)
SIDS	Sudden infant death syndrome	Death in an infant <1 y that cannot be explained after thorough investigation, including • Complete autopsy • Examination of the death scene • Review of the clinical history
SUDC	Sudden unexplained death in childhood	Death in a child >12 mo of age that remains unexplained after a thorough investigation, including • Complete autopsy • Examination of the death scene • Review of the clinical history

The most common pediatric SCD etiologies include congenital heart defects, cardiomyopathies, and inherited arrhythmia syndromes. Their recognition following a resuscitated sudden cardiac arrest (SCA) allows secondary prevention and family screening. Many have autosomal dominant inheritance and thus convey a 50% risk in first-degree relatives.

The true incidence of pediatric SCD is not well understood, limiting the ability to estimate risk and create policies for pre-event diagnosis and prevention. Identifying children at risk before a tragedy remains elusive for numerous reasons:

• Studying SCD in the young prospectively is difficult with rare events in disparate communities with varying reporting practices.
• Etiologies and incidence vary by age, requiring awareness and index of suspicion.
• Many diseases are silent until a sudden fatal event.
• Special pediatric populations raise complexity in evaluation and/or risk.
• Broad screening programs, although ostensibly detect children at risk and prevent SCD, remain in clinical equipoise with debated methods, efficacy, and outcomes.
• Postmortem evaluations vary in pediatric autopsies.
• Cascade screening after heritable SCD diagnosis is not always performed.

EPIDEMIOLOGY

The loss of a previously healthy child shocks a community; grief is propagated via news reports and social media, igniting fear and calls to action to prevent further tragedy. The emotional impact of a child's death is enormous, as are life-years lost. Despite the publicity, however, childhood SCD remains a relatively rare occurrence. According to the Centers for Disease Control and Prevention (CDC), heart disease in general accounts for far fewer childhood deaths than injuries, suicide, and malignancy (**Fig. 1**).[3]

Multiple studies have attempted to define the incidence of childhood SCD, estimated at 0.7 to 6.4 per 100,000 patient-years, far less than in adults.[2,4–6] In 1999, there were 5000 to 7000 childhood sudden deaths in the United States, compared with 300,000 to 400,000 adults,[4] whereas in 2005 the CDC estimated that 2000 people younger than 25 years die per year.[7] Approximately 60% to 75% of childhood SCD victims are male,[2,5,8–14] perhaps due to hormonal differences, level of athletic exertion, and other presumed variables.

One limitation in interpreting SCD studies in the young is lack of a uniform upper age limit. There is general consensus that infant death is a separate phenomenon; therefore, the lower cutoff is 1 year. Studies loosely define young people as those younger than the age at which atherosclerotic disease predominates, and thus includes individuals up to 30 to 45 years.

Existing data are largely based on regional populations in areas with disparate tracking of sudden deaths, thus affecting the incidence numerator. Most regions lack comprehensive health records with mandatory reporting of sudden deaths and rely on multiple and often less reliable sources: media and Internet searches, catastrophic

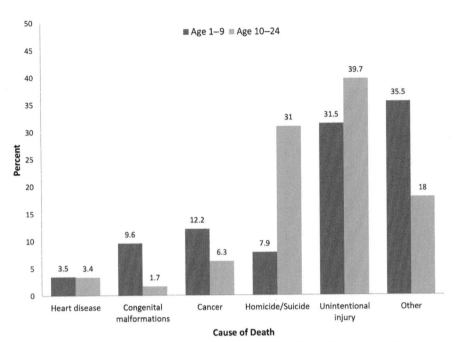

Fig. 1. Distribution of all causes of death in young people, United States 2014. Heart disease in general was responsible for <4% of deaths among young people 1 to 24 years of age. (*Adapted from* Heron M. Deaths: leading causes for 2014. Natl Vital Stat Rep 2016;65(5):1–96.)

insurance claims, local public health records, and population-specific databases. Outside of focused registries or regions with mandatory reporting, the denominator is dependent on estimated populations. Incidence is also affected by the inclusion or exclusion of successfully resuscitated SCAs. Exclusion of SCA underestimates the frequency of SCD. With the launch of the Sudden Death in the Young Registry, knowledge of the prevalence, causes, and risk factors for pediatric SCD should improve.[15]

ETIOLOGIES

SCD can be due to structural and functional problems, primary electrical disorders, or uncommon conditions, such as trauma or infection. Some may be "silent" before presentation with cardiac arrest. **Table 2** describes etiologies responsible for pediatric SCD.

Structural Heart Disease

Structural heart disease includes congenital heart defects (CHD), cardiomyopathies, and aortopathies. Following surgical CHD repair or palliation, there is increased risk of arrhythmic SCD, estimated at 100 per 100,000 patient-years.[16] SCD accounts for at least 20% of deaths in adults with complex CHD.[17]

Cardiomyopathies include hypertrophic, dilated, restrictive, noncompaction, and arrhythmogenic. Macroscopic and/or microscopic myopathic alterations result in ventricular dysfunction and proarrhythmic conditions. Patients may have vague or no symptoms before clinical presentation with heart failure, arrhythmia, or SCD. When cardiomyopathy develops slowly, children can compensate phenomenally well. Routine review of symptoms and family history is paramount. Family history in a first-degree relative should prompt presymptomatic evaluation in children. Anatomic changes may develop later in life; therefore, early cardiac imaging may not rule out future disease development. Additionally, arrhythmias may precede dysfunction or gross manifestations.

Certain congenital anatomic abnormalities may not result in ventricular dysfunction or hemodynamic disturbance until a certain age or activity. One example is anomalous coronary artery origin, present in 0.05% to 0.7% of the population.[18,19] Anomalous left coronary artery from the pulmonary artery presents predominantly with symptoms in infancy. Conversely, anomalous left coronary artery from the right sinus of Valsalva with a slitlike orifice and intramural or interarterial course can be asymptomatic until coronary obstruction provokes myocardial ischemia. Coronary anomalies may be found after SCD or identified incidentally during evaluation of unrelated

Table 2
Most common cardiac etiologies of sudden cardiac death (SCD)

Diagnosis	Incidence	Diagnostic Utility						Autopsy Findings, %	Therapeutic Utility			
		ECG	Echo	CT/MRI	ETT	Drug Testing	Gene Testing		Medical	Surgical	ICD	OHT
Structural												
Cardiomyopathies												
Hypertrophic	1:500	✓	✓	✓	✓		✓	6–50	✓	✓	✓	
Dilated	1:250–500	✓	✓				±	4	✓	✓	✓	✓
Noncompaction	Rare		✓	✓			✓	4			✓	✓
Arrhythmogenic	1:1000–2500	✓	✓	✓	✓		✓	5–16			✓	
Restrictive	Rare	✓	✓	✓								
Coronary anomalies	1:100–1:500		✓	✓	✓			1.3–27	✓	✓		
Aortopathies	Varied		✓	✓			✓	4–5	✓	✓		
Arrhythmia syndromes												
Long QT	1:2000	✓			✓	✓	✓	15–25	✓	LCSD	✓	
Short QT	Rare	✓				✓	✓		✓		✓	
Brugada	1:2000	✓			✓	✓	✓	Rare			✓	
CPVT	1:10,000	✓			✓	✓	✓	12	✓	LCSD	✓	
WPW	1:250–750	✓	✓		✓		✓	3–5	✓	Ablation		
Idiopathic VF	Rare	✓	✓		✓	✓					✓	
Other												
Myocarditis	1:20,000–1:100,000	✓	✓	✓				3–12	✓			
Commotio cordis	Rare											
1° pulmonary HTN	Not defined		✓		✓		✓		✓			

Abbreviations: CPVT, catecholaminergic polymorphic ventricular tachycardia; CT, computed tomography; ECG, electrocardiogram; ETT, exercise tolerance testing; HTN, hypertension; ICD, implantable cardioverter defibrillator; LCSD, left cardiac sympathetic denervation; OHT, orthotopic heart transplant; VF, ventricular fibrillation; WPW, Wolff-Parkinson-White; ✓, a test that should be done; ±, possible test for the given diagnosis.

symptoms. Once identified, coronary reimplantation or unroofing is generally indicated. Although it has been broadly accepted that "left from right" abnormal coronary origin presents risk of SCD, there remains debate about the implications, risks, and indication for surgery for right coronary artery from the left sinus of Valsalva.

Aortopathies include connective tissue disorders that may result in weakening of the arterial walls with risk of aortic aneurysm and rupture. Marfan syndrome has a reported risk of SCD of 0.2% to 0.3% annually.[20] SCD in Marfan syndrome also may result from arrhythmias, as high as 4%.[21] In the vascular form of Ehlers-Danlos syndrome, 25% of patients have a major vascular event by age 20.[22] Loeys-Dietz syndrome is a diffuse aortopathy with mean age of death at 26 years due to dissection.[23] Fortunately, aortopathies are typically diagnosed before disease progression to severe phenotype or aneurysm rupture.

Arrhythmia Syndromes

Inherited arrhythmia syndromes are electrical disorders, typically in individuals with normal cardiac anatomy and function. Mainly caused by alterations in the function of ion channels, these are collectively referred to as ion channelopathies. Most follow Mendelian genetics with autosomal dominant inheritance, although de novo mutations occur, with variable penetrance and expressivity. Pathophysiology and frequency are similar to those seen in adult populations (see **Table 2**), although some have particular malignancy during childhood.

One of the most common heritable arrhythmia syndromes is LQTS. Outside of the neonatal period, standard definitions of QT prolongation generally apply to children and adolescents: greater than 450 to 460 ms in boys and greater than 460 to 470 ms in girls, and the diagnosis of LQTS made according to established guidelines. Clinical phenotype and risk profiles vary throughout childhood in relation to gender and hormonal influences on repolarization, with prepubertal boys having a higher risk of cardiac events than girls, and postpubertal female individuals having a longer QT interval than male individuals.

Catecholaminergic polymorphic ventricular tachycardia (CPVT), a less common inherited arrhythmia syndrome, is of particular importance due to the early onset of malignant symptoms, including syncope, seizure, and SCA. With a mortality rate of up to 50% by age 20,[24] recognizing this condition early can be life-saving for the child and potentially for relatives. Although resting electrocardiogram (ECG) and cardiac imaging are normal, CPVT can be diagnosed on ambulatory ECG, exercise stress testing, or catecholamine provocation.

Arrhythmogenic right ventricular cardiomyopathy (ARVC) is a progressive disease that evolves during young life, with arrhythmic manifestations potentially preceding detectable cardiomyopathy. Diagnostic criteria are based on adult manifestations, creating ambiguity in children:

- Early precordial T-wave inversion is a normal finding in pediatrics.
- Epsilon waves are rare in the young.
- Assessment of global and regional dysfunction by cardiac imaging modalities has not been validated in children.[25]

Two rare forms of autosomal recessive ARVC present early in life: Carvajal syndrome (ARVC8) and Naxos disease (ARVC12), associated with woolly hair and palmoplantar keratoderma. Naxos disease has nearly 100% penetrance by adolescence and 2.3% annual SCD.[26]

Brugada and Brugada[27] described an autosomal dominant life-threatening syndrome in structurally normal hearts characterized by right precordial ST segment elevation, right bundle branch block, and susceptibility to ventricular tachyarrhythmias. Symptoms occur more commonly in male individuals, typically between 13 and 40 years of age, although can rarely manifest in younger children. More commonly, a child is identified presymptomatically after an adult presents with SCD.

Wolff-Parkinson-White (WPW), unlike many life-threatening arrhythmia syndromes, is common, does not involve ion channel dysfunction, is largely not inherited, and may be readily identified on a resting ECG. A bidirectional WPW pathway allows for atrioventricular reentrant tachycardia and, less commonly but more importantly, may support rapid anterograde propagation of atrial fibrillation leading to ventricular fibrillation and SCA. Catheter ablation is curative, eliminating the risk of SCD. With established guidelines on pediatric WPW and the increasing use of ablation for first-line therapy, WPW has become largely a problem of pediatrics with ablative cure before adulthood.

Idiopathic ventricular fibrillation typically presents in the fourth decade of life but is seen in children. A diagnosis of exclusion, this is difficult to confirm in a resuscitated pediatric patient, as cardiomyopathy may become evident years later. Treatment with secondary prevention implantable cardioverter defibrillators (ICDs) remains the mainstay of therapy, although implantation in the youngest victims can be challenging.

A challenge in arrhythmia syndromes is the difficulty in identifying the condition before a fatal event, as SCD is the first manifestation in up to 50%.[28] Symptoms may be present, although vague: palpitations, chest pain, dyspnea, syncope, and seizures. Prodromal symptoms occurring within 24 hours before death have been reported in 15% to 32% of pediatric SCDs, whereas antecedent symptoms more than 24 hours premortem have been reported in 25% to 53%.[2,8,10,11,13] Because symptoms are often nonspecific, recognition and referral for cardiac evaluation may be delayed.

A standard ECG may be insufficient in establishing a diagnosis; advanced and provocative testing is required, although may be technically challenging in young patients. Arrhythmia syndrome diagnoses are difficult to conceptualize, particularly when an individual is asymptomatic. Beyond the fear associated with the risk of sudden death, children may feel "different" and socially isolated by the diagnosis and by imposed restrictions. Clinical evaluation and discussions must be customized to physical and cognitive developmental stages. Parents of children with SADS diagnoses also suffer anxiety and distress.[29] Clear communication with the patient, family, and community resources are critical in providing appropriate education, recommendations, and psychosocial support.

Other

Multiple other causes of SCD exist, including the following:

- Myocarditis, typically due to a viral infection, results in ventricular dysfunction and potential arrhythmias. Diagnosis often requires a strong index of suspicion to avoid a fatal outcome.
- Primary pulmonary hypertension is rare with a poor prognosis when diagnosed clinically.
- Commotio cordis is a rare cause of ventricular fibrillation and SCD induced by high-velocity blunt trauma to the chest area overlying the cardiac silhouette during early ventricular repolarization. This is most commonly related to sports with smaller, nonpneumatic spheres.

AUTOPSY FINDINGS

When a child dies suddenly and without obvious cause, a postmortem evaluation can identify the structural cardiac diseases that predispose to SCD. Results of autopsies in young SCD victims vary greatly in the distribution of diagnoses found (see **Table 2**).[2,5,10,12,30–33] Autopsy-negative SCD has been reported in 6% to 51% of individuals younger than 40 years, with most studies reporting at least 30% due to SADS (**Fig. 2**).[5,9,10,34–36] In a large cohort of young military persons, SUDS represented 41% of SCD in individuals younger than 35 years, compared with 11% of soldiers older than 35 years.[37]

GENETIC TESTING

In autopsy-negative presumed arrhythmic death, genetic testing on the deceased's DNA (molecular autopsy) can provide closure for a family, enhance understanding of SADS etiologies, and improve health outcomes for family members. Many structural and arrhythmic SCD syndromes are genetically determined; identifying a gene mutation is invaluable in screening relatives. Expert consensus by the Heart Rhythm Society (HRS), European Heart Rhythm Association (EHRA) and Asia Pacific Heart Rhythm Society (APHRS) defines the collection of blood and/or tissue collection for molecular autopsy as a Class I indication in SADS cases.[38]

There are evolving complexities in molecular genetic diagnosis with rapidly expanding technology. The yield of pathogenic mutations by molecular autopsy may be as low as 7% to 9% when focused genetic mutations are evaluated and as high as 30% with broader panels.[5,8,34,39–42] It has become technically possible and economically feasible to perform whole exome or whole genome sequencing. Although evaluating the entire genome provides hope of catching a needle in the haystack, this also opens Pandora's box: variants of uncertain significance (VUS). The ensuing diagnostic purgatory increases the uncertainty surrounding a tragic death, is difficult for families to comprehend, and increases complexity of managing living relatives.

When mutations are found through molecular autopsy, targeted DNA testing can be done in conjunction with clinical screening of relatives. Although useful, molecular autopsy is not standard practice and is fraught with challenges:

- Awareness of the importance and implications of genetic testing may be limited.
- Tissue retention may be hindered by costs and space for storage.
- DNA testing on a deceased patient is not covered by insurance.
- Selection of the optimal genetic test is increasingly complex.
- Dissemination of results to family and/or primary care providers may leave uncertainty with how to proceed.

CASCADE SCREENING

Cascade screening is stepwise clinical and genetic testing of relatives of SCD or SCA victims.

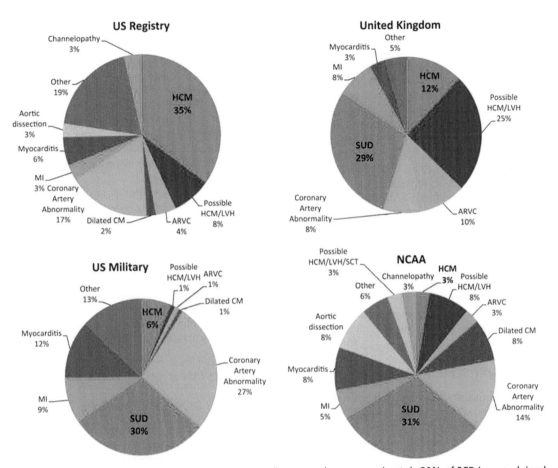

Fig. 2. Causes of SCD are heterogeneous. Among 4 studies, most show approximately 30% of SCD is unexplained. CM, cardiomyopathy; LVH, left ventricular hypertrophy; MI, myocardial infarction; NCAA, National Collegiate Athletic Association; SCT, sickle cell trait; SUD, sudden unexplained death. (*From* Harmon KG, Drezner JA, Maleszewski JJ, et al. Pathogeneses of sudden cardiac death in national collegiate athletic association athletes. Circ Arrhythm Electrophysiol 2014;7(2):202; with permission.)

This sequential evaluation may be initiated by any provider (**Fig. 3**), begins with first-degree relatives, and should be done in a center with expertise in SADS where advanced diagnostic testing is available.[38] Detailed personal and family history, targeted cardiac examination and testing, and consideration of genetic testing should be performed by an interdisciplinary team, including

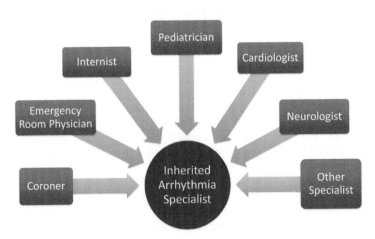

Fig. 3. Recognition of the heritability of sudden cardiac death diagnoses is critical. Following sudden cardiac arrest or death in an individual <50 years old, referral for cascade screening of first-degree relatives may be initiated by any provider. With autopsy-negative sudden death, the cardiologist should be an inherited arrhythmia specialist.

cardiologists, geneticists, and genetic counselors. Clinical testing typically includes baseline and specialized ECGs, echocardiogram, exercise stress testing, and ambulatory monitoring. Additional diagnostic evaluation may include event recorders, provocative drug testing, cardiac MRI, and electrophysiology studies (although rarely used in pediatric screening). Cascade screening results in diagnostic yield of 13% to 50% of SADS families[5,11,38,43–45] and increases to 62% of families when evaluating relatives of survivors of unexplained cardiac arrest.[43]

Like cardiomyopathies, SADS diagnoses present at varying stages of life and may not be manifest in children despite genetic predisposition. The current yield of genetic testing varies by diagnosis, but ranges from 25% to 75%; negative genetic testing does not rule out disease. Thus, an initial negative clinical and genetic evaluation does not preclude future phenotype development. Therefore, when initial screening cannot definitively rule out a diagnosis, periodic clinical evaluations are warranted.

COMMUNITY SCREENING

Community-based screening programs have been highly debated with regard to potential benefit and harm, cost-efficacy, and logistics of implementation. Challenges include the following:

- Rare event rate and unknown incidence of SCD in young people results in unclear and often unfavorable cost-effectiveness when diagnostic testing is added to history and examination.
- Diseases may be silent, with no symptoms or physical findings, resulting in difficulty structuring comprehensive yet simple and cost-effective screening.
- False-positive screening leads to anxiety, unnecessary changes in lifestyle or activities, and increased health care utilization and costs.
- False-negative results artificially reassure and can result in a tragic outcome.

Much of the debate concerns ECG screening programs. Experts in interpreting pediatric ECGs and identifying cardiac diagnoses are relatively scarce, raising the question of accuracy of ECG interpretation. Among pediatricians, more than 70% surveyed responded that their ability to interpret an ECG was a barrier to utilization.[46] One area of general misunderstanding relates to accurate QTc calculation.[47,48] Additionally, normal ECGs may provide false reassurance, as some SCD diseases display no resting ECG changes.

SPECIAL POPULATIONS
Athletes

SCD in athletes has been highly studied, as millions of children participate in sports, deaths are highly publicized, and certain conditions pose a higher risk with adrenergic states. Reported incidences of death among young athletes range widely from 1:23,000 to 1:971,000.[12,13,49–52] The relative risk of SCD in athletes is 2.5 to 4.5 higher than in nonathletes, with disproportionate risks in male and black athletes.[12,53–56]

Many screening programs target competitive athletes and high school children, missing younger children at risk and those who will die outside of competitive sports participation. The median age of diagnosis of LQTS, hypertrophic cardiomyopathy (HCM), CPVT, and anomalous left coronary artery was 10.1 years, with more than 70% presenting at age ≤13 years.[57] Although publicized SCD is often of athletes during sporting events, many studies have shown that most childhood SCD is unrelated to exertion[2,5,8–10]:

- 32% to 41% in sleep
- 27% to 41% at rest or during activities of daily living
- 9% to 38% during moderate to vigorous exercise

Stimulant Medications

Screening has been debated in attention deficit hyperactivity disorder (ADHD). There is a theoretic concern about proarrhythmia with stimulant medications. In a large population-based study, very low risk of sudden death or ventricular arrhythmia was found in children receiving stimulants.[58] Additional studies found no SCD events among 32,807 and 5351 stimulant users.[59,60] One possible exception is patients with confirmed LQTS: those on ADHD medications had increased cardiac events (62%) compared with patients with LQTS not on ADHD medications (28%, $P<.001$).[61]

TREATMENT

Treatments for SCD diagnoses are disease-specific and similar to those of adult patients:

- Lifestyle modifications, including reporting of symptoms, attention to hydration, avoidance of exacerbating medications, and minimizing situations or activities that promote ischemia or arrhythmia
- Heart failure and antiarrhythmic medications
- Cardiac rhythm devices, such as pacemakers, ICDs, and cardiac resynchronization therapy (CRT)

- Surgical interventions, including septal myomectomy, mitral valve replacement, and, less commonly in pediatrics, septal alcohol ablation for HCM, coronary artery reimplantation, or cardiac sympathectomy
- Rarely, consideration of cardiac transplantation

The primary challenges in the treatment of pediatric SCD are twofold: compliance with recommended therapies and precautions, and the short-term and long-term risks of certain therapies. Developmental ability to comply with medications can be difficult in toddlers who may refuse medications or in teenagers who may consciously decide not to take medications as they become more autonomous in their medical care. Parents may be averse to chronic medications due to concerns about side effects. Cardiac rhythm device implantation may not be straightforward. In the smallest patients, devices are implanted via epicardial approach and may require subcutaneous leads. Pacemakers and ICDs are implanted with the knowledge that these individuals will require decades of revisions and replacements. Devices in pediatrics and young adults are known to have 25% or greater adverse events, including need for reoperation, infection, venous occlusion, lead failure, ICD storms, and inappropriate shocks.[62,63]

Exercise

Exercise recommendations are contended for patients with SCD risk. In patients with inherited arrhythmia syndromes, there has been a shift from restrictive to permissive exercise recommendations in some patients under care of a specialist. Historically, limited knowledge of diseases and fear of cardiac events led to expert consensus for restriction. With increasing understanding and longer follow-up demonstrating lower risk of exertional arrhythmias, specialists have moved from paternalistic restrictions toward shared parental/coach/teacher/physician decision making, allowing exercise with strict medical therapy compliance and appropriate precautions in place. Despite permission from a specialist, however, fear of SCD and general lack of understanding in the community often leaves children excluded from team sports, leading to social isolation and physical deconditioning.

Certain conditions warrant exercise restrictions, including ARVC due to activity-related disease progression, CPVT due to adrenergic arrhythmias often despite medications, and obstructive HCM due to the risk of myocardial ischemia. It is critical to have a thorough discussion on the risks and benefits of physical activity with a family to create an individualized plan based on a patient's diagnosis, phenotype, and specific circumstances.

SUMMARY

Contemporary challenges in pediatric SCD are plentiful. Understanding the incidence and number of children at risk of SCD remains difficult despite decades of attention due to lack of mandatory reporting, historical paucity of registries for prospective data collection, ascertainment bias, and lack of consensus on inclusion criteria for evaluation of SCD in the young.

Many pediatric SCD conditions are silent before the fatal event, thus preemptively identifying an at-risk individual is challenging. Physical examination and resting ECG may be normal. With awareness, however, clues are often present and should trigger additional inquiry and evaluation. Although symptoms can be nonspecific and may be benign, they may uncover a critical diagnosis. Complaints of palpitations, chest pain, unexplained or exertional syncope, near-drowning, or atypical seizures should alert a provider to look further. Interval review of a child's family history can identify clues to a heritable cardiac condition, such as pacemakers or defibrillator implantation, heart failure, or SCA or death in a young relative.

Prospective data collection, cascade screening of relatives, awareness of the etiologies of childhood SCD, and vigilance for warning signs are crucial in preventing this rare but devastating event.

Key point: warning signs

- Unexplained fainting or seizures, particularly with exertion or emotions
- Relative with SCA or unexplained death before age 50

REFERENCES

1. Lown B. Sudden cardiac death: the major challenge confronting contemporary cardiology. Am J Cardiol 1979;43(2):313–28.
2. Pilmer CM, Kirsh JA, Hildebrandt D, et al. Sudden cardiac death in children and adolescents between 1 and 19 years of age. Heart Rhythm 2014;11(2):239–45.
3. Heron M. Deaths: leading causes for 2014. Natl Vital Stat Rep 2016;65(5):1–96.
4. Berger S, Dhala A, Friedberg DZ. Sudden cardiac death in infants, children, and adolescents. Pediatr Clin North Am 1999;46(2):221–34.
5. Bagnall RD, Weintraub RG, Ingles J, et al. A prospective study of sudden cardiac death among children and young adults. N Engl J Med 2016;374(25):2441–52.
6. Ackerman M, Atkins DL, Triedman JK. Sudden cardiac death in the young. Circulation 2016;133(10):1006–26.

7. Kung HC, Hoyert DL, Xu J, et al. Deaths: final data for 2005. Natl Vital Stat Rep 2008;56(10):1–120.

8. Winkel BG, Risgaard B, Sadjadieh G, et al. Sudden cardiac death in children (1-18 years): symptoms and causes of death in a nationwide setting. Eur Heart J 2014;35(13):868–75.

9. Meyer L, Stubbs B, Fahrenbruch C, et al. Incidence, causes, and survival trends from cardiovascular-related sudden cardiac arrest in children and young adults 0 to 35 years of age: a 30-year review. Circulation 2012;126(11):1363–72.

10. Glinge C, Jabbari R, Risgaard B, et al. Symptoms before sudden arrhythmic death syndrome: a nationwide study among the young in Denmark. J Cardiovasc Electrophysiol 2015;26(7):761–7.

11. Giudici V, Spanaki A, Hendry J, et al. Sudden arrhythmic death syndrome: diagnostic yield of comprehensive clinical evaluation of pediatric first-degree relatives. Pacing Clin Electrophysiol 2014;37(12):1681–5.

12. Harmon KG, Drezner JA, Wilson MG, et al. Incidence of sudden cardiac death in athletes: a state-of-the-art review. Br J Sports Med 2014; 48(15):1185–92.

13. Holst AG, Winkel BG, Theilade J, et al. Incidence and etiology of sports-related sudden cardiac death in Denmark–implications for preparticipation screening. Heart Rhythm 2010;7(10):1365–71.

14. Mellor G, Raju H, de Noronha SV, et al. Clinical characteristics and circumstances of death in the sudden arrhythmic death syndrome. Circ Arrhythm Electrophysiol 2014;7(6):1078–83.

15. Burns KM, Bienemann L, Camperlengo L, et al. The sudden death in the young case registry: collaborating to understand and reduce mortality. Pediatrics 2017;139(3) [pii:e20162757].

16. Jortveit J, Eskedal L, Hirth A, et al. Sudden unexpected death in children with congenital heart defects. Eur Heart J 2016;37(7):621–6.

17. Walsh EP. Sudden death in adult congenital heart disease: risk stratification in 2014. Heart Rhythm 2014;11(10):1735–42.

18. Fedoruk LM, Kern JA, Peeler BB, et al. Anomalous origin of the right coronary artery: right internal thoracic artery to right coronary artery bypass is not the answer. J Thorac Cardiovasc Surg 2007; 133(2):456–60.

19. Young ML, McLeary M, Chan KC. Acquired and congenital coronary artery abnormalities. Cardiol Young 2017;27(S1):S31–5.

20. Chiu HH, Wu MH, Chen HC, et al. Epidemiological profile of Marfan syndrome in a general population: a national database study. Mayo Clin Proc 2014; 89(1):34–42.

21. Yetman AT, Bornemeier RA, McCrindle BW. Long-term outcome in patients with Marfan syndrome: is aortic dissection the only cause of sudden death. J Am Coll Cardiol 2003;41(2):329–32.

22. Pepin M, Schwarze U, Superti-Furga A, et al. Clinical and genetic features of Ehlers-Danlos syndrome type IV, the vascular type. N Engl J Med 2000; 342(10):673–80.

23. Loeys BL, Schwarze U, Holm T, et al. Aneurysm syndromes caused by mutations in the TGF-beta receptor. N Engl J Med 2006;355(8):788–98.

24. van der Werf C, Wilde AA. Catecholaminergic polymorphic ventricular tachycardia: from bench to bedside. Heart 2013;99(7):497–504.

25. Deshpande SR, Herman HK, Quigley PC, et al. Arrhythmogenic right ventricular cardiomyopathy/dysplasia (ARVC/D): review of 16 pediatric cases and a proposal of modified pediatric criteria. Pediatr Cardiol 2016;37(4):646–55.

26. Protonotarios N, Tsatsopoulou A, Anastasakis A, et al. Genotype-phenotype assessment in autosomal recessive arrhythmogenic right ventricular cardiomyopathy (Naxos disease) caused by a deletion in plakoglobin. J Am Coll Cardiol 2001;38(5): 1477–84.

27. Brugada P, Brugada J. Right bundle branch block, persistent ST segment elevation and sudden cardiac death: a distinct clinical and electrocardiographic syndrome. A multicenter report. J Am Coll Cardiol 1992;20(6):1391–6.

28. Chugh SS, Kelly KL, Titus JL. Sudden cardiac death with apparently normal heart. Circulation 2000; 102(6):649–54.

29. Hendriks KS, Grosfeld FJ, van Tintelen JP, et al. Can parents adjust to the idea that their child is at risk for a sudden death? Psychological impact of risk for long QT syndrome. Am J Med Genet A 2005; 138A(2):107–12.

30. Stojanovska J, Garg A, Patel S, et al. Congenital and hereditary causes of sudden cardiac death in young adults: diagnosis, differential diagnosis, and risk stratification. Radiographics 2013;33(7):1977–2001.

31. Berger S, Kugler JD, Thomas JA, et al. Sudden cardiac death in children and adolescents: introduction and overview. Pediatr Clin North Am 2004;51(5): 1201–9.

32. Hill SF, Sheppard MN. A silent cause of sudden cardiac death especially in sport: congenital coronary artery anomalies. Br J Sports Med 2014;48(15):1151–6.

33. Behere SP, Weindling SN. Catecholaminergic polymorphic ventricular tachycardia: an exciting new era. Ann Pediatr Cardiol 2016;9(2):137–46.

34. Mazzanti A, Priori SG. Molecular autopsy for sudden unexplained death? Time to discuss pros and cons. J Cardiovasc Electrophysiol 2012;23(10):1099–102.

35. Harmon KG, Asif IM, Klossner D, et al. Incidence of sudden cardiac death in National Collegiate Athletic Association athletes. Circulation 2011;123(15): 1594–600.

36. Harmon KG, Drezner JA, Maleszewski JJ, et al. Pathogeneses of sudden cardiac death in National

Collegiate Athletic Association athletes. Circ Arrhythm Electrophysiol 2014;7(2):198–204.

37. Eckart RE, Shry EA, Burke AP, et al. Sudden death in young adults: an autopsy-based series of a population undergoing active surveillance. J Am Coll Cardiol 2011;58(12):1254–61.

38. Priori SG, Wilde AA, Horie M, et al. HRS/EHRA/APHRS expert consensus statement on the diagnosis and management of patients with inherited primary arrhythmia syndromes: document endorsed by HRS, EHRA, and APHRS in May 2013 and by ACCF, AHA, PACES, and AEPC in June 2013. Heart Rhythm 2013;10(12):1932–63.

39. Skinner JR, Crawford J, Smith W, et al. Prospective, population-based long QT molecular autopsy study of postmortem negative sudden death in 1 to 40 year olds. Heart Rhythm 2011;8(3):412–9.

40. Winkel BG, Larsen MK, Berge KE, et al. The prevalence of mutations in KCNQ1, KCNH2, and SCN5A in an unselected national cohort of young sudden unexplained death cases. J Cardiovasc Electrophysiol 2012;23(10):1092–8.

41. Tester DJ, Medeiros-Domingo A, Will ML, et al. Cardiac channel molecular autopsy: insights from 173 consecutive cases of autopsy-negative sudden unexplained death referred for postmortem genetic testing. Mayo Clin Proc 2012;87(6):524–39.

42. Semsarian C, Ingles J, Wilde AA. Sudden cardiac death in the young: the molecular autopsy and a practical approach to surviving relatives. Eur Heart J 2015;36(21):1290–6.

43. Kumar S, Peters S, Thompson T, et al. Familial cardiological and targeted genetic evaluation: low yield in sudden unexplained death and high yield in unexplained cardiac arrest syndromes. Heart Rhythm 2013;10(11):1653–60.

44. McGorrian C, Constant O, Harper N, et al. Family-based cardiac screening in relatives of victims of sudden arrhythmic death syndrome. Europace 2013;15(7):1050–8.

45. Tan HL, Hofman N, van Langen IM, et al. Sudden unexplained death: heritability and diagnostic yield of cardiological and genetic examination in surviving relatives. Circulation 2005;112(2):207–13.

46. Leslie LK, Rodday AM, Saunders TS, et al. Cardiac screening prior to stimulant treatment of ADHD: a survey of US-based pediatricians. Pediatrics 2012; 129(2):222–30.

47. Viskin S, Rosovski U, Sands AJ, et al. Inaccurate electrocardiographic interpretation of long QT: the majority of physicians cannot recognize a long QT when they see one. Heart Rhythm 2005;2(6):569–74.

48. Taggart NW, Haglund CM, Tester DJ, et al. Diagnostic miscues in congenital long-QT syndrome. Circulation 2007;115(20):2613–20.

49. Drezner J, Pluim B, Engebretsen L. Prevention of sudden cardiac death in athletes: new data and modern perspectives confront challenges in the 21st century. Br J Sports Med 2009;43(9):625–6.

50. Roberts WO, Stovitz SD. Incidence of sudden cardiac death in Minnesota high school athletes 1993-2012 screened with a standardized pre-participation evaluation. J Am Coll Cardiol 2013;62(14):1298–301.

51. Corrado D, Basso C, Pavei A, et al. Trends in sudden cardiovascular death in young competitive athletes after implementation of a preparticipation screening program. JAMA 2006;296(13):1593–601.

52. Steinvil A, Chundadze T, Zeltser D, et al. Mandatory electrocardiographic screening of athletes to reduce their risk for sudden death: proven fact or wishful thinking. J Am Coll Cardiol 2011;57(11):1291–6.

53. Corrado D, Basso C, Rizzoli G, et al. Does sports activity enhance the risk of sudden death in adolescents and young adults? J Am Coll Cardiol 2003; 42:1959–63.

54. Maron BJ, Haas TS, Ahluwalia A, et al. Incidence of cardiovascular sudden deaths in Minnesota high school athletes. Heart Rhythm 2013;10(3):374–7.

55. Toresdahl BG, Rao AL, Harmon KG, et al. Incidence of sudden cardiac arrest in high school student athletes on school campus. Heart Rhythm 2014;11(7): 1190–4.

56. Marijon E, Tafflet M, Celermajer DS, et al. Sports-related sudden death in the general population. Circulation 2011;124(6):672–81.

57. Dalal A, Czosek RJ, Kovach J, et al. Clinical presentation of pediatric patients at risk for sudden cardiac arrest. J Pediatr 2016;177:191–6.

58. Schelleman H, Bilker WB, Strom BL, et al. Cardiovascular events and death in children exposed and unexposed to ADHD agents. Pediatrics 2011; 127(6):1102–10.

59. Winterstein AG, Gerhard T, Shuster J, et al. Cardiac safety of central nervous system stimulants in children and adolescents with attention-deficit/hyperactivity disorder. Pediatrics 2007;120(6):e1494–1501.

60. McCarthy S, Cranswick N, Potts L, et al. Mortality associated with attention-deficit hyperactivity disorder (ADHD) drug treatment: a retrospective cohort study of children, adolescents and young adults using the general practice research database. Drug Saf 2009;32(11):1089–96.

61. Zhang C, Kutyifa V, Moss AJ, et al. Long-QT syndrome and therapy for attention deficit/hyperactivity disorder. J Cardiovasc Electrophysiol 2015;26(10): 1039–44.

62. Czosek RJ, Meganathan K, Anderson JB, et al. Cardiac rhythm devices in the pediatric population: utilization and complications. Heart Rhythm 2012;9(2): 199–208.

63. Alexander ME, Cecchin F, Walsh EP, et al. Implications of implantable cardioverter defibrillator therapy in congenital heart disease and pediatrics. J Cardiovasc Electrophysiol 2004;15(1):72–6.

Sudden Cardiac Death in Genetic Cardiomyopathies

Gourg Atteya, MD, Rachel Lampert, MD*

KEYWORDS

- Dilated cardiomyopathy • Genetic cardiomyopathy • Hypertrophic cardiomyopathy
- Arrhythmogenic right ventricular cardiomyopathy

KEY POINTS

- Sudden cardiac death (SCD) caused by ventricular arrhythmias is common in patients with genetic cardiomyopathies (CMs) including dilated CM, hypertrophic CM, and arrhythmogenic right ventricular CM (ARVC).
- Phenotypic features can identify individuals at high enough risk to warrant placement of an implantable cardioverter-defibrillator (ICD), although risk stratification schemes remain imperfect.
- Genetic testing is valuable for family cascade screening but with few exceptions (eg, LMNA mutations) do not identify higher risk for SCD.
- Medical therapies have not been shown to prevent SCD. Although randomized trials are lacking, observational data suggest that ICDs can be beneficial.
- Vigorous exercise can exacerbate ARVC disease progression and increase likelihood of ventricular arrhythmias. The risks of exercise are less well defined in hypertrophic cardiomyopathy and dilated cardiomyopathy.

DILATED CARDIOMYOPATHY

Epidemiology

Dilated cardiomyopathy (DCM) is defined as left ventricular dilatation and systolic dysfunction in the absence of coronary artery disease or abnormal loading conditions proportionate to the degree of left ventricle (LV) impairment.[1] It is one of the leading causes of heart failure (HF), predominantly affects young adults, and is the most frequent indication for cardiac transplant. The condition is best regarded not as a single disease entity but as a nonspecific phenotype, the final common response of myocardium to several genetic and environmental insults (genetic, toxins, infectious, metabolic, inflammatory, infiltrative, autoimmune, neuromuscular, pregnancy, and arrhythmias).[2] However, in a high proportion of cases, the cause remains unsolved and it is classified as idiopathic. Idiopathic DCM is defined as an enlarged LV with systolic function depressed in the absence of pressure or volume overload, or ischemic disease.[3] DCM has an estimated prevalence of 40 cases per 100,000 individuals and an annual incidence of 7 cases per 100,000 individuals.[4,5] Racial differences are reported,[6] whereas sex-related differences are less consistent.[6]

Within the group of idiopathic DCM, 30% to 50% of diagnosed cases affect multiple family members, implying a genetic origin.[7–10] However, pathogenic mutations have been found in only 20% to 30% of patients.[11,12]

Genetic Causes of Dilated Cardiomyopathy

Molecular genetic analysis has uncovered causal mutations for DCM in more than 60 genes.[2] These genes involve the function of the sarcomere (myosin and troponin), cytoskeleton, desmosomes (desmoplakin), nuclear envelope (Lamin A/C), ion channels (SCN5A), and others[2,11,13] (**Fig. 1**). Cytoskeleton mutations (truncating mutations in the

Yale School of Medicine, New Haven, CT, USA
* Corresponding author. Section of Cardiology, Yale School of Medicine, New Haven, CT 06520.
E-mail address: Rachel.lampert@yale.edu

Card Electrophysiol Clin 9 (2017) 581–603
http://dx.doi.org/10.1016/j.ccep.2017.07.009
1877-9182/17/© 2017 Elsevier Inc. All rights reserved.

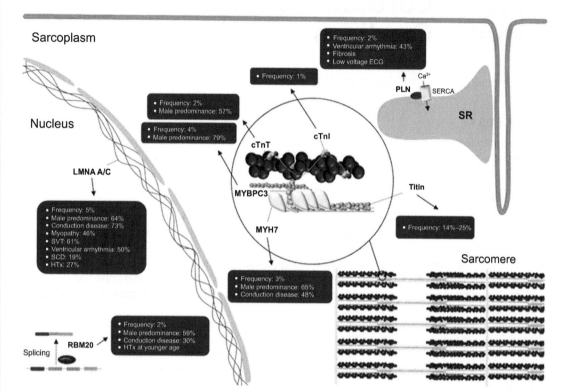

Fig. 1. DCM: genetic bases. Summary of predominant phenotypic features in patients with DCM with mutations in LMNA, PLN, RBM20, MYBPC3, MYH7, TNNT2, TNNI3, and TTN genes. cTnI, cardiac troponin I; cTnT, cardiac troponin T; ECG, electrocardiogram; HTx, heart transplant; LMNA A/C, lamin A/C; MYBPC3, myosin-binding protein C; MYH7, myosin heavy chain; PLN, phospholamban; RBM20, RNA-binding motif protein 20; SCD, sudden cardiac death; SVT, supraventricular tachycardia; SR, sarcoplasmic reticulum. (*From* Kayvanpour E, Sedaghat-Hamedani F, Amr A, et al. Genotype-phenotype associations in dilated cardiomyopathy: meta-analysis on more than 8000 individuals. Clin Res Cardiol 2017;106:135; with permission.)

Titin gene [TTN]) have been found in 25% of familial or severe transplant DCM cases and up to 13% of unselected nonfamilial DCM cases.[2] At present, the identification of a causal mutation carries few implications for prognosis or treatment of the index case, and the principal rationale for testing is to allow mutation-specific cascade screening of family members. An exception is LMNA mutations, which are associated with high rates of conduction system disease, ventricular arrhythmias, and sudden cardiac death (SCD) and may consequently lower the threshold for prophylactic implantable cardioverter-defibrillator (ICD) implantation.[14,15] At present, routine genetic testing is only recommended in familial disease (≥2 affected family members).[6]

Clinical Presentation

HF, sudden death, or thromboembolism may be the presenting manifestation of DCM. Alternatively, patients may be diagnosed with subclinical DCM identified in the process of family evaluations.[16] Clinical manifestations vary substantially even within an individual family. In families in which the pathogenic mutation has been identified, most, but not all, carriers of the disease mutation ultimately develop overt cardiomyopathy (ie, incomplete penetrance). DCM caused by mutations in the sarcomere genes MYH7, TNNT2, and TPM1 may present at any age; however, adverse outcomes seem to be more common with pediatric presentations. TTN-associated DCM typically does not present until adulthood, although adverse outcomes occur earlier in male patients. Alternatively, LMNA-associated heart disease typically does not manifest until the third decade, usually with conduction disease or arrhythmia that precedes DCM.

Incidence of Sudden Cardiac Death in Dilated Cardiomyopathy

Sudden death, which occurs in up to 12% of patients with this disorder and accounts for 25% to 30% of all deaths,[17] can be caused by electromechanical dissociation or ventricular arrhythmias. Survival in patients with idiopathic DCM has improved substantially over the last decades when treated according to current guidelines.[18]

Risk Stratification for Sudden Cardiac Death in Dilated Cardiomyopathy

Risk stratification for SCD in DCM is primarily based on clinical factors but genetic testing can play a limited role.

Genetic risk-stratifying features in dilated cardiomyopathy

Although most identified DCM mutations do not affect SCD risk, LMNA mutations are associated with high rates of conduction system disease, ventricular arrhythmias, and SCD and may consequently lower the threshold for prophylactic ICD implantation.[14,15,19] In a recent study, pooled analysis of available genotype-phenotype data totaling 8097 genotyped patients with DCM with a total of 1% to 5% of pooled frequency of different gene mutations showed a higher prevalence of SCD, cardiac transplant, or ventricular arrhythmias in LMNA (lamin A/C) and phospholamban (PLN) mutation carriers compared with sarcomeric gene mutations in patients with DCM.[20] In another study of 28 families affected by Filamin C (FLNC) gene truncating mutations, an overlapping phenotype of dilated and left-dominant arrhythmogenic cardiomyopathies was observed. This phenotype was complicated by frequent premature sudden death and accordingly prompt implantation of an ICD should be considered in those patients.[21] Another study of a large Spanish family affected by DCM showed that a novel frameshift mutation in the BAG3 gene was correlated with a more severe phenotype of the disease, mainly in younger individuals.[22] Other specific mutations have not been predictive of SCD risk.

Clinical risk-stratifying features in dilated cardiomyopathy

Looking ahead, the correlation of distinctive phenotypic features with rare alleles and elucidation of the molecular pathways responsible could revolutionize the approach to treatment, as recently exemplified by a study in patients with a variant of the SCN5A gene.[23] This cohort showed a striking DCM phenotype associated with multiple arrhythmias. Functional characterization of the mutation in vitro revealed an activating effect on the Nav1.5 sodium channel, predicted to cause rate-dependent ventricular ectopy.

In a recent meta-analysis of SCD risk stratification in all-comers with DCM, several LV remodeling and electrophysiologic variables, such as baroreflex sensitivity, heart rate turbulence, heart rate variability, left ventricular end-diastolic diameter (LVEDD), left ventricular ejection fraction (LVEF), electrophysiology study, nonsustained ventricular tachycardia (NSVT), QRS/left bundle branch block (LBBB), signal-averaged electrocardiogram (ECG), fragmented QRS, spatial QRS-T angle, and T-wave alternans, were associated with an increased risk of arrhythmic outcomes. With the exception of fragmented QRS complexes, none of the variables individually provided more than modest predictive power.[24]

A recent meta-analysis focusing on MRI parameters, including 2948 patients from 29 studies, showed that, across a wide spectrum of patients with DCM, late gadolinium enhancement (LGE), a marker of fibrosis, was strongly and independently associated with ventricular arrhythmia or SCD. LGE, present in 44%, quadrupled the risk of ventricular arrhythmia or SCD, from 1.6% annually without, to 6.9% with[25] (**Fig. 2**). Smaller studies have evaluated other MRI parameters, finding that, among those with moderate LV dysfunction, right ventricle (RV) dysfunction was a strong, independent predictor of arrhythmic events,[26] as was left ventricular long-axis strain in another study.[27]

Treatment of Sudden Cardiac Death Prevention

Medical treatment

Few studies have addressed treatment of genetic DCM specifically, and, for the most part, treatment is identical to that for other forms of DCM based on the phenotype of LV dysfunction. This topic is discussed in more detail in Daniel P. Morin and colleagues' article, "Prediction and Prevention of Sudden Cardiac Death," in this issue. One exception is a unique cohort of patients with genetic DCM: those with SCN5A mutation. In 1 small study of 42 individuals from 2 related large kindreds, these patients responded poorly to conventional HF therapy, but treatment with sodium channel blocking drugs produced a dramatic reduction in ectopy and normalization of LV function.[23] Paradigms describing therapies most beneficial at different stages of disease progression have been described, as shown in **Fig. 3**.

Role of implantable cardioverter-defibrillators

For the most part, patients with genetic DCM receive ICDs based on current criteria for nonischemic CM in general, as discussed in detail in Daniel P. Morin and colleagues' article, "Prediction and Prevention of Sudden Cardiac Death," in this issue. Current guidelines recommend ICD implantation in patients with DCM who

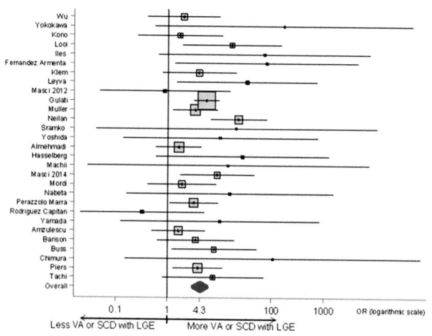

Fig. 2. DCM: risk stratification for ICD, emerging markers. Meta-analysis data showing correlation between LGE on cardiac magnetic resonance (CMR) and SCD in patients with DCM. VA, ventricular arrhythmia. (*From* Di Marco A, Anguera I, Schmitt M, et al. Late gadolinium enhancement and the risk for ventricular arrhythmias or sudden death in dilated cardiomyopathy: systematic review and meta-analysis. JACC Heart Fail 2017;5(1):35; with permission.)

CENTRAL ILLUSTRATION: Potential for Detailed DCM Assessment to Guide Therapy

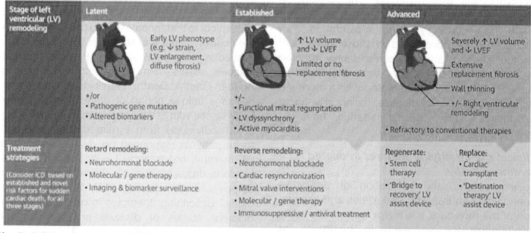

Fig. 3. DCM: treatment paradigm. Potential for detailed DCM assessment to guide therapy. (*Left*) Detection of latent DCM through enhanced screening and surveillance of at-risk patients may permit targeted treatment measures to arrest the myopathic process and prevent remodeling. (*Middle*) For patients with an established DCM phenotype, a combination of pharmacologic, genetic, device, and mechanical strategies may be deployed to promote reverse remodeling. (*Right*) In advanced disease, particularly with widespread myocardial fibrosis, emerging regenerative treatments, such as cell-based therapies or intensive mechanical unloading, may offer an alternative to transplant or long-term LV assist device. Novel risk prediction tools integrating multiple prognostic variables may allow individualized SCD risk assessment for patients at all stages of remodeling to guide optimal use of ICD implantation. (*From* Japp AG, Gulati A, Cook SA, et al. The diagnosis and evaluation of dilated cardiomyopathy. J Am Coll Cardiol 2016;67:3005; with permission.)

have survived ventricular fibrillation (VF) or symptomatic ventricular tachycardia (VT) (secondary prevention) or in patients at increased risk of SCD (primary prevention) with LVEF and HF class as the basis of selection of these patients. Landmark studies of the ICD in nonischemic cardiomyopathy did not evaluate potential genetic causes and there are few reports of use of ICDs specifically in genetic DCM. Paradigms for combining ejection fraction with other risk markers such as LGE have been described,[28] as shown in **Fig. 4**.

Among genetic causes, LMNA mutations are associated with high rates of conduction system disease, ventricular arrhythmias, and SCD. In light of these known high risks, French investigators looked into the role of prophylactic ICD implantation in 47 LMNA mutation carriers with significant conduction disorders. Ventricular arrhythmias were common in this population (even with normal EF), occurring in 30% of patients, and the ICD was an effective treatment.[19] ICD should be considered in this population for primary prevention. Whether ICD should be considered in other genetic populations beyond the standard risk factors has not yet been evaluated. The recent "2013 Appropriate Use Criteria for Implantable Cardioverter-defibrillators and Cardiac Resynchronization Therapy" describes ICD use for primary prevention in those with familial dilated/nonischemic cardiomyopathy associated with SCD as appropriate for those with structural heart disease, and may be appropriate for those with normal

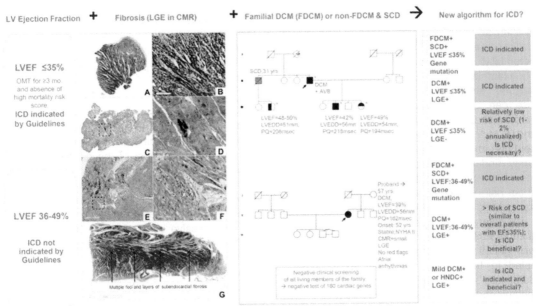

Fig. 4. DCM: risk stratification for ICD. The possible polyparametric integration of criteria selectively useful for clinical decision making regarding implantable cardioverter-defibrillator therapy for primary prevention of sudden cardiac death in patients with nonischemic DCM. The 2 left panels summarize the indications for ICD implantation in primary prevention, according to current guidelines. The pathology panels show a spectrum of myocardial fibrosis in nonischemic DCM: (A and B) Low-magnification and high-magnification views of an endomyocardial biopsy from a patient with dilated cardiolaminopathy; (C and D) Low-magnification and high-magnification views of dilated cardiotroponinopathy and single-myocyte necrosis; (E and F) low-magnification and high-magnification views of a myocardial sample from the heart of a patient with dilated cardiodystrophinopathy and focal myocardial inflammation; (G) low-magnification view of a left ventricular wall sample from a previously asymptomatic and unrecognized patient who died suddenly. (A–F) Some of the different patterns of interstitial fibrosis, likely detectable by CMR in (C) to (F) and likely undetectable in (A) and (B). The true diagnostic resolution of CMR is one of the key issues to be resolved to prevent or limit underestimation of mild interstitial fibrosis. The pedigree panels show 2 paradigmatic examples of DCM: familial, autosomal dominant dilated cardiolaminopathy (top) and nonfamilial, sporadic DCM (bottom). The right panel highlights the conditions in which ICD therapy is indicated (green-filled cells) and those in which ICD therapy may not currently be indicated by guidelines but probably needs revision (yellow-filled cells) (modified with permission from Disertori and colleagues J Cardiovasc Med, 2016). AVB, atrioventricular block; FDCM, familial DCM; HNDC, hypokinetic nondilated cardiomyopathy (as described by Pinto and colleagues Eur Heart J, 2016.); NYHA, New York Heart Association; OMT, optimal medical therapy. (From Arbustini E, Disertori M, Narula J. Primary prevention of sudden arrhythmic death in dilated cardiomyopathy: current guidelines and risk stratification. JACC Heart Fail 2017;5:40; with permission.)

hearts but carrying the implicated gene (Table 2.5 in that article).[29]

Exercise and Sudden Cardiac Death Risk in Dilated Cardiomyopathy

In general, the 2013 American Heart Association (AHA) guidelines for management of HF[6] recommend exercise training (or regular physical activity) as safe and effective for patients with HF who are able to participate, to improve functional status (class I; level of evidence, A). It also states that cardiac rehabilitation can be useful in clinically stable patients with HF to improve functional capacity, exercise duration, health-related quality of life, and mortality (class IIa; level of evidence, B). Although not specifically directed toward genetic DCM, these recommendations are likely to apply.

Although no studies have investigated the effect of exercise in patients with genetic DCM specifically, some studies of structured exercise have potentially included those with genetic cause. For example, in one study by Dougherty and colleagues[30] showing that prescription of home exercise can be safe and effective in improving cardiovascular performance in patients with ICDs and DCM,[31] 48 patients (30% of the study population) had idiopathic DCM.[30] The larger HF-Action study, finding a modest but sustained improvement in their quality of life with exercise, included about half nonischemic CM, although how many had genetic or idiopathic DCM is not described.[32]

The safety versus risk of more vigorous exercise such as athletic training or competition for those with genetic DCM has not been described, as noted in the 2015 AHA–American College of Cardiology (ACC) eligibility and disqualification recommendation for competitive athletes.[33] Their recommendation is that symptomatic athletes with DCM should not participate in most competitive sports, with the possible exception of low-intensity (class 1A) sports, at least until more information is available (class III; level of evidence, C). It is unclear whether asymptomatic patients with DCM are at risk for sudden death during competitive athletics, because ventricular tachyarrhythmias are most common in patients with more advanced disease; that is, with cardiac symptoms and lower ejection fraction.[33] There are no data regarding exercise in patients with positive genotype and negative phenotype.[33]

HYPERTROPHIC CARDIOMYOPATHY
Epidemiology

Hypertrophic cardiomyopathy (HCM) is the most common genetic cardiomyopathy. It is a global disease, with epidemiologic studies from several parts of the world reporting a similar prevalence of about 0.2% (ie, 1 in 500) in the general population, which is equivalent to at least 600,000 people affected in the United States.[34] HCM can be complicated by SCD, HF, or cardioembolic stroke resulting from atrial fibrillation (AF), which affects up to 28% of patients with HCM.[35]

Clinical Presentation and Clinical Diagnosis

Suspicion of HCM usually follows the onset of symptoms or a cardiac event but can also arise from recognition of a heart murmur or abnormal 12-lead ECG during routine or preparticipation sports examinations, or in family cascade screening. Clinical diagnosis is confirmed conventionally by imaging the HCM phenotype with two-dimensional echocardiography, cardiovascular MRI, or both. Imaging findings show an absolute increase in left ventricular wall thickness. Other common findings, such as mitral valve systolic anterior motion or hyperdynamic LV, are not obligatory for a diagnosis of HCM.[36]

Genetic Diagnosis

In most cases, HCM is inherited as an autosomal dominant genetic trait with a 50% risk of transmission to offspring. Most of the genetic mutations happen in the sarcomere.[37] Some cases are explained by de novo mutations, but apparently sporadic cases can arise because of incomplete penetrance in a parent and, less commonly, autosomal recessive inheritance. In patients fulfilling HCM diagnostic criteria, sequencing of sarcomere protein genes identifies a disease-causing mutation in up to 60% of cases. Sarcomeric and non-sarcomeric gene mutations have been studied, with mutations in 2 sarcomeric genes (MYH7 and MYBPC3) accounting for almost three-quarters of clinical cases of HCM with an identified underlying mutation[37] **Fig. 5**. The likelihood of finding a causal mutation is highest in patients with familial disease and lowest in older patients and individuals with nonclassic features.[38]

Incidence of Sudden Cardiac Death in Hypertrophic Cardiomyopathy

Incidence of sudden death in HCM varies by age, with highest risk in children and decreasing into older adulthood. In early series, based on data from tertiary referral centers, mortality in children, mostly caused by sudden death, was reported at up to 6%/y. However, more recent data show a much lower death rate, with one study of 474 patients aged 7 to 29 years showing a mortality of 0.54%/y. In that study, the rate of aborted life-threatening events, including ICD-treated

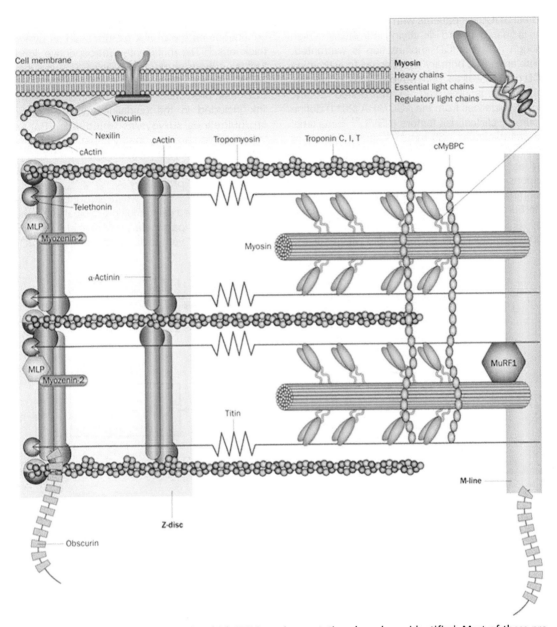

Fig. 5. HCM: genetic bases. Proteins in which HCM-causing mutations have been identified. Most of these proteins are components of the sarcomere. Notably, mutations in 2 genes, MYH7 and MYBPC3 (encoding myosin-7 and cMyBPC, respectively), account for up to three-quarters of all clinical cases of HCM in which the underlying mutation has been defined. Mutations in nonsarcomeric proteins, such as vinculin, can also result in HCM. cActin, α-cardiac muscle actin 1; cMyBPC, cardiac myosin-binding protein C; MLP, cysteine and glycine-rich protein 3 (also known as muscle LIM protein); MuRF1, E3 ubiquitin-protein ligase TRIM63 (also known as muscle-specific RING finger protein 1). (*From* Frey N, Luedde M, Katus HA. Mechanisms of disease: hypertrophic cardiomyopathy. Nat Rev Cardiol 2011;9:93; with permission.)

ventricular arrhythmias, resuscitated arrest, or heart transplant, was close to 2%/y, suggesting that current therapies are significantly improving survival in this population.[39] However, in older patients, for those more than 60 years of age, even with conventional risk factors, mortality was low, at 0.64%/y.[40]

Risk Stratification of Sudden Cardiac Death in Hypertrophic Cardiomyopathy

HCM is an important cause of arrhythmic SCD. Estimation of SCD risk is an integral part of the clinical management of HCM. Although there are no randomized controlled trials showing mortality benefit of ICDs in patients with HCM, SCD prevention is geared toward identifying individuals at high enough risk that ICD implantation is warranted. There are now 2 primary approaches to estimating SCD risk, as well as more novel risk factors whose importance is emerging. In the United States, recent guidelines from the ACC/AHA (2011) define 4 primary clinical risk factors (NSVT,[41,42] maximal LV wall thickness $\geq$30 mm,[43–46] family history of SCD,[43,47,48] and unexplained syncope[41,43,45]) as well as 1 minor factor (abnormal blood pressure response to exercise[41,43,48,49]) to determine recommendation for ICD[34] (**Fig. 6**).

In Europe, recent European Society of Cardiology (ESC) guidelines (2014) take a different approach, designed to take into account the different effect size of individual risk factors and continuous nature of risk factors such as LV wall thickness.[38] The multicenter, retrospective, longitudinal cohort study HCM-Risk-SCD, including 3675 patients, developed and validated a new SCD risk prediction model. The model, with a link included in the guidelines (www.escardio. org/guidelines-surveys/esc-guidelines/Pages/ hypertrophic-cardiomyopathy.aspx), provides an individualized 5-year risk estimate and recommends ICD if risk is greater than 5%. The formula is as follows: $\text{probability}_{SCD \text{ at 5 years}} = 1 - 0.998^{\exp(\text{prognostic index})}$, where prognostic index can be calculated using multiple clinical and echocardiographic parameters (maximal LV wall thickness, left ventricular outflow tract [LVOT]

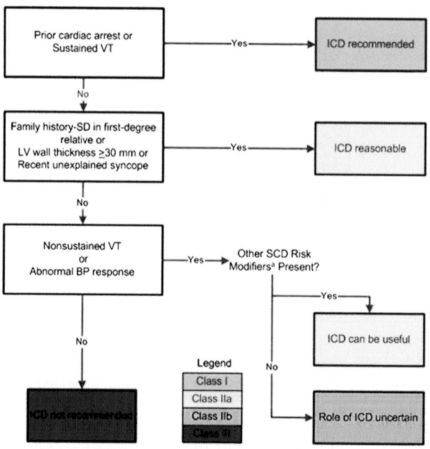

Fig. 6. HCM: risk stratification for ICD, AHA guidelines. Flow chart for ICD implantation in HCM according to the 2011 AHA guidelines. Indications for ICDs in HCM. Regardless of the level of recommendation put forth in these guidelines, the decision for placement of an ICD must involve prudent application of individual clinical judgment, and thorough discussions of the strength of evidence, the benefits, and the risks (including but not limited to inappropriate discharges, lead and procedural complications) to allow active participation of the fully informed patient in ultimate decision making. [a] SCD risk modifiers include established risk factors and emerging risk modifiers. BP, blood pressure; SD, sudden death. (*From* Gersh BJ, Maron BJ, Bonow RO, et al. 2011 ACCF/AHA guideline for the diagnosis and treatment of hypertrophic cardiomyopathy: a report of the American College of Cardiology Foundation/American Heart Association Task Force on Practice Guidelines. Circulation 2011;124:e783–831; with permission.)

gradient, left atrium diameter, and so forth). In the European guidelines, HCM Risk-SCD is recommended as a method of estimating risk of sudden death at 5 years in patients aged at least 16 years without a history of life-threatening arrhythmia (class I; level of evidence, B. **Fig. 7**). In one head-to-head comparison with a model using the 4 major risk factors, the European prediction model

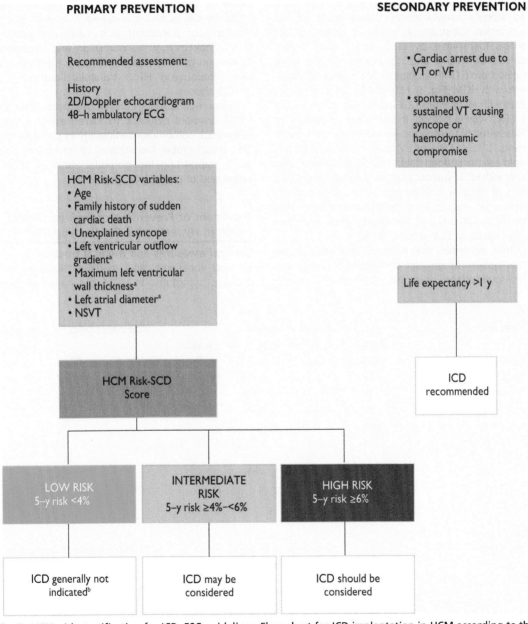

PRIMARY PREVENTION

Recommended assessment:

History
2D/Doppler echocardiogram
48–h ambulatory ECG

HCM Risk-SCD variables:
• Age
• Family history of sudden cardiac death
• Unexplained syncope
• Left ventricular outflow gradient[a]
• Maximum left ventricular wall thickness[a]
• Left atrial diameter[a]
• NSVT

HCM Risk-SCD Score

LOW RISK
5–y risk <4%

INTERMEDIATE RISK
5–y risk ≥4%–<6%

HIGH RISK
5–y risk ≥6%

ICD generally not indicated[b]

ICD may be considered

ICD should be considered

SECONDARY PREVENTION

• Cardiac arrest due to VT or VF

• spontaneous sustained VT causing syncope or haemodynamic compromise

Life expectancy >1 y

ICD recommended

Fig. 7. HCM: risk stratification for ICD, ESC guidelines. Flow chart for ICD implantation in HCM according to the 2014 ESC guidelines. NSVT recorded during 24-hour to 48-hour ambulatory ECG monitoring. [a] Use absolute values for LVOT gradient, maximum left ventricular wall thickness (MLVWT), and left atrial dimension. [b] ICD not recommended unless there are other clinical features of potential prognostic importance and when the likely benefit is greater than the lifelong risk of complications and the impact of an ICD on lifestyle, socioeconomic status, and psychological health. 2D, two-dimensional. (*From* Authors/Task Force members, Elliott PM, Anastasakis A, Borger MA, et al. 2014 ESC guidelines on diagnosis and management of hypertrophic cardiomyopathy: the Task Force for the Diagnosis and Management of Hypertrophic Cardiomyopathy of the European Society of Cardiology (ESC). Eur Heart J 2014;35:2766; with permission.)

improved risk prediction.[50] However, other head-to-head comparisons have not confirmed the predictive ability of the risk-score model.[51]

Other clinical markers of risk are emerging. Most promising of these is contrast-enhanced cardiac magnetic resonance (CMR), which has emerged as a powerful, advanced imaging technique that can identify structurally abnormal areas of the myocardial substrate; in particular, replacement fibrosis identifiable by LGE. In a recent meta-analysis by Weng and colleagues,[52] data were pooled from 5 CMR studies with a total of 3000 patients with HCM (**Fig. 8**). Fifty-five percent of the patients with HCM were LGE positive and the extent of LGE was a strong independent predictor of disease-related outcome, including sudden death events. LGE ($\geq$15% of LV mass) also conferred a 2-fold greater sudden death risk compared with patients with HCM without LGE, even when taking into account other variables associated with sudden death risk, including systolic dysfunction. This study also showed a similar strong relationship between extent of LGE and HF death.

Other potential risk markers are also under investigation. Magri and colleagues[53] performed cardiopulmonary exercise tolerance testing (CPETT) in 623 patients with HCM and found that ventilation versus carbon dioxide relation during exercise (VE/Vco$_2$ slope) might improve SCD risk stratification, particularly in those HCM categories classified at low-intermediate SCD risk according to contemporary 2014 ESC guidelines. In a larger study of use of CPETT in 1898 patients with HCM by Coats and colleagues,[54] annual rate of mortality or transplant was 1.6% per person-year. Peak oxygen consumption and ventilation to carbon dioxide production were predictors of death because of HF or transplant but not SCD or ICD shocks.

In an echocardiogram study, peak exercise LVOT gradient evaluation showed additive value to predict outcomes, particularly in patients with rest mean global longitudinal strain greater than 15%, supporting the potential value of resting strain and of peak LVOT gradient.

Treatment of Prevention of Sudden Cardiac Death in Hypertrophic Cardiomyopathy

General measures and medical treatment
General measures and medical therapies may improve symptoms in HCM but have not been

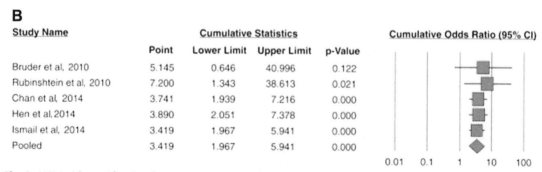

Fig. 8. HCM: risk stratification for ICD, emerging markers. Meta-analysis data showing correlation between LGE on CMR and SCD in patients with HCM. (*A*) Cumulative analysis using all 7 studies; (*B*) cumulative analysis using 5 studies. CI, confidence interval. (*From* Weng Z, Yao J, Chan RH, et al. Prognostic value of LGE-CMR in HCM: a meta-analysis. JACC Cardiovasc Imaging 2016;9(12):1397; with permission.)

shown to improve overall survival or freedom from SCD to date. Patients with symptomatic LVOT obstruction (LVOTO) are treated initially with nonvasodilating β-blockers titrated to maximum tolerated dose with very few studies comparing individual β-blockers (recommendation I-B). If β-blockers alone are ineffective, disopyramide (class IA antiarrhythmic drug), titrated up to a maximum tolerated dose, may be added (recommendation I-B),[55,56] which can abolish basal LV outflow pressure gradients, and improve exercise tolerance and functional capacity without proarrhythmic effects or an increased risk of SCD.[55,56] Calcium blockers, including verapamil[57] or diltiazem for those who are intolerant or have contraindications to β-blockers and verapamil,[58] can be used. Low-dose loop or thiazide diuretics may be used cautiously to improve dyspnea associated with LVOTO, but it is important to avoid hypovolemia.

Ongoing studies are evaluating the impact of novel medications on symptoms, quality of life, and progression of disease, including Liberty-HCM (evaluating the effect of eleclazine [GS-6615] on exercise capacity, quality of life, and safety and tolerability), VANISH (evaluating whether treatment with valsartan will have beneficial effect in early HCM by assessing many domains that reflect myocardial structure, function, and biochemistry), HALT (a phase 1 trial of N-acetylcysteine tolerability and safety), treatment of preclinical HCM with diltiazem (evaluating whether early administration will decrease the progression of HCM in individuals with sarcomere gene mutations), and RHYME (evaluating ranolazine in patients with HCM with chest pain or dyspnea).

Invasive treatment of left ventricular outflow tract obstruction

Medications, surgical myectomy, and alcohol ablation are approaches to relieving LVOTO and improving symptoms for patients with obstructive HCM. There are no randomized trials comparing the impact of these modalities on mortality, sudden death, or arrhythmias, although observational studies have favored surgical myectomy. In one early comparison, symptomatic patients who underwent myectomy had an improved total survival and freedom from sudden death compared with those who did not, and a similar survival to the general population.[59] Although surgical myectomy is the primary treatment option for most patients with severe symptoms of obstructive HCM, alcohol septal ablation (ASA) has also been recommended as a selective alternative for older patients, those with comorbidities, or patients with reluctance toward surgery.[36] Since the introduction of ASA, there have been concerns regarding

the arrhythmogenic effect of the ablation scar in patients already at an increased risk of life-threatening arrhythmias. In a recent European study of more than 1000 patients with HCM (including 566 with either myectomy or ablation), there was a 2-fold increase in sudden death risk with alcohol ablation over the duration of the study as well as a higher number of appropriate ICD shocks for VT or VF, despite a greater risk profile in the myectomy patients,[60] with similar findings in other studies.[61] Based on these data, international consensus and guideline recommendations from the United States and Europe state that septal myectomy should be considered the treatment of choice for most patients with HCM and severe drug-refractory HF symptoms attributable to LV outflow obstruction.[62]

However, other studies of long-term outcome after ASA versus surgical myectomy showed survival and clinical outcomes to be comparable after both procedures, with no difference in SCD/appropriate ICD shocks,[63] with 2 meta-analyses showing long-term mortality and (aborted) SCD rates after ASA and myectomy to be similarly low (0.41% and 0.49%/y) after ASA and myectomy respectively.[64,65]

Role of implantable cardioverter-defibrillators to reduce sudden cardiac death

There are no randomized controlled trials on the role of ICDs in patients with HCM, although observational studies have shown effectiveness. Patients with HCM who survive VF or sustained VT are at very high risk of subsequent lethal cardiac arrhythmias and should receive an ICD (secondary prevention).[66–70] Risk stratification and indications for primary prevention ICDs are described earlier.

Observational studies show that ICDs are effective at treating ventricular arrhythmias in patients with HCM. Rates of appropriate therapy for ventricular arrhythmias range from 10% to 11% yearly for patients receiving the device for secondary prevention, and from 3% to 5% yearly for primary prevention patients.[66,71] In a longitudinal registry of 224 unrelated children and adolescents with HCM judged at high risk for SCD,[72] defibrillators were activated appropriately to terminate VT or VF in 43 patients (19%) over a mean of 4 years. In one of the larger studies, the multinational registry study of ICDs implanted between 1986 and 2003, 506 unrelated patients with HCM were enrolled and had a mean follow-up of 3.7 years.[11] Almost 20% of patients experienced appropriate device therapy for VT/VF. Discharge rates were 5.5%/y overall, 11%/y for secondary prevention (after cardiac arrest or sustained VT), and 4%/y for primary prevention (≥1 risk factor). ICD therapy was most common in young patients (average, 40 years of age), with the highest rates in children and adolescents (11%/y).

Exercise and Sudden Cardiac Death Risk in Hypertrophic Cardiomyopathy

The risk of SCD associated with exercise in individuals with HCM is a topic of active research, and how much exercise in these individuals is safe is not yet delineated. Retrospective series suggest that HCM underlies a significant percentage of sudden death in athletes,[73] and one report-based study suggests that many of these athletes die during exercise.[74] Based on these data, disease-specific guidelines on HCM from both the 2014 ESC[42] and the 2011 AHA,[34] and sports-specific guidelines for eligibility for competitive sports from both Europe[75] and the United States,[33] recommend against competitive sports participation for patients with HCM. One study has shown that, in a series of athletes with ICDs who did choose to compete, including 75 patients with HCM, there were no deaths or resuscitated arrests or arrhythmia-related or shock-related injuries related to sports.[76,77]

Recommendations for participation in competitive athletics for asymptomatic, genotype-positive patients with HCM without evidence of LV hypertrophy by two-dimensional echocardiography and CMR varies, with US guidelines permitting sports participation for this group, whereas European guidelines do not. There are no data on the safety of sports for athletes who are genotype positive but phenotype negative for HCM.

Further research is needed to establish the long-term safety of exercise at moderate and higher levels of intensity. The LIVE_HCM (Lifestyle and Exercise in Hypertrophic Cardiomyopathy) study is currently enrolling patients to determine the risks versus safety of more vigorous exercise for individuals with HCM, aged 8 to 60 years, with or without ICDs, as well as the impact of exercise on quality of life for these individuals (http://livehcm.org/).

Although determining safe levels of athletic participation and vigorous exercise is an important question for a minority of patients with HCM, for most, understanding how to increase activity for the sedentary may be a more important issue. A recent survey by Reineck and colleagues[78] compared patients with HCM with NHANES (National Health and Nutrition Examination Survey) participants, finding that the patients with HCM reported less time engaged in physical activity at work and for leisure, as well as higher body mass index. An Australian study[79] similarly found that most patients with HCM did not meet physical activity recommendations. In that study, many participants reported that they had been advised not to exercise at all.

Several studies have evaluated the safety of exercise programs to increase fitness for patients with HCM, finding improved exercise capacity and no increase in arrhythmias. In a small pilot study, Klempfner and colleagues[80] investigated the benefits and feasibility of increasing exercise in 20 symptomatic patients with HCM who were significantly limited in their everyday activity. Patients exercised in a cardiac rehabilitation center twice a week, using treadmill, arm ergometer, and upright cycle exercise, with exercise prescription based on heart rate reserve determined from a symptom-limited graded exercise stress test. Exercise intensity was gradually increased from 50% to 85% of the heart rate reserve over the training period. Functional capacity, assessed by a graded exercise test, improved significantly, and New York Heart Association (NYHA) functional class improved from baseline by greater than or equal to 1 grade in 10 patients (50%). During the study period and the following 12 months, none of the patients experienced clinical deterioration or significant adverse events. This study suggests that moderate exercise may be not just safe but beneficial in decreasing symptom burden. There are several possible pathways through which exercise could improve symptoms: exercise improves diastolic function[81] and improves endothelial function.

The recently published RESET-HCM study, the first randomized clinical trial of exercise for patients with HCM, sheds further light on the safety of exercise in those patients. Moderate-intensity, unsupervised aerobic training after consultation with an exercise physiologist versus usual activity was investigated in 136 adults with HCM over a 4-month follow-up period. There was a statistically significant increase in the primary end point of change in mean peak oxygen consumption (peak Vo_2) (+1.35 mL/kg/min) among patients in the exercise group (n = 67) compared with those in the usual-activity group (n = 66) (+0.08 mL/kg/min). Exploratory secondary end points showed reduced premature ventricular contraction burden and improved quality-of-life scores in the exercise group. The moderate exercise regimen used in this study increased exercise capacity at 16 weeks without increase, and with possible decrease, in the likelihood of arrhythmia.[82]

ARRHYTHMOGENIC RIGHT VENTRICULAR CARDIOMYOPATHY
Epidemiology

Arrhythmogenic right ventricular cardiomyopathy (ARVC), also known as arrhythmogenic right ventricular dysplasia, is a leading cause of sudden death in young people in some areas.[83] It is a heritable heart muscle disorder that predominantly affects the RV. Progressive loss of right ventricular myocardium and its replacement by fibrofatty tissue is the pathologic hallmark of the disease.[83] The prevalence of ARVC is estimated to range from 1 case in 5000 persons in the general population to 1 in 2000 in some European countries, including Italy and Germany.[84,85]

Clinical Presentation and Clinical Diagnosis

Clinically overt disease is preceded by a preclinical phase characterized by minimal or no structural abnormalities (so-called concealed disease). SCD may be the first clinical manifestation of the disease.[83] The most common clinical presentation is palpitations or effort-induced syncope in an adolescent or young adult with T-wave inversion in the right precordial leads (V1–V4) on the ECG, ventricular arrhythmias with an LBBB pattern, and right ventricular abnormalities on imaging tests. In a study by Bhonsale and colleagues,[86] late diagnosis was seen in 21% of patients with ARVC.

Ventricular arrhythmias range from frequent premature ventricular beats to VT, which may degenerate into VF. Diagnostic alterations of the RV on imaging studies consist of global dilatation and dysfunction and regional wall-motion abnormalities such as systolic akinesia or dyskinesia or diastolic bulging; the LV and the septum are usually involved to a lesser extent, if at all. Cardiac MRI (CMR) has become the preferred imaging technique because it combines the evaluation of structural and functional ventricular abnormalities with noninvasive tissue characterization with the use of LGE, which provides information about the presence and amount of fibrofatty myocardial scarring.[87,88]

To standardize the clinical diagnosis of ARVC, in 1994 an international task force proposed guidelines in the form of a qualitative scoring system with major and minor criteria.[89] In 2010, the task force revised the guidelines to improve diagnostic sensitivity, mostly for the clinical screening of family members, by providing quantitative criteria for diagnosing right ventricular abnormalities and adding molecular genetic criteria.[90] However, the diagnosis remains problematic because of the low specificity of electrocardiographic abnormalities, multiple causes of right ventricular arrhythmias, difficulties in the use of imaging to assess right ventricular structure and function, and the sometimes puzzling results of genetic testing.

Genetic Diagnosis

Mutations in the gene encoding plakoglobin (JUP) were the first disease-causing variants to be identified in patients with Naxos disease.[91] Plakoglobin is a major constituent of desmosomal complexes. Mutations in genes encoding other desmosomal proteins were subsequently shown to cause the more common (nonsyndromic) autosomal dominant form of ARVC. These proteins include desmoplakin (DSP), plakophilin 2 (PKP2), desmoglein 2 (DSG2), and desmocollin 2 (DSC2). A recessive mutation in the *DSP* gene was shown to cause another cardiocutaneous syndrome, the Carvajal syndrome. Autosomal dominant ARVC has also been linked to rare pathogenic mutations in genes unrelated to cell-to-cell junctional apparatus[92–96] (**Fig. 9**).

From pooled data from major studies of molecular genetic screening for desmosomal gene mutations, the estimated overall rate of identified pathologic mutations among patients meeting the diagnostic criteria for ARVC established by the international task force is approximately 50%.[97–100]

Incidence of Sudden Cardiac Death in Arrhythmogenic Right Ventricular Cardiomyopathy

The estimated overall mortality varies among studies, ranging from 0.08%/y to 3.6%/y.[101] The mortality was initially overestimated because it was based on studies at tertiary referral centers, which predominantly included high-risk patients. Recent studies of community-based patient cohorts have shown that the long-term outcome for treated index patients and family members is more favorable (annual mortality <1%).[102–104]

Risk Stratification of Sudden Cardiac Death in Arrhythmogenic Right Ventricular Cardiomyopathy

As described in a recent review by Corrado and colleagues,[83] the prognosis for patients with ARVC depends largely on the severity of arrhythmias and ventricular dysfunction, as shown in **Fig. 10**.[14,101,105–109] Prior cardiac arrest caused by VF and sustained VT are the most important predictors of life-threatening arrhythmic events during follow-up. Moderate-sized studies (50–150 patients) identifying risks for arrhythmia have predominantly focused on populations with ICDs in place, focusing on fast VT (>240 beats/min [bpm]) or VF (ie, lifesaving ICD interventions). Risk factors with the most data supporting an association with arrhythmia include unexplained syncope[106,110]; nonsustained VT on

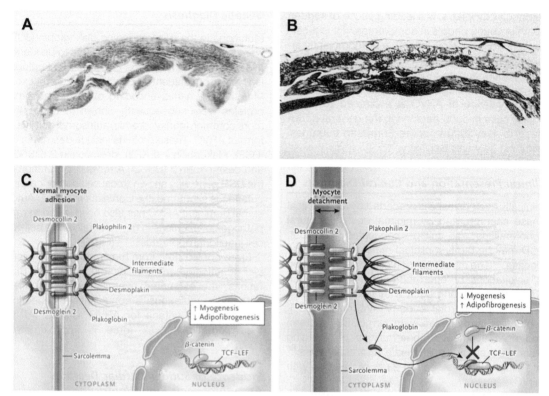

Fig. 9. ARVC: genetic bases. Histopathologic features and pathogenesis of ARVC. The distinctive histopathologic feature of ARVC is the loss of right ventricular myocardium and the substitution of fibrous and fatty tissue. (*A*) A full-thickness histologic section (azan trichrome stain) of the anterior right ventricular wall in a normal heart; (*B*) a similar section from the heart of a patient with ARVC who died suddenly. With the azan trichrome stain, myocytes appear red, fibrous tissue appears blue, and fatty tissue appears white. ARVC is caused by genetically defective desmosomes, which are cell-to-cell adhesive structures. The desmosome contains 3 major components: desmoplakin, which binds to intermediate filaments (ie, cardiac desmin); transmembrane proteins (ie, desmosomal cadherins), including desmocollin 2 and desmoglein 2; and linker proteins (ie, proteins of the armadillo family), including plakoglobin and plakophilin 2, which mediate interactions between the desmosomal cadherin tails and desmoplakin, as shown in (*C*). Abnormal desmosomes confer a predisposition over time to disruption of the intercellular junction, as shown in (*D*; *double-headed arrow*), mostly under conditions of increased mechanical stress, such as sports activity. A parallel pathogenic mechanism involves the canonical Wnt–β-catenin signaling pathway. This evolutionarily conserved pathway plays a pivotal role in cardiac development, myocyte differentiation, and normal myocardial architecture. During canonical Wnt–β-catenin signaling, β-catenin forms complexes with members of the TCF–LEF (T-cell factor–lymphocyte-enhancing factor) family of transcription factors in the nucleus to prevent the differentiation of mesodermal precursors into adipocytes and fibrocytes by suppressing the expression of adipogenic and fibrogenic genes (*C*). Impairment of desmosomal assembly by genetically defective proteins causes the translocation of plakoglobin from the sarcolemma to the nucleus (*arrows* in *D*), where it may antagonize the effects of β-catenin. By competing with β-catenin, intranuclear plakoglobin suppresses Wnt–β-catenin signaling and induces a gene transcriptional switch from myogenesis to adipogenesis and fibrogenesis (*D*). (*From* Corrado D, Link MS, Calkins H. Arrhythmogenic right ventricular cardiomyopathy. N Engl J Med 2017;62, with permission.)

ambulatory monitoring or exercise testing[105,106]; and severe dilatation or dysfunction of RV, LV, or both.[107–114] Other risk factors shown to predict arrhythmia in smaller studies include male gender[97], young age at the time of diagnosis,[107,108] amount of electroanatomic scar,[115] electroanatomic scar–related fractionated electrograms,[116] extent of T-wave inversion across precordial and inferior leads,[108,117,118] low QRS amplitude,[118] and QRS fragmentation.

Although some studies have shown predictive value of inducible arrhythmias on programmed ventricular stimulation at electrophysiology study,[105] others have shown a low predictive accuracy for receiving appropriate ICD therapy.[106,108]

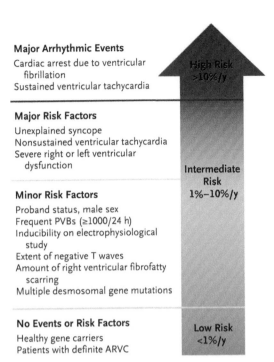

Major Arrhythmic Events
Cardiac arrest due to ventricular
   fibrillation
Sustained ventricular tachycardia

High Risk
>10%/y

Major Risk Factors
Unexplained syncope
Nonsustained ventricular tachycardia
Severe right or left ventricular
   dysfunction

Intermediate
Risk
1%–10%/y

Minor Risk Factors
Proband status, male sex
Frequent PVBs (≥1000/24 h)
Inducibility on electrophysiological
   study
Extent of negative T waves
Amount of right ventricular fibrofatty
   scarring
Multiple desmosomal gene mutations

No Events or Risk Factors
Healthy gene carriers
Patients with definite ARVC

Low Risk
<1%/y

Fig. 10. Risk stratification in ARVC. Proposed scheme for prognostic stratification of patients with ARVC according to the clinical presentation. The risk subgroups shown have been defined by the estimated probability of a major arrhythmic event (SCD, cardiac arrest caused by VF, sustained VT, or an event requiring defibrillator intervention) during follow-up, in relation to previous arrhythmic events or risk factors. An estimated annual risk of more than 10% defines the high-risk group, a risk between 1% and 10% the intermediate risk group, and a risk less than 1% the low-risk group. PVB, premature ventricular beats. (*From* Corrado D, Link MS, Calkins H. Arrhythmogenic right ventricular cardiomyopathy. N Engl J Med 2017;376:67; with permission.)

Genetic Risk Stratification

Although some mutations have been identified that carry higher risk for SCD, specifically compound heterozygous mutations and single truncating mutations in the desmoplakin gene (DSP),[97] ICD is not recommended based on genetic testing alone, because of the variable phenotypic expression.[101] One exception may be the nondesmosomal missense mutation in TMEM43, which is highly penetrant and highly lethal, but this is a very rare variant.[119,120]

Treatment for Prevention of Sudden Cardiac Death in Arrhythmogenic Right Ventricular Cardiomyopathy

Medical treatment

Despite limited supportive data, agents with antiadrenergic activity are currently recommended for all clinically affected persons, for both prevention of arrhythmias and reduction of right ventricular wall stress.[101] Current practice is based largely on anecdote, extrapolation from other conditions, and studies that did not necessarily differentiate between different agents.[121] One early study of individuals with ARVC who had inducible VT during programmed ventricular stimulation and those who had noninducible VT found that[122] sotalol was effective at decreasing arrhythmias in both groups, with efficacy of 68.4% and 82.8% respectively, whereas amiodarone was less effective. However, in a more recent report from the North American ARVC registry, both sotalol and β-blockers were not protective against clinically relevant ventricular arrhythmias, whereas amiodarone was more effective.[123] However, the potential for serious cumulative toxic effects precludes long-term therapy with amiodarone, especially in younger patients. Both studies were small, with fewer than 50 treated patients in any group. No study has addressed the impact of medical therapy on SCD or total mortality.

Role of implantable cardioverter-defibrillators

Although randomized trials of defibrillator therapy in ARVC have not been performed, data from observational studies have consistently shown that they are effective and safe in this population. Patients who benefit most from defibrillators are those who have had an episode of VF or sustained VT. How best to risk-stratify patients with ARVC without a history of arrhythmia to determine benefit from primary prevention ICD remains uncertain, as discussed earlier.[14,101] Based on the data discussed earlier on predictors of arrhythmia, the International Task Force Consensus Statement on Arrhythmogenic Right Ventricular Cardiomyopathy/Dysplasia has recommended a schema for ICDs[101] (**Fig. 11**). For patients with 1 major risk factor, ICD is described as a class IIa recommendation, whereas for those with more than 1 minor criterion, ICD may be considered (class IIB). Those with no risk factors or gene carriers are not recommended to be given ICDs (class III).

Many studies document that the ICD successfully converts lethal ventricular tachyarrhythmias in high-risk patients with ARVC. Overall, between 48% and 78% of patients received appropriate ICD interventions during a mean follow-up period of 2 to 7 years after implantation.[101] In most studies, the survival benefit of the ICD was estimated by comparing the patient survival rate with the projected freedom of ICD interventions for fast VT (>240 bpm) or VF (ie, lifesaving ICD interventions), which were used as a surrogate for aborted SCD, based on the assumption that these

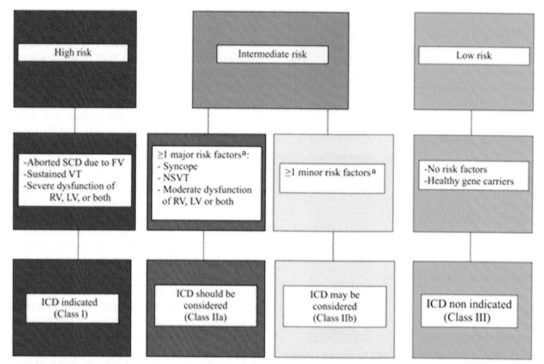

Fig. 11. ARVC: risk stratification for ICD. Flow chart for ICD implantation in patients with ARVC. Flow chart of risk stratification and indications to ICD implantation in ARVC/arrhythmogenic right ventricular dysplasia. Based on the available data on annual mortalities associated with specific risk factors, the estimated risk of major arrhythmic events in the high-risk category is greater than 10%/y, in the intermediate category it ranges from 1% to 10%/y, and in the low-risk category it is less than 1%/y. Indications to ICD implantation were determined by consensus, taking into account not only the statistical risk but also the general health, socioeconomic factors, the psychological impact, and the adverse effects of the device. [a] See the text for distinction between major and minor risk factors. (*From* Corrado D, Wichter T, Link MS, et al. Treatment of arrhythmogenic right ventricular cardiomyopathy/dysplasia: an international task force consensus statement. Circulation 2015;132:449; with permission.)

tachyarrhythmias would have been fatal without termination by the device.

In the largest multicenter series of patients with ARVC with ICDs (132 patients), the fast VT/VF-free survival rate was 72% at 36 months compared with the patient survival of 98%, with an estimated survival benefit of 26%.[107] There were 48% appropriate interventions, with 24% of those considered lifesaving, and 16% inappropriate interventions.[107] The largest single-center experience found an estimated improvement of overall survival of 23%, 32%, and 35% after 1, 3, and 7 years of follow-up, respectively.[109] Despite the short follow-up of the available studies, the time between implantation and the first appropriate discharge was greater than or equal to 1 year in a large proportion of patients, with a maximal interval of 5.5 years.[105,106,124,125]

In asymptomatic patients with no risk factors and in healthy gene carriers, there is generally no indication for prophylactic defibrillator implantation because of the low risk of arrhythmias and the significant risk of device-related and electrode-related complications during long-term follow-up (estimated rate, 3.7%/y).[102–104,109,126]

Exercise and Sudden Cardiac Death in Arrhythmogenic Right Ventricular Cardiomyopathy

Evidence continues to mount that exercise is detrimental in ARVC, leading to increased risk of arrhythmias both acutely and chronically, and to symptomatic progression of RV dysfunction. Acutely, in one early multicenter series of 42 postmortem cases attributed to ARVC, 34 deaths (81%) were sudden, with nearly half of these occurring during exercise.[127] In a study of athletes with ICDs, those with ARVC were the most likely to experience ventricular arrhythmias, and ventricular arrhythmias requiring multiple shocks, during physical activity or sports participation.[77]

Long term, exercise promotes expression of the disease, with endurance exercisers developing symptoms earlier than the sedentary. In the Johns Hopkins ARVC registry, the physical activity of 87 individuals with desmosomal mutations was evaluated.[128] As shown in **Fig. 12**, compared with non-athletes, the endurance athletes were more likely to develop ventricular arrhythmias and HF over a mean follow-up of 8.4 years. Furthermore, 6 of 8 individuals in the top quartile of activity level who continued with significant exercise following their diagnosis experienced their first VT/VF event in follow-up compared with only 1 of 8 individuals who reduced exercise after diagnosis. In a similar study, 108 index cases in the North American multidisciplinary study of ARVC were differentiated into sports participation as competitive, recreational, or inactive.[129] Over 3 years of follow-up, competitive athletes were diagnosed with ARVC at a younger age and had twice the risk of the adverse events, mainly because of increased ventricular arrhythmias. However, there was no difference between the inactive and recreational sports groups.

Physiologic studies support mechanisms through which exercise exacerbates ARVC expression. Physiologically, the hemodynamic impact of exercise was shown in one study of athletes in which RV shear stress increased 125% with prolonged strenuous exercise compared with 14% in the LV.[130] With this increased stretch on the thin-walled RV, the effect of exercise in individuals with ARVC is thought to promote breakdown of the genetically abnormal desmosome that eventually triggers fibrofatty replacement of the RV walls.

Experimental evidence also supports the adverse role of exercise in ARVC. A heterozygous plakoglobin-deficient mouse model was exercised vigorously compared with wild-type control mice. With sustained exercise, the desmosomal mutant mice showed a clear propensity for developing an ARVC phenotype in the form of RV enlargement, systolic dysfunction, and ventricular arrhythmias compared with a wild-type control.[131]

Bases on these data showing detrimental effects of vigorous exercise, in the 2015 AHA-ACC Eligibility and Disqualification Recommendation for Competitive Athletes, it is a class III indication for anyone with a definite, borderline, or possible diagnosis of ARVC to participate in competitive sports except for low-intensity class 1A sports, such as billiards, bowling, and golf.[33] In addition, the 2015 International Task Force Consensus Statement on Treatment of ARVC gave a class IIa recommendation that individuals with definite ARVC restrain from athletic activities beyond recreational low-intensity sports.[101] A class IIa recommendation was also made for asymptomatic genotype carriers to consider avoiding competitive sports.

How much exercise is safe for patients with ARVC is not yet defined. In an interview study of 37 PKP2 mutation carriers from 10 unrelated

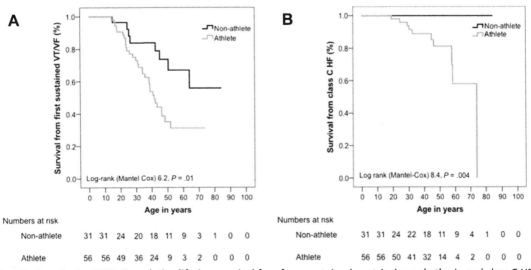

Fig. 12. Exercise in ARVC. Cumulative lifetime survival free from sustained ventricular arrhythmia and class C HF. Cumulative lifetime survival free of sustained ventricular arrhythmias (*A*) and stage C HF (*B*) stratified by participation in endurance athletics. Event-free survival from sustained arrhythmias and stage C HF is significantly lower among endurance athletes. (*From* James CA, Bhonsale A, Tichnell C, et al. Exercise increases age-related penetrance and arrhythmic risk in arrhythmogenic right ventricular dysplasia/cardiomyopathy-associated desmosomal mutation carriers. J Am Coll Cardiol 2013;62:1294; with permission.)

families, participation in both endurance athletics and higher-intensity exercise was associated with adverse outcomes. Family members who restricted exercise at or below the AHA-recommended minimum threshold (450–750 MET-min/wk) had favorable outcomes and no sustained ventricular arrhythmias,[132] suggesting that restricting unaffected desmosomal mutation carriers from endurance and high-intensity athletics but potentially not from AHA-recommended levels of exercise for healthy adults may be safe. How far beyond this level of exercise may be safe has not yet been determined.

REFERENCES

1. Elliott P. Diagnosis and management of dilated cardiomyopathy. Heart 2000;84:106–12.
2. Japp AG, Gulati A, Cook SA, et al. The diagnosis and evaluation of dilated cardiomyopathy. J Am Coll Cardiol 2016;67:2996–3010.
3. Fishman GI, Chugh SS, Dimarco JP, et al. Sudden cardiac death prediction and prevention: report from a National Heart, Lung, and Blood Institute and Heart Rhythm Society workshop. Circulation 2010;122:2335–48.
4. Maron BJ, Towbin JA, Thiene G, et al. Contemporary definitions and classification of the cardiomyopathies: an American Heart Association scientific statement from the Council on Clinical Cardiology, Heart Failure and Transplantation Committee; Quality of Care and Outcomes Research and Functional Genomics and Translational Biology Interdisciplinary Working Groups; and Council on Epidemiology and Prevention. Circulation 2006; 113:1807–16.
5. Taylor MR, Carniel E, Mestroni L. Cardiomyopathy, familial dilated. Orphanet J Rare Dis 2006;1:27.
6. Yancy CW, Jessup M, Bozkurt B, et al. 2013 ACCF/AHA guideline for the management of heart failure: a report of the American College of Cardiology Foundation/American Heart Association Task Force on Practice Guidelines. J Am Coll Cardiol 2013;62: e147–239.
7. Perez-Serra A, Toro R, Sarquella-Brugada G, et al. Genetic basis of dilated cardiomyopathy. Int J Cardiol 2016;224:461–72.
8. McCartan C, Mason R, Jayasinghe SR, et al. Cardiomyopathy classification: ongoing debate in the genomics era. Biochem Res Int 2012;2012: 796926.
9. Burkett EL, Hershberger RE. Clinical and genetic issues in familial dilated cardiomyopathy. J Am Coll Cardiol 2005;45:969–81.
10. Haas J, Frese KS, Peil B, et al. Atlas of the clinical genetics of human dilated cardiomyopathy. Eur Heart J 2015;36:1123–1135a.

11. Herman DS, Lam L, Taylor MR, et al. Truncations of titin causing dilated cardiomyopathy. N Engl J Med 2012;366:619–28.
12. Zimmerman RS, Cox S, Lakdawala NK, et al. A novel custom resequencing array for dilated cardiomyopathy. Genet Med 2010;12:268–78.
13. Roberts AM, Ware JS, Herman DS, et al. Integrated allelic, transcriptional, and phenomic dissection of the cardiac effects of titin truncations in health and disease. Sci Transl Med 2015;7:270ra6.
14. Priori SG, Blomstrom-Lundqvist C, Mazzanti A, et al. 2015 ESC guidelines for the management of patients with ventricular arrhythmias and the prevention of sudden cardiac death: the Task Force for the Management of Patients with Ventricular Arrhythmias and the Prevention of Sudden Cardiac Death of the European Society of Cardiology (ESC). Endorsed by: Association for European Paediatric and Congenital Cardiology (AEPC). Europace 2015;17:1601–87.
15. van Rijsingen IA, Arbustini E, Elliott PM, et al. Risk factors for malignant ventricular arrhythmias in lamin A/C mutation carriers: a European cohort study. J Am Coll Cardiol 2012;59:493–500.
16. Lakdawala NK, Winterfield JR, Funke BH. Dilated cardiomyopathy. Circ Arrhythm Electrophysiol 2013;6:228–37.
17. Dec GW, Fuster V. Idiopathic dilated cardiomyopathy. N Engl J Med 1994;331:1564–75.
18. Broch K, Murbraech K, Andreassen AK, et al. Contemporary outcome in patients with idiopathic dilated cardiomyopathy. Am J Cardiol 2015;116: 952–9.
19. Anselme F, Moubarak G, Savoure A, et al. Implantable cardioverter-defibrillators in lamin A/C mutation carriers with cardiac conduction disorders. Heart Rhythm 2013;10:1492–8.
20. Kayvanpour E, Sedaghat-Hamedani F, Amr A, et al. Genotype-phenotype associations in dilated cardiomyopathy: meta-analysis on more than 8000 individuals. Clin Res Cardiol 2017;106:127–39.
21. Ortiz-Genga MF, Cuenca S, Dal Ferro M, et al. Truncating FLNC mutations are associated with high-risk dilated and arrhythmogenic cardiomyopathies. J Am Coll Cardiol 2016;68:2440–51.
22. Toro R, Perez-Serra A, Campuzano O, et al. Familial dilated cardiomyopathy caused by a novel frameshift in the BAG3 gene. PLoS One 2016;11: e0158730.
23. Mann SA, Castro ML, Ohanian M, et al. R222Q SCN5A mutation is associated with reversible ventricular ectopy and dilated cardiomyopathy. J Am Coll Cardiol 2012;60:1566–73.
24. Goldberger JJ, Subacius H, Patel T, et al. Sudden cardiac death risk stratification in patients with nonischemic dilated cardiomyopathy. J Am Coll Cardiol 2014;63:1879–89.

25. Di Marco A, Anguera I, Schmitt M, et al. Late gadolinium enhancement and the risk for ventricular arrhythmias or sudden death in dilated cardiomyopathy: systematic review and meta-analysis. JACC Heart Fail 2017;5(1):28–38.

26. Mikami Y, Jolly U, Heydari B, et al. Right ventricular ejection fraction is incremental to left ventricular ejection fraction for the prediction of future arrhythmic events in patients with systolic dysfunction. Circ Arrhythm Electrophysiol 2017;10:1–12.

27. Riffel JH, Keller MG, Rost F, et al. Left ventricular long axis strain: a new prognosticator in non-ischemic dilated cardiomyopathy? J Cardiovasc Magn Reson 2016;18:36.

28. Arbustini E, Disertori M, Narula J. Primary prevention of sudden arrhythmic death in dilated cardiomyopathy: current guidelines and risk stratification. JACC Heart Fail 2017;5:39–43.

29. Russo AM, Stainback RF, Bailey SR, et al. ACCF/HRS/AHA/ASE/HFSA/SCAI/SCCT/SCMR 2013 appropriate use criteria for implantable cardioverter-defibrillators and cardiac resynchronization therapy: a report of the American College of Cardiology Foundation Appropriate Use Criteria Task Force, Heart Rhythm Society, American Heart Association, American Society of Echocardiography, Heart Failure Society of America, Society for Cardiovascular Angiography and Interventions, Society of Cardiovascular Computed Tomography, and Society for Cardiovascular Magnetic Resonance. J Am Coll Cardiol 2013;61:1318–68.

30. Dougherty CM, Glenny RW, Burr RL, et al. Prospective randomized trial of moderately strenuous aerobic exercise after an implantable cardioverter defibrillator. Circulation 2015;131:1835–42.

31. Holloway CJ, Dass S, Suttie JJ, et al. Exercise training in dilated cardiomyopathy improves rest and stress cardiac function without changes in cardiac high energy phosphate metabolism. Heart 2012;98:1083–90.

32. Flynn KE, Pina IL, Whellan DJ, et al. Effects of exercise training on health status in patients with chronic heart failure: HF-ACTION randomized controlled trial. JAMA 2009;301:1451–9.

33. Maron BJ, Udelson JE, Bonow RO, et al. Eligibility and disqualification recommendations for competitive athletes with cardiovascular abnormalities: Task Force 3: hypertrophic cardiomyopathy, arrhythmogenic right ventricular cardiomyopathy and other cardiomyopathies, and myocarditis: a scientific statement from the American Heart Association and American College of Cardiology. J Am Coll Cardiol 2015;66:2362–71.

34. Gersh BJ, Maron BJ, Bonow RO, et al. 2011 ACCF/AHA guideline for the diagnosis and treatment of hypertrophic cardiomyopathy: a report of the American College of Cardiology Foundation/American Heart Association Task Force on Practice Guidelines. Circulation 2011;124:e783–831.

35. Alpert C, Day SM, Saberi S. Sports and exercise in athletes with hypertrophic cardiomyopathy. Clin Sports Med 2015;34:489–505.

36. Maron BJ, Maron MS. Hypertrophic cardiomyopathy. Lancet 2013;381:242–55.

37. Frey N, Luedde M, Katus HA. Mechanisms of disease: hypertrophic cardiomyopathy. Nat Rev Cardiol 2011;9:91–100.

38. Authors/Task Force members, Elliott PM, Anastasakis A, Borger MA, et al. 2014 ESC guidelines on diagnosis and management of hypertrophic cardiomyopathy: the task force for the diagnosis and management of hypertrophic cardiomyopathy of the European Society of Cardiology (ESC). Eur Heart J 2014;35:2733–79.

39. Maron BJ, Rowin EJ, Casey SA, et al. Hypertrophic cardiomyopathy in children, adolescents, and young adults associated with low cardiovascular mortality with contemporary management strategies. Circulation 2016;133:62–73.

40. Maron BJ, Rowin EJ, Casey SA, et al. Risk stratification and outcome of patients with hypertrophic cardiomyopathy >=60 years of age. Circulation 2013;127:585–93.

41. Elliott PM, Gimeno JR, Tome MT, et al. Left ventricular outflow tract obstruction and sudden death risk in patients with hypertrophic cardiomyopathy. Eur Heart J 2006;27:1933–41.

42. Gimeno JR, Tome-Esteban M, Lofiego C, et al. Exercise-induced ventricular arrhythmias and risk of sudden cardiac death in patients with hypertrophic cardiomyopathy. Eur Heart J 2009;30:2599–605.

43. Elliott PM, Poloniecki J, Dickie S, et al. Sudden death in hypertrophic cardiomyopathy: identification of high risk patients. J Am Coll Cardiol 2000; 36:2212–8.

44. Spirito P, Bellone P, Harris KM, et al. Magnitude of left ventricular hypertrophy and risk of sudden death in hypertrophic cardiomyopathy. N Engl J Med 2000;342:1778–85.

45. Spirito P, Autore C, Rapezzi C, et al. Syncope and risk of sudden death in hypertrophic cardiomyopathy. Circulation 2009;119:1703–10.

46. Sorajja P, Nishimura RA, Ommen SR, et al. Use of echocardiography in patients with hypertrophic cardiomyopathy: clinical implications of massive hypertrophy. J Am Soc Echocardiogr 2006;19:788–95.

47. Bos JM, Maron BJ, Ackerman MJ, et al. Role of family history of sudden death in risk stratification and prevention of sudden death with implantable defibrillators in hypertrophic cardiomyopathy. Am J Cardiol 2010;106:1481–6.

48. Maki S, Ikeda H, Muro A, et al. Predictors of sudden cardiac death in hypertrophic cardiomyopathy. Am J Cardiol 1998;82:774–8.

49. Sadoul N, Prasad K, Elliott PM, et al. Prospective prognostic assessment of blood pressure response during exercise in patients with hypertrophic cardiomyopathy. Circulation 1997;96:2987–91.

50. O'Mahony C, Jichi F, Pavlou M, et al. A novel clinical risk prediction model for sudden cardiac death in hypertrophic cardiomyopathy (HCM risk-SCD). Eur Heart J 2014;35:2010–20.

51. Maron BJ, Casey SA, Chan RH, et al. Independent assessment of the European Society of Cardiology sudden death risk model for hypertrophic cardiomyopathy. Am J Cardiol 2015;116:757–64.

52. Weng Z, Yao J, Chan RH, et al. Prognostic value of LGE-CMR in HCM: a meta-analysis. JACC Cardiovasc Imaging 2016;9(12):1392–402.

53. Magri D, Limongelli G, Re F, et al. Cardiopulmonary exercise test and sudden cardiac death risk in hypertrophic cardiomyopathy. Heart 2016;102:602–9.

54. Coats CJ, Rantell K, Bartnik A, et al. Cardiopulmonary exercise testing and prognosis in hypertrophic cardiomyopathy. Circ Heart Fail 2015;8: 1022–31.

55. Sherrid MV, Shetty A, Winson G, et al. Treatment of obstructive hypertrophic cardiomyopathy symptoms and gradient resistant to first-line therapy with β-blockade or verapamil. Circ Heart Fail 2013;6:694–702.

56. Sherrid MV, Barac I, McKenna WJ, et al. Multicenter study of the efficacy and safety of disopyramide in obstructive hypertrophic cardiomyopathy. J Am Coll Cardiol 2005;45:1251–8.

57. Epstein SE, Rosing DR. Verapamil: its potential for causing serious complications in patients with hypertrophic cardiomyopathy. Circulation 1981;64: 437–41.

58. Toshima H, Koga Y, Nagata H, et al. Comparable effects of oral diltiazem and verapamil in the treatment of hypertrophic cardiomyopathy: double-blind crossover study. Jpn Heart J 1986;27:701–15.

59. Ommen SR, Maron BJ, Olivotto I, et al. Long-term effects of surgical septal myectomy on survival in patients with obstructive hypertrophic cardiomyopathy. J Am Coll Cardiol 2005;46:470–6.

60. Vriesendorp PA, Liebregts M, Steggerda RC, et al. Long-term outcomes after medical and invasive treatment in patients with hypertrophic cardiomyopathy. JACC Heart Fail 2014;2:630–6.

61. Veselka J, Zemanek D, Jahnlova D, et al. Risk and causes of death in patients after alcohol septal ablation for hypertrophic obstructive cardiomyopathy. Can J Cardiol 2015;31:1245–51.

62. Maron BJ, Nishimura RA. Revisiting arrhythmic risk after alcohol septal ablation: is the pendulum finally swinging...back to myectomy? JACC Heart Fail 2014;2:637–40.

63. Steggerda RC, Damman K, Balt JC, et al. Periprocedural complications and long-term outcome after alcohol septal ablation versus surgical myectomy in hypertrophic obstructive cardiomyopathy: a single-center experience. JACC Cardiovasc Interv 2014;7:1227–34.

64. Singh K, Qutub M, Carson K, et al. A meta analysis of current status of alcohol septal ablation and surgical myectomy for obstructive hypertrophic cardiomyopathy. Catheter Cardiovasc Interv 2016;88: 107–15.

65. Liebregts M, Vriesendorp PA, Mahmoodi BK, et al. A systematic review and meta-analysis of long-term outcomes after septal reduction therapy in patients with hypertrophic cardiomyopathy. JACC Heart Fail 2015;3:896–905.

66. Maron BJ, Spirito P, Shen WK, et al. Implantable cardioverter-defibrillators and prevention of sudden cardiac death in hypertrophic cardiomyopathy. JAMA 2007;298:405–12.

67. O'Mahony C, Lambiase PD, Quarta G, et al. The long-term survival and the risks and benefits of implantable cardioverter defibrillators in patients with hypertrophic cardiomyopathy. Heart 2012;98: 116–25.

68. Syska P, Przybylski A, Chojnowska L, et al. Implantable cardioverter-defibrillator in patients with hypertrophic cardiomyopathy: efficacy and complications of the therapy in long-term follow-up. J Cardiovasc Electrophysiol 2010;21:883–9.

69. Cecchi F, Maron BJ, Epstein SE. Long-term outcome of patients with hypertrophic cardiomyopathy successfully resuscitated after cardiac arrest. J Am Coll Cardiol 1989;13:1283–8.

70. Elliott PM, Sharma S, Varnava A, et al. Survival after cardiac arrest or sustained ventricular tachycardia in patients with hypertrophic cardiomyopathy. J Am Coll Cardiol 1999;33:1596–601.

71. Maron BJ, Shen WK, Link MS, et al. Efficacy of implantable cardioverter-defibrillators for the prevention of sudden death in patients with hypertrophic cardiomyopathy. N Engl J Med 2000;342: 365–73.

72. Maron BJ, Spirito P, Ackerman MJ, et al. Prevention of sudden cardiac death with implantable cardioverter-defibrillators in children and adolescents with hypertrophic cardiomyopathy. J Am Coll Cardiol 2013;61:1527–35.

73. Maron BJ, Doerer JJ, Haas TS, et al. Sudden deaths in young competitive athletes: analysis of 1866 deaths in the United States, 1980-2006. Circulation 2009;119:1085–92.

74. Maron BJ, Shirani J, Poliac LC, et al. Sudden death in young competitive athletes: clinical, demographic, and pathological profiles. JAMA 1996; 276:199–204.

75. Pelliccia A, Corrado D, Bjørnstad HH, et al. Recommendations for participation in competitive sport and leisure-time physical activity in individuals with

cardiomyopathies, myocarditis and pericarditis. Eur J Cardiovasc Prev Rehabil 2006;13:876–85.

76. Lampert R, Olshansky B, Heidbuchel H, et al. Safety of sports for athletes with implantable cardioverter-defibrillators: results of a prospective, multinational registry. Circulation 2013;127:2021–30.

77. Lampert R, Olshansky B, Heidbuchel H, et al. Safety of sports for athletes with implantable cardioverter defibrillators: long-term results of a prospective multinational registry. Circulation 2017; 135(23):2310–2.

78. Reineck E, Rolston B, Bragg-Gresham JL, et al. Physical activity and other health behaviors in adults with hypertrophic cardiomyopathy. Am J Cardiol 2013;111:1034–9.

79. Sweeting J, Ingles J, Timperio I, et al. Physical inactivity in hypertrophic cardiomyopathy: prevalence of inactivity and perceived barriers. Open Heart 2016;3:e000484.

80. Klempfner R, Kamerman T, Schwammenthal E, et al. Efficacy of exercise training in symptomatic patients with hypertrophic cardiomyopathy: results of a structured exercise training program in a cardiac rehabilitation center. Eur J Prev Cardiol 2015;22:13–9.

81. Edelmann F, Gelbrich G, Düngen H-D, et al. Exercise training improves exercise capacity and diastolic function in patients with heart failure with preserved ejection fraction: results of the Ex-DHF (exercise training in diastolic heart failure) pilot study. J Am Coll Cardiol 2011;58:1780–91.

82. Saberi S, Wheeler M, Bragg-Gresham J, et al. Effect of moderate-intensity exercise training on peak oxygen consumption in patients with hypertrophic cardiomyopathy: a randomized clinical trial. JAMA 2017;317:1349–57.

83. Corrado D, Link MS, Calkins H. Arrhythmogenic right ventricular cardiomyopathy. N Engl J Med 2017;376:61–72.

84. Delmar M, McKenna WJ. The cardiac desmosome and arrhythmogenic cardiomyopathies: from gene to disease. Circ Res 2010;107:700–14.

85. Peters S, Trummel M, Meyners W. Prevalence of right ventricular dysplasia-cardiomyopathy in a non-referral hospital. Int J Cardiol 2004;97:499–501.

86. Bhonsale A, Te Riele AS, Sawant AC, et al. Cardiac phenotype and long term prognosis of arrhythmogenic right ventricular cardiomyopathy/dysplasia patients with late presentation. Heart Rhythm 2017;14(6):883–91.

87. Etoom Y, Govindapillai S, Hamilton R, et al. Importance of CMR within the task force criteria for the diagnosis of ARVC in children and adolescents. J Am Coll Cardiol 2015;65:987–95.

88. Sen-Chowdhry S, Prasad SK, Syrris P, et al. Cardiovascular magnetic resonance in arrhythmogenic right ventricular cardiomyopathy revisited: comparison with task force criteria and genotype. J Am Coll Cardiol 2006;48:2132–40.

89. William J, McKenna GT, Nava A, et al. Diagnosis of arrhythmogenic right ventricular dysplasia/cardiomyopathy. Br Heart J 1994;71:215–8.

90. Marcus FI, McKenna WJ, Sherrill D, et al. Diagnosis of arrhythmogenic right ventricular cardiomyopathy/dysplasia: proposed modification of the task force criteria. Eur Heart J 2010;31:806–14.

91. McKoy G, Protonotarios N, Crosby A, et al. Identification of a deletion in plakoglobin in arrhythmogenic right ventricular cardiomyopathy with palmoplantar keratoderma and woolly hair (Naxos disease). Lancet 2000;355:2119–24.

92. Gerull B, Heuser A, Wichter T, et al. Mutations in the desmosomal protein plakophilin-2 are common in arrhythmogenic right ventricular cardiomyopathy. Nat Genet 2004;36:1162–4.

93. Lazzarini E, Jongbloed JD, Pilichou K, et al. The ARVD/C genetic variants database: 2014 update. Hum Mutat 2015;36:403–10.

94. Pilichou K, Nava A, Basso C, et al. Mutations in desmoglein-2 gene are associated with arrhythmogenic right ventricular cardiomyopathy. Circulation 2006;113:1171–9.

95. Rampazzo A, Nava A, Malacrida S, et al. Mutation in human desmoplakin domain binding to plakoglobin causes a dominant form of arrhythmogenic right ventricular cardiomyopathy. Am J Hum Genet 2002;71:1200–6.

96. Syrris P, Ward D, Evans A, et al. Arrhythmogenic right ventricular dysplasia/cardiomyopathy associated with mutations in the desmosomal gene desmocollin-2. Am J Hum Genet 2006;79:978–84.

97. Rigato I, Bauce B, Rampazzo A, et al. Compound and digenic heterozygosity predicts lifetime arrhythmic outcome and sudden cardiac death in desmosomal gene-related arrhythmogenic right ventricular cardiomyopathy. Circ Cardiovasc Genet 2013;6:533–42.

98. Bhonsale A, Groeneweg JA, James CA, et al. Impact of genotype on clinical course in arrhythmogenic right ventricular dysplasia/cardiomyopathy-associated mutation carriers. Eur Heart J 2015; 36:847–55.

99. Quarta G, Muir A, Pantazis A, et al. Familial evaluation in arrhythmogenic right ventricular cardiomyopathy: impact of genetics and revised task force criteria. Circulation 2011;123:2701–9.

100. Sen-Chowdhry S, Syrris P, McKenna WJ. Role of genetic analysis in the management of patients with arrhythmogenic right ventricular dysplasia/cardiomyopathy. J Am Coll Cardiol 2007;50:1813–21.

101. Corrado D, Wichter T, Link MS, et al. Treatment of arrhythmogenic right ventricular cardiomyopathy/dysplasia: an international task force consensus statement. Circulation 2015;132:441–53.

102. Groeneweg JA, Bhonsale A, James CA, et al. Clinical presentation, long-term follow-up, and outcomes of 1001 arrhythmogenic right ventricular dysplasia/cardiomyopathy patients and family members. Circ Cardiovasc Genet 2015;8:437–46.

103. Protonotarios A, Anastasakis A, Panagiotakos DB, et al. Arrhythmic risk assessment in genotyped families with arrhythmogenic right ventricular cardiomyopathy. Europace 2016;18:610–6.

104. Zorzi A, Rigato I, Pilichou K, et al. Phenotypic expression is a prerequisite for malignant arrhythmic events and sudden cardiac death in arrhythmogenic right ventricular cardiomyopathy. Europace 2016;18:1086–94.

105. Bhonsale A, James CA, Tichnell C, et al. Incidence and predictors of implantable cardioverter-defibrillator therapy in patients with arrhythmogenic right ventricular dysplasia/cardiomyopathy undergoing implantable cardioverter-defibrillator implantation for primary prevention. J Am Coll Cardiol 2011;58:1485–96.

106. Corrado D, Calkins H, Link MS, et al. Prophylactic implantable defibrillator in patients with arrhythmogenic right ventricular cardiomyopathy/dysplasia and no prior ventricular fibrillation or sustained ventricular tachycardia. Circulation 2010;122:1144–52.

107. Corrado D, Leoni L, Link MS, et al. Implantable cardioverter-defibrillator therapy for prevention of sudden death in patients with arrhythmogenic right ventricular cardiomyopathy/dysplasia. Circulation 2003;108:3084–91.

108. Link MS, Laidlaw D, Polonsky B, et al. Ventricular arrhythmias in the North American multidisciplinary study of ARVC: predictors, characteristics, and treatment. J Am Coll Cardiol 2014;64:119–25.

109. Wichter T, Paul M, Wollmann C, et al. Implantable cardioverter/defibrillator therapy in arrhythmogenic right ventricular cardiomyopathy: single-center experience of long-term follow-up and complications in 60 patients. Circulation 2004;109:1503–8.

110. Pinamonti B, Dragos AM, Pyxaras SA, et al. Prognostic predictors in arrhythmogenic right ventricular cardiomyopathy: results from a 10-year registry. Eur Heart J 2011;32:1105–13.

111. Lemola K, Brunckhorst C, Helfenstein U, et al. Predictors of adverse outcome in patients with arrhythmogenic right ventricular dysplasia/cardiomyopathy: long term experience of a tertiary care centre. Heart 2005;91:1167–72.

112. Peters S. Long-term follow-up and risk assessment of arrhythmogenic right ventricular dysplasia/cardiomyopathy: personal experience from different primary and tertiary centres. J Cardiovasc Med 2007;8:521–6.

113. Hulot JS, Jouven X, Empana JP, et al. Natural history and risk stratification of arrhythmogenic right ventricular dysplasia/cardiomyopathy. Circulation 2004;110:1879–84.

114. Saguner AM, Vecchiati A, Baldinger SH, et al. Different prognostic value of functional right ventricular parameters in arrhythmogenic right ventricular cardiomyopathy/dysplasia. Circ Cardiovasc Imaging 2014;7:230–9.

115. Migliore F, Zorzi A, Silvano M, et al. Prognostic value of endocardial voltage mapping in patients with arrhythmogenic right ventricular cardiomyopathy/dysplasia. Circ Arrhythm Electrophysiol 2013;6:167–76.

116. Santangeli P, Dello Russo A, Pieroni M, et al. Fragmented and delayed electrograms within fibrofatty scar predict arrhythmic events in arrhythmogenic right ventricular cardiomyopathy: results from a prospective risk stratification study. Heart Rhythm 2012;9:1200–6.

117. Bhonsale A, James CA, Tichnell C, et al. Risk stratification in arrhythmogenic right ventricular dysplasia/cardiomyopathy-associated desmosomal mutation carriers. Circ Arrhythm Electrophysiol 2013;6:569–78.

118. Saguner AM, Ganahl S, Baldinger SH, et al. Usefulness of electrocardiographic parameters for risk prediction in arrhythmogenic right ventricular dysplasia. Am J Cardiol 2014;113:1728–34.

119. Haywood AF, Merner ND, Hodgkinson KA, et al. Recurrent missense mutations in TMEM43 (ARVD5) due to founder effects cause arrhythmogenic cardiomyopathies in the UK and Canada. Eur Heart J 2013;34:1002–11.

120. Hodgkinson KA, Howes AJ, Boland P, et al. Long-term clinical outcome of arrhythmogenic right ventricular cardiomyopathy in individuals with a p.S358L mutation in TMEM43 following implantable cardioverter defibrillator therapy. Circ Arrhythm Electrophysiol 2016;9(3) [pii:e003589].

121. Marcus FI, Fontaine GH, Frank R, et al. Long-term follow-up in patients with arrhythmogenic right ventricular disease. Eur Heart J 1989;10(Suppl D):68–73.

122. Wichter T, Borggrefe M, Haverkamp W, et al. Efficacy of antiarrhythmic drugs in patients with arrhythmogenic right ventricular disease: results in patients with inducible and noninducible ventricular tachycardia. Circulation 1992;86:29–37.

123. Marcus GM, Glidden DV, Polonsky B, et al. Efficacy of antiarrhythmic drugs in arrhythmogenic right ventricular cardiomyopathy: a report from the North American ARVC registry. J Am Coll Cardiol 2009; 54:609–15.

124. Boriani G, Artale P, Biffi M, et al. Outcome of cardioverter-defibrillator implant in patients with arrhythmogenic right ventricular cardiomyopathy. Heart Vessels 2007;22:184–92.

125. Tavernier R, Gevaert S, De Sutter J, et al. Long term results of cardioverter-defibrillator implantation in patients with right ventricular dysplasia and malignant ventricular tachyarrhythmias. Heart 2001;85: 53–6.

126. Schinkel AFL. Implantable cardioverter defibrillators in arrhythmogenic right ventricular dysplasia/cardiomyopathy: patient outcomes, incidence of appropriate and inappropriate interventions, and complications. Circ Arrhythm Electrophysiol 2013; 6:562–8.

127. Corrado D, Basso C, Thiene G, et al. Spectrum of clinicopathologic manifestations of arrhythmogenic right ventricular cardiomyopathy/dysplasia: a multi-center study. J Am Coll Cardiol 1997;30:1512–20.

128. James CA, Bhonsale A, Tichnell C, et al. Exercise increases age-related penetrance and arrhythmic risk in arrhythmogenic right ventricular dysplasia/cardiomyopathy-associated desmosomal mutation carriers. J Am Coll Cardiol 2013;62:1290–7.

129. Ruwald AC, Marcus F, Estes NA 3rd, et al. Association of competitive and recreational sport participation with cardiac events in patients with arrhythmogenic right ventricular cardiomyopathy: results from the North American multidisciplinary study of arrhythmogenic right ventricular cardiomyopathy. Eur Heart J 2015;36:1735–43.

130. La Gerche A, Heidbuchel H, Burns AT, et al. Disproportionate exercise load and remodeling of the athlete's right ventricle. Med Sci Sports Exerc 2011;43:974–81.

131. Kirchhof P, Fabritz L, Zwiener M, et al. Age- and training-dependent development of arrhythmogenic right ventricular cardiomyopathy in heterozygous plakoglobin-deficient mice. Circulation 2006; 114:1799–806.

132. Sawant AC, Te Riele AS, Tichnell C, et al. Safety of American Heart Association-recommended minimum exercise for desmosomal mutation carriers. Heart Rhythm 2016;13:199–207.

Electrocardiographic Markers of Sudden Cardiac Death (Including Left Ventricular Hypertrophy)

Andrés Ricardo Pérez-Riera, MD, PhD[a,b],
Raimundo Barbosa-Barros, MD[c],
Mohammad Shenasa, MD[d,*]

KEYWORDS

- Arrhythmogenic right ventricular dysplasia/cardiomyopathy • Brugada syndrome
- Depolarization markers • Electrocardiogram • Left ventricular hypertrophy • Repolarization markers
- Sudden cardiac death

KEY POINTS

- The electrocardiogram provides significant information regarding the diagnosis and screening for patients at risk of sudden cardiac death.
- Left ventricular hypertrophy is an underestimated cause of sudden cardiac death that can easily be diagnosed by the electrocardiogram.
- The electrocardiogram also provides specific signs of inheritable cardiac disorders such as arrhythmogenic cardiomyopathy, hypertrophic cardiomyopathy, Brugada syndrome, and others.

MAIN CAUSES OF SUDDEN CARDIAC DEATH

The main cause of sudden cardiac death (SCD) is structural heart disease, mostly atherosclerotic heart disease, which represents approximately 85% of all cases (approximately 280,000 SCD per year in the United States). The remaining 15% is caused by cardiopathies without apparent structural heart disease (approximately 53,000 SCD per year). Besides structural heart disease, the other main cause of SCD is atherosclerotic heart disease, which includes coronary artery disease (CAD), followed by others such as nonischemic dilated cardiomyopathy/dilated cardiomyopathy, hypertrophic cardiomyopathy (HCM), arrhythmogenic right ventricular cardiomyopathy/dysplasia (ARVC/D), coronary artery anomalies, myocarditis, mitral valve prolapse, symptomatic moderate to severe calcified aortic stenosis (frequently bicuspid), congenital heart diseases before and after surgical correction, commotio cordis or cardiac concussion, and Wolf–Parkinson–White syndrome. Among the causes of SCD without apparent structural heart disease, channelopathies or "primary electrical" diseases stand out, such as Brugada syndrome and sudden unexplained nocturnal death syndrome. Both sudden

Conflict of Interest: None.
Disclosure: The authors do not report any conflict of interest regarding this work.
[a] Design of Studies and Scientific Writing Laboratory in the ABC School of Medicine, ABC Foundation, Av. Príncipe de Gales, 821 - Vila Principe de Gales, Santo André, São Paulo 09060-650, Brazil; [b] Ambulatorio de cardiologia do Hospital do Coração, R. Des. Eliseu Guilherme, 147 - Paraiso, São Paulo, São Paulo 04004-030, Brazil; [c] Coronary Center of the Hospital de Messejana Dr Carlos Alberto Studart Gomes, Av. Frei Cirilo, 3480, Fortaleza, Ceará 60840-285, Brazil; [d] Department of Cardiovascular Services, Heart and Rhythm Medical Group, O'Connor Hospital, 105 North Bascom Avenue, Suite 204, San Jose, CA 95128, USA
* Corresponding author. 105 North Bascome Ave, Suite 204, San Jose, CA 95128.
E-mail address: mohammad.shenasa@gmail.com

cardiacEP.theclinics.com

unexplained nocturnal death syndrome and Brugada syndrome are phenotypically, genetically, and functionally the same disorder,[1] idiopathic ventricular fibrillation (VF), early repolarization syndrome/J wave syndrome, congenital or acquired long QT syndrome (LQTS), congenital short QT syndrome, catecholaminergic polymorphic ventricular tachycardia (VT), familial progressive cardiac conduction defect/disorder, or Lenègre disease.[2] Genetic screening and identification of the causal mutation are crucial for risk stratification and family counseling. Also, Lev's disease (acquired complete atrioventricular heart block due to idiopathic fibrosis and calcification of the electrical conduction system of the heart, most common in the elderly, and often described as senile degeneration of the conduction system), familial sick sinus syndrome, overlapping syndromes, short-coupled variant of Torsades de Pointes (TdP) with a normal QT interval or Leenhardt syndrome[3] with or without early repolarization on inferolateral leads,[4] sudden infant death syndrome, sudden unexpected death in infancy, and inborn errors of metabolism.[5]

More than 122 years after the discovery of the standard 12-lead electrocardiogram (ECG) by Willem Einthoven,[6] it remains the most common test that is used in the diagnostic armamentarium of the practicing clinician. Because SCD is a complex, multifactorial syndrome, its pathophysiology and triggers are poorly understood. Because SCD has a multifactorial risk profile, it stands to reason that using multiple risk markers, reflecting different facets of the heart's electrical activity, would convey more information than a single marker. At this time, no individual ECG finding has been found to be able to adequately stratify patients with regard to risk for SCD. However, one or more of these candidate surface ECG parameters may become useful components of future multifactorial risk stratification models.[7]

Currently, there is a trend of decreasing the incidence of fast VT/VF. At the same time, there is an increase in pulseless events (ie, cardiac arrest). More people in heart failure have asystole so defibrillation does not work. **Fig. 1** shows the causes of SCD and distribution of arrhythmias.

ELECTROCARDIOGRAPHIC MARKERS OF SUDDEN CARDIAC DEATH: ROLE OF THE ELECTROCARDIOGRAM AS A PART OF A RISK STRATIFICATION OF SUDDEN CARDIAC DEATH

Electrocardiographic depolarization and repolarization disorder and ECG markers of SCD
I. ECG markers of repolarization disorders in SCD
   1. The QT interval or electric systole

- Prolonged QT/QT corrected QT (QT_c) interval
- Short QT–QT_c interval
2. Prolonged JT–corrected JT (JTc)
3. Prolonged QT dispersion
4. Inferolateral early repolarization syndrome/J wave syndrome
5. Interval from the peak to the end of the T-wave ($T_{peak} - T_{end}$) or Tpe
6. $T_{peak} - T_{end}$/QT ratio
7. Macrowave alternans or T wave alternans
8. Microwave alternans or T wave alternans
II. ECG markers of depolarization disorders in SCD
   1. Prolongation of QRS duration (QRS_d)
   2. QRS prolongation in right precordial leads (from V1 to V3).
   3. An S-wave ($\geq$0.1 mV and/or $\geq$40 ms) in lead I
   4. QRS dispersion
   5. Narrow and wide QRS fragmentation (fQRS and fQRS wide)
   6. Epsilon waves
   7. Presence of ventricular late potentials (LPs) using high-resolution or signal-averaged ECG

Electrocardiographic Markers of Repolarization Abnormalities in Sudden Cardiac Death

The QT interval or electric systole

The QT interval is the interval that extends between the first recognizable part of the QRS complex onset up to the last recognizable portion of the T wave (the latter may be hard to determine accurately). The end of T is defined as the return of the T wave to the T-P baseline. The QT interval represents the time between ventricular (electric) depolarization onset and (electric) repolarization offset (terminal part). Therefore, one should correct the QT interval according to the heart rate, the so-called QTc. Several mathematical formulas have been proposed. The most commonly used formula is the one proposed by Bazett in the 1920s.[8] Bazett's formula uses the QTc measurement divided by the square root of RR:

$$QTc = \frac{\text{Measured QT interval}}{\sqrt{RR}}$$

Bazett's formula correction of QT interval has been criticized because it tends to provide an inappropriately short QTc at low heart rates. Consequently, it is inappropriate for QTc measurements at higher rates. Several formulae have been proposed to correct the QT interval for the physiologic effect of heart rate changes (QTc), but none

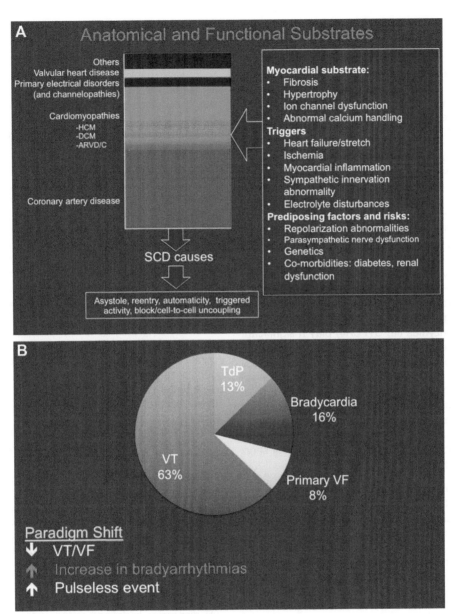

Fig. 1. (*A*) Causes of SCD. (*B*) Distribution of arrhythmias in SCD. ARVD/C, arrhythmogenic right ventricular dysplasia/cardiomyopathy; DCM, dilated cardiomyopathy; HCM, hypertrophic cardiomyopathy; TdP, Torsades de pointes; VT/VF, ventricular tachycardia/ventricular fibrillation. ([A] *From* van der Bijl P, Delgado V, Bax JJ. Noninvasive imaging markers associated with sudden cardiac death. Trends Cardiovasc Med 2016;26(4):348–60; with permission and [B] *Data from* Bayes de Luna A, Coumel P, Leclercq JF. Ambulatory sudden cardiac death: mechanisms of production of fatal arrhythmia on the basis of data from 157 cases. Am Heart J 1989;117:151–9).

of them are perfect. Bazett's correction is used for automated analysis in large clinical trials because it is simple and is incorporated into automatic measurement by most of the commercially available ECG mechanisms. None of the formulas has been shown to be superior to the others, and each carry its own limitations. Bazett's formula is more popular, but Fridericia's correction is preferred because it is more accurate at physiologic heart rate.

Fridericia's formula ($QTcF = \frac{QT}{\sqrt[3]{RR}}$) proposed an alternative correction using the cube root of RR.[9] Apart from heart rate, the duration of the QT interval is also affected by methodological recording and errors of measurement of the QT interval, sympathovagal activity, drugs, genetic abnormalities, electrolyte disorders, cardiac or metabolic diseases, changes in cardiac afterload, and diurnal variation, which can account for 75 to 100 ms.

The normal range of the QT/QTc interval in adults varies between 350 ms and 470 ms or greater (for men) and 480 ms or greater (for women). Both short and long QT intervals can cause a variety of life-threatening ventricular arrhythmias. Other authors consider a QTc "borderline" value to be QTc of 440 ms or greater.[10]

Prolonged corrected QT interval

QT (QT$_C$) interval prolongation is defined as a QTc of 470 ms or greater in men and 480 ms or greater in women, although arrhythmias are most often associated with values of 500 ms or greater. The severity of proarrhythmia at a given QT interval varies from drug to drug and from patient to patient, including their genetic background. Unfortunately, the extent of QT prolongation and risk of TdP with a given drug is not always linearly related to the dose or plasma concentration of the given drug because patient and metabolic factors such as enzymes (ie, CYP3A4) play a significant role (eg, gender, race, electrolyte status, etc). Furthermore, there is not a simple relation between the degree of drug-induced QT prolongation and the likelihood of the development of TdP, which can occasionally occur without any substantial QT interval prolongation. **Table 1** shows the value of QTc to be very prolonged, prolonged, normal, and very short (congenital short QT syndrome).

Measurement of the QT interval

The QT interval should be measured in leads II or V5 or on the lead with the largest T wave. Traditionally, lead II has been used for QT interval measurement because in this lead, the vectors of repolarization usually result in a long single wave rather than discrete T and U waves.[11] Several successive beats should be measured using the maximum interval. U waves 1 mm or greater that are fused to the preceding T wave should be included in the measurement. U waves less than 1 mm and those that are separate from the preceding T wave should be excluded. When measuring the QT interval, the ECG is best recorded at a paper speed of 50 mm/s and at an amplitude of 0.5 mV/cm using a multichannel recorder capable of simultaneously recording all 12 leads. A tangent line to the steepest part of the descending portion of the T wave is then drawn. The intercept between the tangent line and the isoelectric line is defined as the end of the T wave (**Fig. 2**A).

Prolonged JT-JTc

The QTc interval constitutes the classical measurement of ventricular repolarization; however, this parameter also includes ventricular depolarization. Thus, in the presence of wide QRS complex ($\geq$120 ms) such as right or left bundle branch block, nonspecific intraventricular conduction disturbance or Wolff–Parkinson–White syndrome (ventricular preexcitation), the measurement of ventricular repolarization by QTc may be incorrect or is subject to measurement error. In such cases, the measurement of JTc is more accurate than the QTc interval because it excludes depolarization. Additionally, the JTc interval could be a better parameter than the QTc interval for a more accurate measurement of repolarization time in normal healthy subjects, such as physically fit university students.[12] The JT and JTc interval extends from the J-point to the end of the T wave (see **Fig. 2**B).

The JTc interval is calculated by subtracting the QRS duration from the QTc interval in leads II, V2, and V6. The normal JTc value is between 320 and 400 ms. The measurement of JTc may be useful to identify LQTS cases with borderline values, where the QTc interval could be normal at rest on the ECG.

Prolonged QT Dispersion

QT dispersion is defined as the maximum – minimum QT intervals on the 12-lead surface ECG. The normal range for QT dispersion is 40 to 50 ms with a maximum of 65 ms. The QT dispersion values of 65 ms or greater carry a high risk of ventricular arrhythmias and is a risk marker for SCD. An increased QT dispersion reflects inhomogeneity of ventricular action potentials and may be a marker for SCD, which is considered to be an indirect measure of spatial heterogeneity of repolarization, and may be useful in assessing drug efficacy and safety. Patients who received class 1A antiarrhythmic drugs and developed TdP had significantly increased precordial QT dispersion. In contrast, patients receiving amiodarone or class 1A antiarrhythmics without TdP did not have increased QT dispersion, although the QT interval

Table 1
QT/QT$_C$ interval values for men and women

	Men	Women
Normal QT interval (ms)	360–390	370–400
Long QT interval (ms)	450–470	460–480
Very long QT (ms)	$\geq$470	$\geq$480
Congenital short QT syndrome (ms)	<330	<340

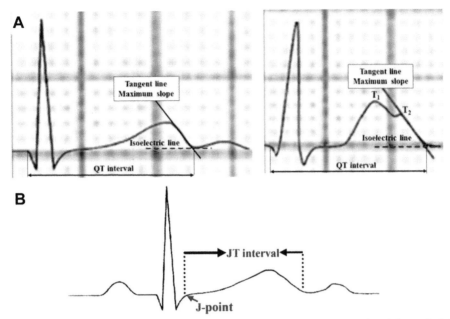

Fig. 2. (*A*) Intersection between the tangent line and the isoelectric line (*T-P*) is considered the end of the wave T. (*B*) The JT interval extends from the J-point to the end of the T wave.

was noticeably prolonged. Thus, spatial heterogeneity/dispersion of the ventricular repolarization may predispose to QT prolongation and increase the risk of TdP.

Early Repolarization

Early repolarization or inferolateral J-point elevation

Early repolarization is defined as QRS–ST junction (J-point) with terminal slurring or notch in at least 2 successive inferior (II, III, aVF) and/or lateral (I, aVL, V4, V5, V6) leads with a value of 1 mV or greater from baseline. The new definition of the early repolarization pattern[13] requires the peak of an end-QRS notch and/or the onset of an end-QRS slur as a measure, denoted Jp, to be determined when an interpretation of early repolarization is being considered. Early repolarization may be present if Jp is 0.1 mV or greater in at least 2 successive leads; however, ST-segment elevation is not a required criterion.

Early Repolarizations Electrocardiographic Variants

I. Classic definition of early repolarization[14–16]
   A. QRS with ST-segment elevation without J wave
   B. QRS with ST-segment elevation with J wave
II. New definition of early repolarization without ST-segment elevation

   C. Slurred QRS downslope without ST-segment elevation (also called lambda-wave)
   D. QRS notching J wave without ST-segment elevation

Inferior J-point elevation is associated with a higher risk of SCD.[17] J-point elevation in patients with idiopathic VF had higher amplitude and wider distribution than those with an established cause of cardiac arrest.

J wave amplitude of 0.2 mV of greater

J wave amplitude was variable on serial ECGs; at least 1 ECG failed to demonstrate early repolarization in 58% of patients.[18] The underlying pathophysiologic mechanism(s) of J wave in anterior leads are different from inferolateral leads because the onset mode of premature ventricular contractions differ between the two groups.[19] **Fig. 3** illustrates the morphology and patterns of malignant J wave: early repolarization in inferior leads or global early repolarization pattern, terminal notching of QRS complex, J wave amplitude of more than 0.2 mV, and horizontal or downward direction of ST-segment elevation signifying higher risk features for SCD in early repolarization patients.

The characteristics of benign early repolarization pattern is predominantly observed in young (<45 years of age), physically active individuals and highly trained athletes, as well as black

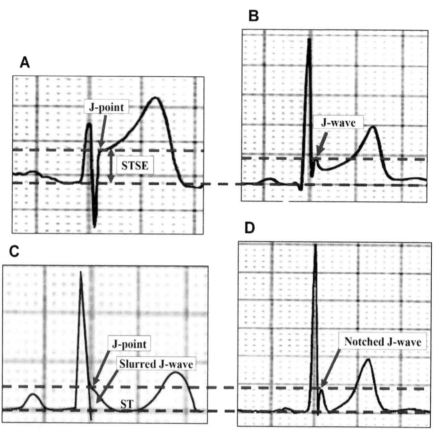

Fig. 3. The 4 different ECG patterns of J wave morphology. The *upper red line* indicates ST-segment elevation degree without (*A*) and with (*B*) J wave, the slur (*C*) or notch (*D*) amplitude, J peak (Jp), whereas the *lower purple line* indicates the baseline used as a reference with respect to which amplitudes should be measured. The *blue line* indicates tangent to the descendant ramp of the R-wave downslope. (*Data from* Macfarlane P, Antzelevitch C, Haissaguerre M, et al. Consensus paper: early repolarization pattern. J Am Coll Cardiol 2015;66(4):470–7.)

men. It is found on the ECG in about 1% of those with chest pain; frequent sinus bradycardia and phasic arrhythmias; axes of QRS orientation in the same direction in the frontal plane; R wave of higher voltage in left precordial leads; notching or slurring of R wave in the terminal descending limb; "fishhook" deformity at the J-point; rapidly ascending ST-segment elevation after the J-point (upwardly concave) followed by tall, pseudosymmetric, broad-based and upright T waves (degree of ST elevation is <25% of the T wave amplitude in V6); deep (≥2 mm) and narrow (<4 ms) Q waves followed by an R wave of great voltage in the left precordial leads; QRS transition in precordial leads of sudden occurrence; J-point and ST-segment modest elevation, usually less than 2 mm (although precordial ST-segment elevation may be up to 5 mm in some instances) concave to the top in middle and/or left precordial leads (V2-V6) and

less than 0.5 mm possibly in the inferior leads; reduction in J-point and ST-segment elevation by sympathetic activity and sympathomimetic drugs; absence of reciprocal changes or mirror image (exception in VR lead); and near symmetric T waves with greater width (duration) and polarity matching QRS and relatively temporal stability (no progression on serial ECGs[20]; **Figs. 4–7**). **Table 2** shows the important characteristics for the differential diagnosis between benign and malignant early repolarization pattern.

Interval from the Peak to the End of the T Wave or Tpe

Analysis of both the QT subintervals $J\text{-}T_{peak}$ and $T_{peak} - T_{end}$ can differentiate drugs that selectively block hERG K^+ channels (high TdP risk) from drugs that block hERG and late Na^+ or Ca^{++}

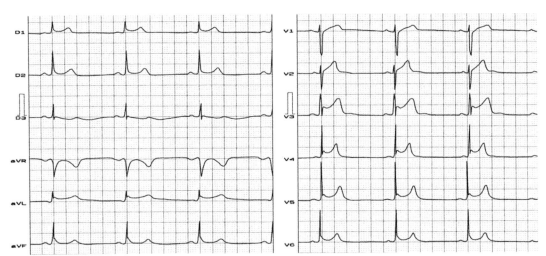

Fig. 4. Example of a typical electrocardiogram (ECG) in a 24-year-old African American professional basketball player with benign early repolarization pattern. His height and weight are 1.91 m and 82 kg. The ECG diagnosis is sinus bradycardia (heart rate, 50 beats/min). J-point and ST-segment elevation concave upward followed by tall T waves (with elevation > 4 mm), notch or slurring of terminal portion of the QRS complex (J-point) and mirror image only in aVR. Interpretation is sinus bradycardia with early repolarization syndrome (pattern).

currents (low TdP risk). Tpe becomes relatively shorter after I_{Kr} inhibition by dl-sotalol. The most pronounced repolarization changes were present in the ascending segment of the minimal T wave representation.[21]

The Tpe interval in the precordial leads was highly related to malignant ventricular arrhythmias in a large cohort of patients with Brugada syndrome. This simple ECG parameter could be used for risk stratification in high-risk patients. The Tpe interval from lead V1 to lead V4, maximum value of the Tpe interval, and Tpe dispersion in all precordial leads were significantly higher in patients with SCD or appropriate implantable cardioverter-defibrillator (ICD) therapy, and those with syncope compared with asymptomatic patients. A maximum value of the Tpe interval of 100 ms or greater was present in 47 of 226 asymptomatic patients (21%), in 48 of 73 patients with syncope (66%), and in 22 of 26 patients with SCD or appropriate ICD therapy (85%), respectively. In a multivariate analysis, a maximum value of the Tpe interval of 100 ms or greater was independently related to arrhythmic events.[22] **Fig. 8** shows a representation of this case.

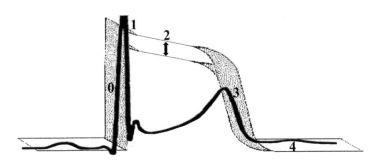

Fig. 5. Theoretic electrophysiologic explanation of ST-segment elevation on electrocardiograms in athletes. In "benign" early repolarization, there is a voltage gradient; however, no dispersion of duration of action potentials in ventricular wall thickness is observed. Therefore, these patients demonstrate notching or slurring in the R wave in the descending branch, ST-segment elevation concave upward, followed by T waves of greater voltage and polarity matching QRS with no risk of developing arrhythmias.

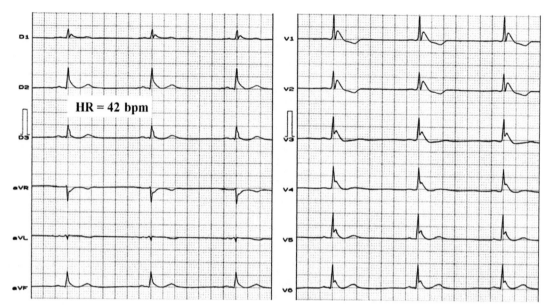

Fig. 6. Typical example of "malignant" early repolarization pattern in a patient with symptomatic idiopathic ventricular fibrillation. Sinus bradycardia (heart rate [HR], 42 beats/min), and J wave (slurred and notched) across precordial leads and inferior leads are present.

RISK PREDICTION OF VENTRICULAR ARRHYTHMIAS AFTER MYOCARDIAL INFARCTION

Prolonged QTc is a known risk marker for mortality and ventricular arrhythmias. QTc does not constitute a high predictive value for arrhythmic events in patients after myocardial infarction. The terminal part of the QT interval, T_{peak} to T_{end}, or Tpe may have a more accurate value in predicting adverse outcomes. Tpe predicts malignant arrhythmias in patients after myocardial infarction independent of the left ventricular ejection fraction (LVEF). Tpe may contribute in the risk

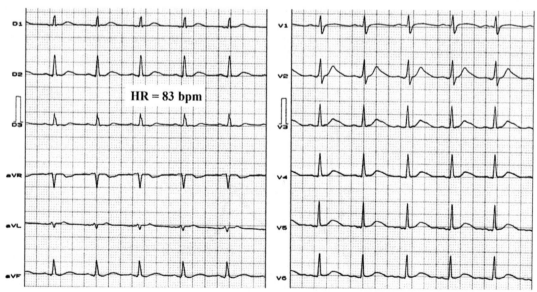

Fig. 7. Electrocardiogram of the same patient as in **Fig. 6** preformed 2 days after oral quinidine administration (1500 mg/d). Interpretation is sinus rhythm with a heart rate (HR) of 83 beats/min. The J wave disappeared because quinidine reduced the magnitude of the I_{to} channel, a mediator of phase 1 of action potential.

Table 2
Important characteristics for the differential diagnosis between a benign and a malignant ERP

	Malignant ERP	Benign ERP
Resuscitation from cardiac arrest or documented VF	Very suggestive	Asymptomatic
Positive family history for SCD in young relative	Possible	Absent
Sinus bradycardia	Absent	Common
Axes of QRS, ST segment, and T wave morphology	Frequently discordant	Often concordant
Mirror or reciprocal image	Frequently in several leads	Only aVR
Transient augmentation of J waves	Characteristic (present)	Absent
Short coupled PVCs	Frequent (present)	Absent
Coexisting channelopathies such as Brugada syndrome, SQTS, idiopathic VF	Frequent (present)	Rare
Degree of ST segment elevation/ high-amplitude J waves in the inferior leads	J waves >2 mm[28]	<2 mm
Widespread J waves in inferolateral leads and/or globally across all the leads	Strong signal[29,30]	Absent
ST segment upstroke (positive) convex or lambda wave shape (sharp monophasic or biphasic waveforms)	It is the rule[31]	Absent; the ST segment is concave upward followed by a T wave of high voltage and polarity matching QRS (concordance)
J waves in the inferior leads	Also present	Possible
J waves in lateral leads, tall R waves, rapidly ascending ST segments followed by tall T waves	Absent	Characteristic[32,33]
In a population of athletes, ERP is associated with increased QRS voltages, ST-segment elevation, and LV remodeling	Absent	Characteristic[34]
T wave voltage +	Lower[35] (T wave amplitude of ≤10% of the R-wave voltage in the same lead)	Higher
Lower $^T/_R$ ratio in II or V5 +	Yes	No
Longer QTc interval	Yes	No

Abbreviations: ERP, early repolarization pattern; LV, left ventricle; PVC, premature ventricular contraction; SCD, sudden cardiac death; SQTS, short QT syndrome; VF, ventricular fibrillation.

stratification to identify patients after myocardial infarction with malignant arrhythmias and an indication for ICD therapy.[23]

The T_{peak}–T_{end}/QT Ratio

The T_{peak}–T_{end}/QT ratio is measured in leads V2 and V6, which are considered to reflect the transmural axis of the left ventricle in Brugada syndrome and other channelopathies.[24]

In patients with inducible VT/VF at electrophysiology study (EPS), the mean ± standard deviation values are: V2 = 0.227 ± 0.034; V6 = 0.206 ± 0.012. In patients with noninducible VT/VF at EPS the mean ± standard deviation values are: V2 = 0.206 ± 0.012; V6 = 0.180 ± 0.014.

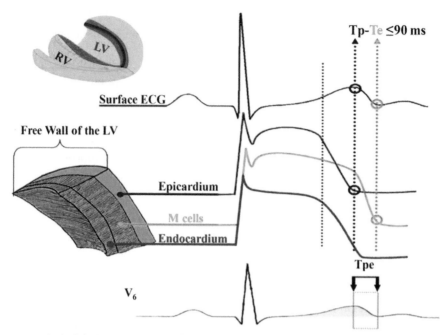

Fig. 8. Representation of the T_{peak}/T_{end} interval (Tpe). This is the interval between the apex to the end of the T wave ($T_{peak} - T_{end}$ interval or Tpe). The wall of the heart consists of 3 layers: the epicardium (external layer), the myocardium (middle layer with M cells) and the endocardium (inner layer). Tpe may correspond to transmural dispersion of repolarization and, consequently, the amplification of this interval is associated to malignant ventricular arrhythmias. The normal value of the T_{peak}/T_{end} interval (Tpe) is 94 ms in men and 92 ms in women when measured in lead V5. In congenital short QT syndrome this parameter is greater than 92 ms in women and greater than 94 ms in men (measurement in V5). ECG, electrocardiogram.

$T_{peak}-T_{end}/QT$ ratio was associated with VT/VF inducibility in Brugada syndrome. The utility of $T_{peak}-T_{end}/QT$ ratio as a new marker of arrhythmogenesis in Brugada syndrome warrants a large patient cohort.[25]

Macrowave T Wave Alternans or Macroscopic T Wave Alternans

Macrowave T wave alternans or macroscopic T wave alternans is a beat-to-beat variation in the polarity and shape/morphology of the ST segment and T wave in 12-lead ECG as shown in **Fig. 9**. In long lead II, a T wave with positive polarity followed by of the next negative T wave polarity, that alternates sequentially. This variety was described for the first time by Schwartz and Malliani,[26] in patient carriers of congenital LQTS. These authors showed that changes in T wave

polarity may be reproduced experimentally, by stimulation of the left stellate ganglion. T wave alternans consist of polarity or voltage modifications in the ST segment, T wave or ST–T wave, which represents ventricular repolarization (T wave) along with the ST segment preceding it and the U wave. The phenomena corresponds to ST segment (phase 2), T wave (phase 3), and U wave (phase 4) of an action potential.

Micro T Wave Alternans

Micro T wave alternans are a variant of T wave alternan that detects T wave alternans signals as small as one-millionth of a volt (millivolt). Although T wave alternans seems to be a useful marker of susceptibility for malignant ventricular arrhythmias and cardiovascular death, so far there is no sufficient evidence from randomized clinical trials to

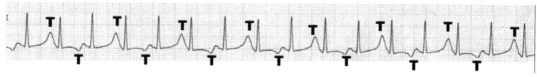

Fig. 9. Macrowave T wave alternans.

support its use in guiding therapy.[27] It is not used in daily clinical practice except for academic centers. A T wave alternan level of 1.9 µV or greater with sufficient signal-to-noise ratio for greater than 2 minutes is defined as a positive test result, whereas a T wave alternan level of less than 1.9 µV is considered negative. Recently, Takasugi and colleagues[28] reported that µV T wave alternans is far more prevalent in LQTS patients than previously reported and is strongly associated with a history of TdP. T wave alternans should be monitored from precordial leads in LQTS patients. Highest T wave alternan levels were recorded in precordial leads (V1-V6) in 93.8% of patients, most frequently in lead V2 (43.8%). A single ECG lead detected only 63.6% or less of T wave alternans of 42 µV or greater episodes, whereas the combined leads V2 to V5 detected 100% of T wave alternans of 42 µV or greater. None of the healthy subjects had T wave alternans of 42 µV or greater. The use of a limited set of ECG leads in conventional monitoring has led to an underestimation of T wave alternans and its association with TdP.

ELECTROCARDIOGRAPHIC MARKERS OF SUDDEN CARDIAC DEATH: DEPOLARIZATION ABNORMALITIES
Prolongation QRS Duration

There is conflicting data regarding the relationship between prolonged QRSd and arrhythmic events, including SCD in heart failure patients with or without ICDs. Dhar and colleagues[29] studied the prognostic significance of prolonged QRSd relative to arrhythmic outcomes in medically and ICD-treated patients enrolled in the MADIT II trial (Multicenter Automatic Defibrillator Implantation Trial). Using a Cox proportional hazards model adjusting for ejection fraction, heart failure class, and blood urea nitrogen, the authors estimated the association of prolonged QRSd of 140 ms or greater with SCD in the medically treated arm and SCD or first appropriate ICD therapy for rapid VT/VF (ie, cycle length ≤260 ms) in the ICD-treated arm. In the medically treated arm, prolonged QRSd was a significant independent predictor of SCD. However, in the ICD-treated arm, prolonged QRSd did not predict SCD or rapid VT/VF. The authors concluded that in patients with prior myocardial infarction and an LVEF of 30% or less, a prolonged QRSd does not predict SCD, VT, or VF in ICD-treated patients; however, it does predict SCD in medically treated patients. This highlights the noncorrespondence of VT/VF and SCD and the need for caution in the risk

stratification of SCD when using nonrandomized databases that include only patients with ICDs.

To assess the potential improvement in SCD risk prediction, one should add ECG risk markers from the 12-lead ECG (resting heart rate, QRSd, and JTc intervals) to the LVEF. From the ongoing Oregon Sudden Unexpected Death Study, SCD cases with available pre-event LVEF were compared with matched control subjects with CAD. The authors concluded that combining these 3 selected 12-lead ECG markers with LVEF improves SCD risk prediction. In other words, when the ECGs markers are combined, it has cumulative effects on the risk of SCD prediction.[30]

In Brugada syndrome, a prolonged QRSd, measured from QRS onset to the J-point in leads V2 and II from a standard 12-lead ECG, is associated with symptoms and could serve as a simple noninvasive ECG risk marker of vulnerability to life-threatening ventricular arrhythmias.[31] The mean QRS interval is 129.0 ± 23.9 ms in symptomatic patients with Brugada syndrome versus 108.3 ± 15.9 ms in asymptomatic patients[32] (**Figs. 10 and 11**).

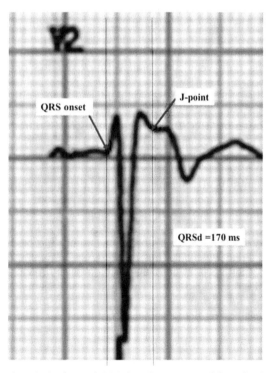

Fig. 10. Prolonged QRS duration measured from lead II or lead V2 of 120 ms or greater in a patient with Brugada syndrome.

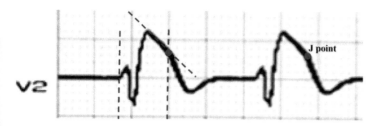

Fig. 11. *Vertical dotted lines* show the onset and termination of the QRS complex in lead V2. In this case the QRS duration is 165 ms. The oblique line is the tangent line that we use to determinate the end of QRS and the beginning of repolarization (J-point).

Right Precordial QRS Duration Prolongation (Parietal Block)

When the equation QRSd in (V1 + V2 + V3)/(V4 + V5 + V6) is 1.2 or greater, in carriers of ARVC/D genes, this ECG sign constitutes a sign of high sensitivity for ARVC/D diagnosis and is present in 98% of subjects. Selective prolongation of QRSd is considered typical of ARVC/D, but it is also observed in Brugada syndrome.[33] This author identified selective prolongation of QT interval duration in the right precordial leads (V1–V3) in comparison with the left ones (V4–V6); thus, it is not a specific marker. This longer QRSd complex in the right precordial leads is due to the so-called right parietal (focal or right divisional) block characteristic of ARVC/D: QRSd of (V1 + V2 + V3)/(V4 + V5 + V6) of 1.2 or greater. Because the QT interval is the result of ventricular depolarization (QRS) plus ventricular repolarization (ST/T), we believe that this selective prolongation represents a certain degree of parietal (intramural) or partial (QRSd ≤120 ms) block in the right ventricular outflow track, as the one observed in ARVC/D.

A QRSd of (V1 + V2 + V3)/(V4 + V5 + V6) of 1.2 or greater is observed in approximately 65% of cases of ARVC/D.[34] The presence of QRSd from V1 to V3 greater than V4 to V6 has 91% sensitivity, 90% specificity that predicts VT in patients carriers of ARVC/D[35] **(Fig. 12)**.

In ARVC/D, there is evidence of peripheral right bundle branch block, as it was initially reported by Guy Fontaine, topographic incomplete or complete right bundle branch block occurs in the fascicular portion of the right branch and/or in the right ventricular free wall after the trunk of the branch splits at the base of the papillary muscle of the tricuspid valve. This mechanism seems to be due to the presence of dysplasia in the free wall, in the right ventricular outflow tract, in the right ventricular inflow tract, or in the apical region (triangle of dysplasia), an area where there is dysplasia. The mechanism of the right conduction defect is not a disease of the bundle branch itself, but a distal block probably situated at the junction of the right bundle to the right ventricular wall. This

hypothesis is supported by the histologic appearances of the dysplastic zones.[34]

In ARVC/D, among those without right bundle branch block, a prolonged S-wave upstroke in V1 through V3 of 55 ms or greater was the most prevalent ECG feature (95%) and correlated with disease severity and induction of VT on EPS. This ECG feature also best distinguished ARVC/D (diffuse and localized) from right ventricular outflow tract.[34,36] **Fig. 13**.

An S-Wave 0.1 mV or Greater and/or 40 ms or Greater in Lead I

Calò and colleagues[37] analyzed data from 347 consecutive patients with spontaneous type 1 Brugada syndrome by ECG parameters but

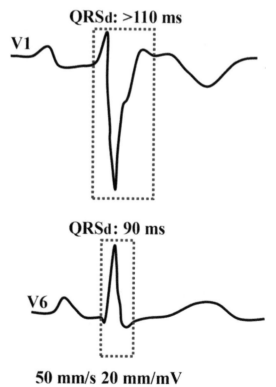

Fig. 12. Electrocardiographic measurement in a patient with arrhythmogenic right ventricular cardiomyopathy/dysplasia.

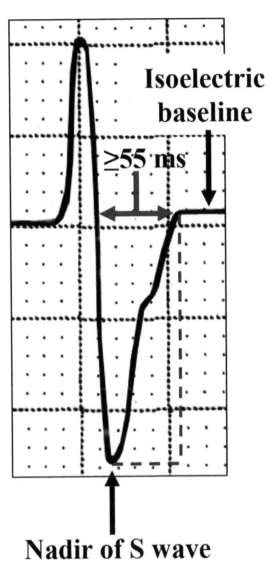

Isoelectric baseline

≥55 ms

Nadir of S wave

Fig. 13. Prolonged S-wave upstroke in leads V1 through V3 of 55 ms or greater.

with no history of cardiac arrest (including 91.1% asymptomatic at presentation, 5.2% with a history of atrial fibrillation, and 4% with a history of arrhythmic syncope). The most powerful marker for VF/SCD was the presence of S-wave (≥0.1 mV and/or ≥40 ms) in lead I. In the multivariate analysis, the duration of S-wave in lead I of 40 ms or greater and atrial fibrillation were independent predictors of VF/SCD during follow-up. Electroanatomic mapping in 12 patients showed an endocardial activation time significantly longer in patients with an S-wave in lead I, mostly because of a significant delay in the anterolateral right ventricular outflow tract.[37]

QT Dispersion

QT dispersion is an indirect measure of spatial heterogeneity of repolarization, which may be useful in assessing drug efficacy and safety. In an important study, patients who received class 1a antiarrhythmic drugs and developed TdP had significantly increased QT interval dispersion. In contrast, patients receiving amiodarone or class 1A antiarrhythmics without TdP did not have increased QT dispersion, although the QT interval was noticeably prolonged. Thus, spatial heterogeneity/dispersion of ventricular repolarization may be promoted in addition to QT prolongation for the genesis of TdP. The most critical adverse effects of class III drugs are marked QT interval prolongation and TdP.[38] Although the use of QT dispersion in the assessment of drugs that prolong the QT interval needs further confirmation, it may provide information about the clinical significance of QT prolongation. Thus, the use of QT dispersion in the assessment of drugs that prolong the QT interval needs further confirmation, and may provide information about the clinical significance of QT prolongation to identify individual patients at risk of TdP and SCD.

Narrow QRS, Fragmented QRS Complex/Wide QRS Fragmentation

Narrow QRS fragmentation definition

The presence of notched R or S waves without accompanying typical bundle branch blocks, or the existence of an additional wave like RSR′ pattern within the QRS complex 1 or more R′ or notching of S or R wave with a normal QRSd (<120 ms) present in at least 2 contiguous (successive) leads. This has been defined as narrow fQRS. fQRS includes various morphologies of the QRS (<120 ms), which included an additional R wave (R′) or notching in the nadir (lowest point) of the S wave, or greater than 1 R′ (fragmentation) in 2 contiguous leads, corresponding with a major coronary artery territory. fQRS can be caused by zigzag conduction around the scarred myocardium, resulting in multiple spikes within the QRS complex.[39,40] Narrow fQRS is a simple, inexpensive, and readily available noninvasive ECG parameter.

Wide fQRS definition

Fragmentation of wide complex QRS (≥120 ms) consists of various RSR patterns, with more than 2 R waves (R″) or more than 2 notches in the R wave, or more than 2 notches in the downstroke or upstroke of the S wave **(Fig. 14)**.

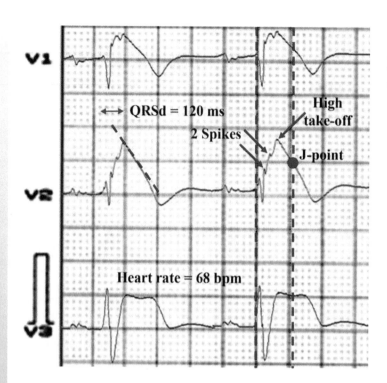

Fig. 14. Wide QRS fragmentation in a symptomatic patient with Brugada syndrome. *Dotted lines* show the onset and the end of the QRS complex.

Observation

For both narrow and wide fQRS, it is necessary to exclude typical bundle branch block (right bundle branch block or left bundle branch block) pattern (QRS ≥ 120 ms) and incomplete right bundle branch block. The presence of fQRS has been investigated among the patients with ischemic and nonischemic cardiomyopathy, suggesting that this ECG parameter may suggest an adverse prognosis and risk of SCD, risk of ICD therapy, and response to cardiac resynchronization therapy. In addition, there is evidence that fQRS could play an important role as a screening and prognostic tool among the patients with tetralogy of Fallot, channelopathies, hereditary cardiomyopathies such as ARVC/D, HCM, several scenarios of CAD, hypertension, collagenopathies, cardiomyopathies such as chronic Chagas myocarditis (in Latin America), sarcoidosis, amyloidosis, and so on (**Fig. 15**). However, fQRS is not specific for any cardiac pathology. Rather, it is a marker of slow conduction that could be present.

Technical problems that affect fragmented QRS complexes

A low-pass filter (35 Hz) is usually used to reduce electrical and musculature noises when recording the ECG, but the cutoff frequency of the low-pass filter influences detection of fQRS. When a low-pass filter is used, the number of spikes within the QRS complex could be reduced. Increasing the cutoff frequency of the low-pass filter from 35 to 150 Hz unmasked 3 additional spikes within the QRS complex that are frequently observed.[41]

Major causes of fragmented QRS complexes
Congenital heart disease
Tetralogy of Fallot in adults Although a QRSd of 180 ms or greater has a prognostic value in adults with tetralogy of Fallot, its sensitivity to predict mortality is low. Fragmented QRS complexes are related to myocardial fibrosis scar or site of ventriculotomy and dysfunction in patients with tetralogy of Fallot. The extent of fQRS is superior to QRSd in predicting mortality in adult patients with tetralogy of Fallot and may be used in risk stratification.[42] The presence of fQRS on ECG may be a useful tool in daily clinical practice to identify patients at risk for developing ventricular tachyarrhythmia and those with congenital heart disease, in addition to known predictors of ventricular tachyarrhythmias.[43]

Channelopathies
- Brugada syndrome: Fragmented QRS and early repolarization pattern are common ECG findings in patients at a high risk of Brugada syndrome, occurring in up to 27% of cases. When combined, fQRS and an early repolarization pattern confer a higher risk of

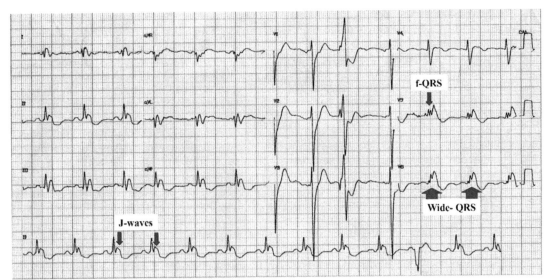

Fig. 15. Electrocardiogram (ECG) in a patient with severe coronary artery disease. Association of QRS fragmentation in at least 2 contiguous leads on the 12-lead ECG plus wide QRS complexes plus J waves of 0.1 mV or greater combined with a descending/horizontal ST segment and inverted T waves in left precordial leads (V5-V6) constitute a malignant early repolarization pattern, because they identify patients with a higher risk of fatal arrhythmias after coronary artery bypass grafting. All of these are components of multifactorial risk for increased morbidity and mortality, sudden cardiac death, and recurrent cardiovascular events.

appropriate ICD interventions during a long-term follow-up.[44,45] The presence or absence of inferolateral early repolarization and fQRS predicted a worse or better prognosis.[46]

- Idiopathic VF: Patients with idiopathic VF with the combined appearance of fQRS and J wave in resting ECG are at an increased risk of VF and SCD. This subgroup of patients with idiopathic VF has a unique clinical feature and is discussed elsewhere.[47]
- Early repolarization syndrome.[48]
- LQTS: Acquired predisposing factors promoted repolarization abnormality (especially prolongation of QT and Tpe intervals), and the existence of fQRS plays an important role in the development of TdP in patients with acquired LQTS.[49]

Hereditary cardiomyopathies

- HCM: HCM is the most common cause of SCD in the young, particularly among athletes. Identifying high-risk individuals is very important for SCD prevention. QRS may have a substantially higher sensitivity and diagnostic accuracy compared with pathologic Q waves for detecting myocardial fibrosis in HCM.[40,50] In patients with HCM and apical aneurysm, fQRS is associated with an increased risk of VT.[51] fQRS predicts heart failure progression in patients with HCM.[52] Fragmented QRS and T wave

inversion in multiple leads are more common in high-risk patients.[53] The presence of a fQRS may be a good candidate marker for prediction of nonsustained or sustained VT, SCD, or appropriate ICD therapies in patients with HCM.[54] fQRS predicts arrhythmic events in patients with obstructive HCM and should be implemented in the risk stratification model.[55]

- ARVC/D: The fQRS complex on standard 12-lead ECG predicts fatal and nonfatal arrhythmic events in patients with ARVC/D. Therefore, large-scale and prospective studies are needed to confirm those findings.[56] fQRS in ARVC/D has a high diagnostic value, similar to epsilon wave potentials by a highly amplified and modified recording technique.[57]
- Idiopathic dilated cardiomyopathy: In idiopathic dilated cardiomyopathy, approximately 30% of cases have a genetic background and, like HCM, fQRS plays an important marker in identifying high-risk patients.

Acquired diseases

- CAD: Based on current evidence, fQRS is associated with increased major adverse cardiovascular events, mortality, Q wave myocardial infarction, anterior wall myocardial infarction, and decreased LVEF in CAD. fQRS is a reliable marker in patients with CAD who may be at risk of arrhythmic events.[58]

- Acute myocardial infarction
  - ST-segment elevation myocardial infarction: The number of leads with fQRS on ECG is an independent predictor of in-hospital all-cause mortality in patients with ST-segment elevation myocardial infarction treated by primary percutaneous coronary intervention.[59]
  - Non–ST-segment elevation myocardial infarction: The fQRS complexes are commonly present in non–ST-segment elevation myocardial infarction and the fQRS complexes are an independent predictor of major adverse cardiac events in non–ST-segment elevation myocardial infarction patients.[60]
  - Remote myocardial infarction: Defined fQRS has higher sensitivity and negative predictive value compared with the Q wave.[39]
- Coronary slow flow: This phenomenon is a delayed anterograde progression of contrast agent to the distal branch of a coronary artery in the absence of obstructive CAD; a narrow fQRS may be a potential indicator of myocardial damage in patients with coronary slow flow.[61]
- Left ventricular aneurysm: fQRS in V5 to V6 in the absence of bundle branch block suggests left ventricular aneurysm.[62]
- Hypertensive heart disease: The left ventricular mass index in hypertensive patients who had fQRS on their ECGs was significantly higher than that of the patients who did not, and fQRS on ECG was an important indicator of left ventricular hypertension in hypertensive patients.[63] Carboxy-terminal propeptide of type 1 procollagen is a marker of extracellular collagen synthesis. fQRS on the ECG has been demonstrated as a marker of myocardial fibrosis. Serum propeptide of type 1 procollagen level is a strong and independent predictor of fQRS. Discriminative performance of serum propeptide of type 1 procollagen levels for the presence of fQRS is high. The fQRS may indicate myocardial fibrosis in patients with hypertension.[64]
- Chronic Chagas' cardiomyopathy: The fQRS is highly prevalent among patients with chronic Chagas' cardiomyopathy. It is a poor predictor of appropriate therapies delivered by ICD in this population.[65]
- Obstructive sleep apnea: Patients with obstructive sleep apnea show leftward shift of electrical axis, low QRS voltage, QRSd prolongation, and fQRS, suggestive of depolarization disturbance and indicative of electrical remodeling.[66] Both

parameters (fQRS and QRSd prolongation) are related to an increased cardiovascular mortality. Consequently, it seems reasonable to recommend a more detailed evaluation of patients with obstructive sleep apnea with fQRS or prolonged QRS complexes with respect to the presence of cardiovascular diseases.[67]
- Systemic lupus erythematosus: Cardiac involvement is present in more than one-half of the patients with systemic lupus erythematosus. The frequency of fQRS is higher in patients with systemic lupus erythematosus (41% of cases). fQRS may be used for the early detection in patients with systemic lupus erythematosus.[68]
- Ankylosing spondylitis: Inflammatory diseases may cause fibrosis. The presence of fQRS may be a simple and cost-effective method for predicting cardiac fibrosis in ankylosing spondylitis patients. fQRS can be a predictive marker for fibrosis in patients with this disease.[69]
- Extracardiac sarcoidosis: fQRS is associated with cardiac events in extracardiac sarcoidosis.[70]
- Light-chain cardiac amyloidosis: The presence of fQRS may improve diagnosis and prognostic risk stratification in this entity.[71]
- Psoriasis vulgaris: It was suggested that the presence of fQRS in the ECG may be related to myocardial fibrosis in patients with psoriasis who do not have cardiovascular disease. fQRS could be used as a predictive marker for myocardial fibrosis in patients with psoriasis.[72]

In summary, fQRS reflects intramyocardial conduction delay owing to myocardial fibrosis and/or the presence of scar tissue. Thus, it is conceivable that it increases the risk of malignant arrhythmias, but is a non-specific marker.

Epsilon Wave or Fontaine Wave

In approximately 30% of the severe cases of ARVC/D, a small deflection or zigzag may be observed at the end of the QRS in the V1 to V4 leads. They are delayed potentials, which appear after the end of ventricular depolarization (at the end of the QRS complex; Fig. 16) or postexcitation phenomenon that may be demonstrated by epicardial mapping, intracavitary electrode mapping, ECG, and signal-averaged ECG (SA-ECG).[73,74] It was reported for the first time by Dr Guy Fontaine,[75] using the Greek letter epsilon (epsilon waves). Other terms include epsilon potentials,[76] ventricular postexcitation waves,[77] postexcitation (epsilon) waves,[78] or with the eponymous Fontaine wave[79]; however, we

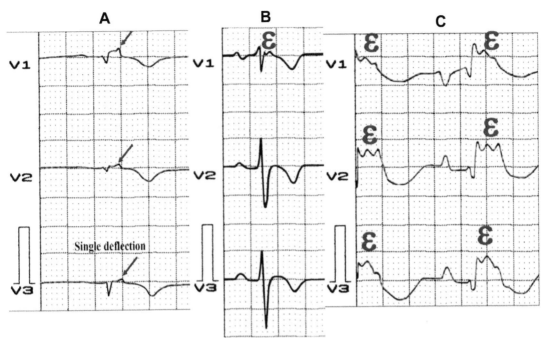

Fig. 16. Epsilon wave with single deflection. (*A*) Prominent upright deflections (*red arrows*) after the QRS complex in right precordial leads V1 through V3, associated with negative T waves. Epsilon waves are one of the major depolarization diagnostic criteria of arrhythmogenic right ventricular cardiomyopathy/dysplasia (ARVC/D) following the task force. Epsilon waves can be recorded using a 12-lead electrocardiogram during sinus rhythm, and are useful for establishing a diagnosis of ARVC/D. (*B*) Sinus rhythm, right atrial enlargement, bizarre complete right bundle branch block, and a terminal notch located in the J-point (epsilon wave). The epsilon wave could be the result of delayed activation in the right ventricle. It is visible in leads V1 to V3 and in the frontal plane leads. T wave inversion is observed in leads V1 to V3, characteristic of ARVC/D. (*C*) Epsilon wave with multiple deflections inside of the QRS complex. ([*A*] *Data from* Anan R, Takenaka T, Tei C. Epsilon waves in a patient with arrhythmogenic right ventricular cardiomyopathy. Heart 2002;88(5):444.)

recommend using Epsilon wave to avoid confusion. It is a late depolarization of right ventricular fibers of right ventricular free wall (dysplastic triangle), registered mainly in leads V1 to V4. Epsilon waves are not the direct counterpart of late potentials, but reflect the delay in peripheral activation in the right ventricular free wall; therefore, it seems to be responsible for much of the genesis of negative T waves.[78] If we consider that epsilon waves are located after the J-point at the beginning of ST-segment only, the phenomenon theoretically could not be a depolarization criterion because ST segment occurs during the repolarization. **Fig. 16** explains depolarization and repolarization intervals on ECG.

Classification of Epsilon Waves by the Number of Deflections

We classified the epsilon waves according to the number of deflections: 1 (see **Fig. 16**), 2, or multiple deflections. **Fig. 17** shows an ECG of an 18-year-old Caucasian man with ARVC/D and severe right heart failure.

Sensitivity of Electrocardiography for the Detection of Epsilon Wave Frequency in Arrhythmogenic Right Ventricular Cardiomyopathy/Dysplasia With Standard 12-Lead Electrocardiogram With F-ECG and With R-ECG

Epsilon waves are observed in approximately 15% to 30% of the most severe cases of ARVC/D when the S-ECG is used.

Prognostic Significance of the Epsilon Wave in Arrhythmogenic Right Ventricular Cardiomyopathy/Dysplasia

Epsilon waves aid in the prognosis and risk stratification of patients with ARVC/D.[80] The detection of epsilon waves on the 12-lead ECG reflects significant right ventricular outflow tract involvement, which was associated with episodes of sustained VT, but not SCD or heart failure.[81] The fQRS complex on S-ECG predicts fatal and nonfatal arrhythmic events in patients with ARVC/D.[82]   Therefore,   large-scale   and

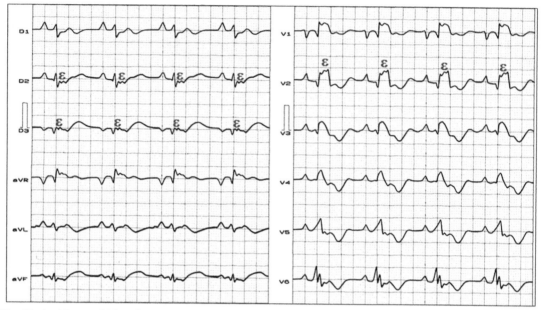

Fig. 17. An 18-year-old female Caucasian with a weight of 53 Kg and height of 1.52 m. Electrocardiographic diagnosis, sinus rhythm; heart rate, 60 beats/min; P wave, SAQRS near 0°; voltage, 3 mm; duration, 130 ms; negative polarity in V1 and positive in V2, q wave in V1 and V2, biatrial enlargement? Or a significant right ventricular enlargement? QRSd: 230 ms (complete right bundle branch block); epsilon waves are observed in numerous leads inside and outside of the QRS (*arrows*).

prospective studies are needed to confirm these findings.[56] fQRS is a valuable marker to predict total mortality and major adverse cardiac events in patients with CAD.[83]

Sarcoidosis
Multivariate analyses revealed that fQRS complexes are an associated risk factor for developing cardiac events in extracardiac sarcoidosis.[70]

Brugada syndrome
In Brugada syndrome, the presence of fQRS and early repolarization correlates with increased risk in several studies.[84,85] On multivariable analysis, a history of VF and syncope episodes, an inferolateral early repolarization pattern, and fQRS were independent predictors of documented VF and SCD.[46] In a large multicenter, observational, long-term study, the ECG findings that were useful for predicting adverse outcome in patients with ARVC/D were: T wave inversion in the inferior leads, a precordial QRS amplitude ratio of 0.48 or greater, and fQRS.[86]

Pathognomonic Features
Despite being characteristic of ARVC/D, epsilon waves are not pathognomonic, because they have been described in other pathophysiologic conditions associated with myocardial damage.

Physiologic Epsilon Waves

Ventricular hypertrophy in elite endurance senior athletes
Epsilon wave was found in 3 senior athletes (1.57%) from 347 elite endurance athletes (seniors, 190; juniors, 157), with a mean age of 20 years and 200 subjects with a mean age of 21 years, belonging to a control group of 505 normal sedentary population.[87] Bizarre QRS, ST-T patterns suggestive of abnormal impulse conduction in the right ventricle, including the right outflow tract, associated with prolonged QTc interval in some cases were observed in highly trained endurance athletes. The genetic analyses, negative in most athletes, identified surprising mutations in SCN5A and KCN genes in some cases.[87]

Pathologic Epsilon waves

1. Giant cell myocarditis: Epsilon waves are a major diagnostic criterion for ARVC/D, but also other cardiac pathologies such as giant cell myocarditis can cause severe right

ventricular conduction disturbances manifesting with epsilon waves and VT on surface ECG.[88]

2. Sickle cell anemia.[89]

3. Brugada syndrome: It is believed that Brugada syndrome and ARVC/D are different clinical entities with respect to the clinical presentation and the genetic predisposition. The coexistence of these 2 relatively rare clinical entities was also reported.[90] In clinical practice, there may be cases where the dividing line is not so clear.[91,92] Epsilon waves seem to be rare in patients with Brugada syndrome and were found in 2 of 47 patients by Letsas and colleagues,[93] and in 1 patient from a total of 12 unrelated index patients with Brugada syndrome that were included in the study by Yu and colleagues.[94]

4. Idiopathic VF in the absence of Brugada syndrome phenotype with loss-of-function mutation of the SCN3B-encoded sodium channel beta-3 subunit.[95]

5. During exercise testing or treadmill stress testing in asymptomatic gene carriers: Depolarization abnormalities during exercise testing in asymptomatic gene carriers were found to develop more frequently compared with healthy controls; epsilon waves appeared in 4 of 28 (14%).[96] Recently, Adler and colleagues[85] uncovered epsilon waves in asymptomatic patients carrying mutations in the PKP2 gene. This finding suggests that exercise testing may be valuable for the diagnosis of ARVC/D and that exercise-induced epsilon waves may be found in various genetic subtypes of this disease.

6. Postoperative tetralogy of Fallot.[97]

7. Right ventricular myocardial infarction.[98]

8. Inferior or lateral old (remote) posterior myocardial infarction.[99]

9. Infiltrative diseases, such as cardiac sarcoidosis[100]: Increasing evidence suggests that cardiac sarcoidosis might produce the pathologic substrate of myocardial inhomogeneity causing epsilon waves. Therefore, differentiating these 2 entities is of paramount clinical importance.[101]

Epsilon Wave and Relationship to Ventricular Tachycardia

The presence of these waves indicate slow and fragmented conduction, which favors reentry circuits, which in turn result in sustained VT runs with complete left bundle branch block morphology, suggesting origination in the right ventricle.[89,102] The tracing should run at a double velocity (50 mm/s) and voltage (20 mm/s) to compare the duration of QRS complexes (QRSd) in different leads, as well as to try to record epsilon waves. **Fig. 18** shows more clearly the epsilon wave with double velocity and double voltage. The rate of widespread T wave inversion (exceeding V3) was significantly higher in patients with epsilon waves than in those without. Because these waves are of relatively low voltage, they may go undetected by S-ECG or unnoticed by the interpreter.[99]

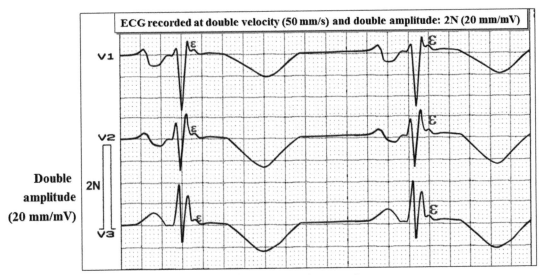

Fig. 18. Epsilon wave with double velocity and voltage. ECG, electrocardiogram.

PRESENCE OF VENTRICULAR LATE POTENTIALS USING HIGH-RESOLUTION OR SIGNAL-AVERAGED ELECTROCARDIOGRAPHY

Sufficient data are available to recommend the use of high-resolution or SA-ECG in patients recovering from myocardial infarction without bundle branch block to help determine the risk for developing sustained ventricular tachyarrhythmias.[40] However, no data are available about the extent to which pharmacologic or nonpharmacologic interventions in patients with LPs have an impact on the incidence of SCD. Therefore, controlled, prospective studies are required before this issue can be resolved.

Value of the Signal-Averaged Electrocardiogram in the Diagnosis of Arrhythmogenic Right Ventricular Cardiomyopathy/Dysplasia

SA-ECG or high-resolution ECG is observed more frequently by using this method in cases of ARVC/D. In ARVC/D, SA-ECG frequently is associated to LPs. The epsilon wave may be observed in surface ECG; however, it is seen much more frequently in SA-ECG. SA-ECG is used to detect LPs and epsilon waves in ARVC/D carriers. Patients with positive SA-ECG (presence of LPs) have a significantly increased risk of sustained VT and/or SCD in comparison with those with normal SA-ECG or branch block.

Electrocardiographic predictor of sudden death in left ventricular hypertrophy

The association of SCD/LVH diagnosed from the 12-lead ECG was first reported 47 years ago in a prospective study. A population-based study from Michigan showed an association of LVH by ECG with 98 coronary heart disease deaths (45 SCD events) observed over a 6-year duration, and predicted an SCD rate of 48 per 1000 over this time frame, compared with 2.6 per 1000 with a normal ECG.[40,103,104]

Advantages of the electrocardiograph for the diagnosis of left ventricular hypertrophy

- Low cost.
- Easily available to perform at any medical facility globally.
- High specificity (close to 99%).
- Simple diagnostic criteria.
- Possibility of identifying ischemia, necrosis, arrhythmias, and associated dromotropic disorders immediately.
- Independent from the experience of the observer and the quality of the equipment.

- Irreplaceable in apical HCM when revealing the typical giant negative T waves from V2 to V5 accompanied by positive voltage criteria.
- Preparticipation screening is a life-saving and cost-effective strategy in young athletes in whom SCD is mostly caused by ECG-detectable myocardial diseases.[105] The addition of an ECG to preparticipation screening saves 2.06 life-years per 1000 athletes at an incremental total cost of $89 per athlete and yields a cost effectiveness ratio of $42 900 per life-year saved (95% CI, $21 200–$71 300 per life-year saved) compared with cardiovascular-focused history and physical examination alone.[106] However, controversies continue on the role and value of ECG screening in the preparticipation of athletes.

The main method to diagnose LVH is echocardiography, which allows measuring the thickness of the muscle of the heart. Two-dimensional echocardiography can produce images of the left ventricle. The thickness of the left ventricle as visualized in echocardiography correlates with its actual mass. A normal thickness of the left ventricular myocardium is from 6 to 11 mm (as measured at the very end of diastole). If the myocardium is more than 1.1 cm thick, the diagnosis of LVH can be made by echocardiography. Echocardiography, if available, should be the test of choice to assess for LVH. It is much more sensitive than ECG and can also detect other abnormalities such as left ventricular dysfunction and valvular disease.

Cardiac MRI is the gold standard test for LVH, because it is even more accurate and reproducible than echocardiography.[107] It can precisely estimate a patient's left ventricular mass and assess for other structural cardiac abnormalities. The use of MRI, however, is significantly restricted in clinical practice owing to its high cost and limited availability and expertise to evaluate the test.

A QRS-T angle between 90° and 180° (QRS/ST-T angle broadening: ST-segment depression and T wave inversion in the left precordial leads and in the limb leads in which major QRS deflections are upright) is associated with an increased risk of SCD, independent of the LVEF[108] (Fig. 19). Prolonged QTc is an independent marker of SCD among subjects with LVH.[109] In the setting of aggressive antihypertensive therapy, a prolonged QRSd identifies hypertensive patients at higher risk for SCD.[110] The presence of cardiac sympathetic hyperactivity may predict SCD in the asymptomatic hemodialysis patients with LVH.[111]

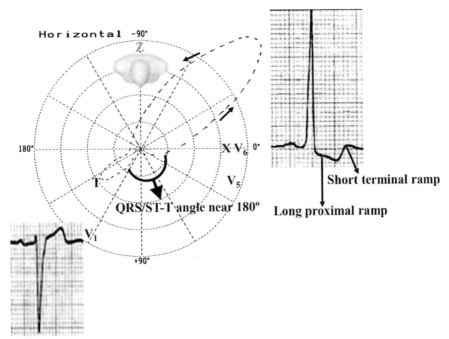

Fig. 19. Left ventricular strain pattern. Deviation of the ST-segment and the T wave/loop in the opposite direction to the main QRS vector causes widening QRS amplitude and wide QRS/T angle between 90° and 180°. This is called left ventricular strain pattern. A $^{QRS}/_{ST-T}$ angle of 90° or greater and a T wave upright in V2 and more negative than −01 mV in V6, and ST segment depression with upward convexity and T wave inversion in the left precordial leads.

SUMMARY

Although the ECG was invented more than 100 years ago, it remains the most commonly used test in clinical medicine. It is easy to perform, relatively cheap, and results are readily available. Interpretation of the ECG, however, needs expertise and knowledge. Amazingly, new data, phenomenon, and syndromes are continuously discovered by the ECG. It is important to differentiate between normal and abnormal ECGs first and then try to correlate the findings with clinical pathologies. Today, the ECG is also an integral part of the screening model for a variety of conditions such as channelopathies, athletes, preoperative risk profile, and remains the cardiologist's best friend.[112]

ACKNOWLEDGMENTS

We wish to thank Mariah Smith for her assistance in preparing this article.

REFERENCES

1. Vatta M, Dumaine R, Varghese G, et al. Genetic and biophysical basis of sudden unexplained nocturnal death syndrome (SUNDS), a disease allelic to Brugada syndrome. Hum Mol Genet 2002;11(3):337–45.

2. Baruteau AE, Probst V, Abriel H. Inherited progressive cardiac conduction disorders. Curr Opin Cardiol 2015;30(1):33–9.

3. Leenhardt A, Glaser E, Burguera M. Short-coupled variant of torsade de pointes. A new electrocardiographic entity in the spectrum of idiopathic ventricular tachyarrhythmias. Circulation 1994;89(1):206–15.

4. Kondo H, Shinohara T, Takahashi N. A case of short-coupled premature ventricular beat-induced ventricular fibrillation with early repolarization in the inferolateral leads. J Arrhythm 2015;31(1):60–3.

5. Rubio-Gozalbo ME, Bakker JA, Waterham HR, et al. Carnitine-acylcarnitine translocase deficiency, clinical, biochemical and genetic aspects. Mol Aspects Med 2004;25(5–6):521–32.

6. Einthoven W. Ueber die Form des menschlichen Electrocardiogramms. Pflugers Arch Eur J Physiol 1895;60:101–2.

7. Abdelghani SA, Rosenthal TM, Morin DP. Surface electrocardiogram predictors of sudden cardiac arrest. Ochsner J 2016;16(3):280–9.

8. Bazett HC. An analysis of the time-relations of electrocardiograms. Heart 1920;7:353–70.

9. Fridericia LS. The duration of systole in the electrocardiogram of normal subjects and of patients with heart disease. Acta Med Scand 1920;53:469–86.

10. Johnson JN, Ackerman MJ. QTc: how long is too long? Br J Sports Med 2009;43(9):657–62.

11. Garson A Jr. How to measure the QT interval – what is normal? Am J Cardiol 1993;72(6):14B–6B.

12. Misigoj-Durakovic M, Durakovic Z, Prskalo I. Heart rate-corrected QT and JT intervals in electrocardiograms in physically fit students and student athletes. Ann Noninvasive Electrocardiol 2016;21(6): 595–603.

13. Macfarlane PW, Antzelevitch C, Haissaguerre M, et al. The early repolarization pattern: a consensus paper. J Am Coll Cardiol 2015;66(4):470–7.

14. Surawicz B, Macfarlane P. Inappropriate and confusing electrocardiographic terms. J Am Coll Cardiol 2011;57(15):1584–6.

15. Antzelevitch C, Yan G, Viskin S. Rationale for the use of the terms J-wave syndromes and early repolarization. J Am Coll Cardiol 2011;57(15):1587–90.

16. Macfarlane P, Antzelevitch C, Haissaguerre M, et al. Consensus paper: early repolarization pattern. J Am Coll Cardiol 2015;66(4):470–7.

17. Tikkanen JT, Anttonen O, Junttila MJ, et al. Long-term outcome associated with early repolarization on electrocardiography. N Engl J Med 2009; 361(26):2529–37.

18. Derval N, Simpson CS, Birnie DH, et al. Prevalence and characteristics of early repolarization in the CASPER registry: cardiac arrest survivors with preserved ejection fraction registry. J Am Coll Cardiol 2011;58(7):722–8.

19. Kamakura T, Wada M, Ishibashi K, et al. Differences in the onset mode of ventricular tachyarrhythmia between patients with J wave in anterior leads versus inferolateral leads. Heart Rhythm 2017;14(4):553–61.

20. Shenasa M, Josephson M, Estes NAM. The ECG handbook of contemporary challenges. Minneapolis (MN): Cardiotext; 2015.

21. Shakibfar S, Graff C, Kanters JK, et al. Minimal T-wave representation and its use in the assessment of drug arrhythmogenicity. Ann Noninvasive Electrocardiol 2017;22(3):e12413.

22. Maury P, Sacher F, Gourraud JB, et al. Increased Tpeak-Tend interval is highly and independently related to arrhythmic events in Brugada syndrome. Heart Rhythm 2015;12(12):2469–76.

23. Hetland M, Haugaa KH, Sarvari SI, et al. A novel ECG-index for prediction of ventricular arrhythmias in patients after myocardial infarction. Ann Noninvasive Electrocardiol 2014;19(4):330–7.

24. Lambiase PD. Tpeak-Tend interval and Tpeak-Tend/QT ratio as markers of ventricular tachycardia inducibility in subjects with Brugada ECG phenotype. Europace 2010;12(2):158–9.

25. Letsas KP, Weber R, Astheimer K, et al. Tpeak-Tend interval and Tpeak-Tend/QT ratio as markers of ventricular tachycardia inducibility in subjects with Brugada ECG phenotype. Europace 2010; 12(2):271–4.

26. Schwartz PJ, Malliani A. Electrical alternation of the T-wave: clinical and experimental evidence of its relationship with the sympathetic nervous system and with the long Q-T syndrome. Am Heart J 1975;89(1):45–50.

27. Aro AL, Kenttä TV, Huikuri H. Microvolt T-wave alternans: where are we now? Arrhythm Electrophysiol Rev 2016;5(1):37–40.

28. Takasugi N, Goto H, Takasugi M, et al. Prevalence of microvolt T-wave alternans in patients with long QT syndrome and its association with Torsade de Pointes. Circ Arrhythm Electrophysiol 2016;9(2): e003206.

29. Dhar R, Alsheikh-Ali AA, Estes NA 3rd, et al. Association of prolonged QRS duration with ventricular tachyarrhythmias and sudden cardiac death in the Multicenter Automatic Defibrillator Implantation Trial II (MADIT-II). Heart Rhythm 2008; 5(6):807–13.

30. Reinier K, Narayanan K, Uy-Evanado A, et al. Electrocardiographic Markers and the left ventricular ejection fraction have cumulative effects on risk of sudden cardiac death. JACC Clin Electrophysiol 2015;1(6):542–50.

31. Junttila MJ, Brugada P, Hong K, et al. Differences in 12-lead electrocardiogram between symptomatic and asymptomatic Brugada syndrome patients. J Cardiovasc Electrophysiol 2008;19(4): 380–3.

32. Ohkubo K, Watanabe I, Okumura Y, et al. Prolonged QRS duration in lead V2 and risk of life-threatening ventricular arrhythmia in patients with Brugada syndrome. Int Heart J 2011;52(2):98–102.

33. Pitzalis MV, Anaclerio M, Iacoviello M, et al. QT-interval prolongation in right precordial leads: an additional electrocardiographic hallmark of Brugada syndrome. J Am Coll Cardiol 2003;42(9):1632–7.

34. Nasir K, Bomma C, Tandri H, et al. Electrocardiographic features of arrhythmogenic right ventricular dysplasia/cardiomyopathy according to disease severity: a need to broaden diagnostic criteria. Circulation 2004;110(12):1527–34.

35. Nasir K, Tandri H, Rutberg J, et al. Filtered QRS duration on signal-averaged electrocardiography predicts inducibility of ventricular tachycardia in arrhythmogenic right ventricle dysplasia. Pacing Clin Electrophysiol 2003;26(10):1955–60.

36. Fontaine G, Frank R, Guiraudon G, et al. Significance of intraventricular conduction disorders observed in arrhythmogenic right ventricular dysplasia. Arch Mal Coeur Vaiss 1984;77(8):872–9.

37. Calò L, Giustetto C, Martino A. New electrocardiographic marker of sudden death in Brugada syndrome: the S-wave in lead I. J Am Coll Cardiol 2016;67(12):1427–40.

38. Kotake Y, Kurita T, Akaiwa Y, et al. Intravenous amiodarone homogeneously prolongs ventricular

repolarization in patients with life-threatening ventricular tachyarrhythmia. J Cardiol 2015;66(2): 161–7.

39. Das MK, Khan B, Jacob S, et al. Significance of a fragmented QRS complex versus a Q wave in patients with coronary artery disease. Circulation 2006;113(21):2495–501.

40. Shenasa M, Shenasa H. Electrocardiographic markers of sudden cardiac death in different substrates. In: Shenasa M, Josephson M, Estes M, editors. ECG handbook of contemporary challenges. Cardiotext; 2015.

41. Das MK, Saha C, El Masry H, et al. Fragmented QRS on a 12-lead ECG: a predictor of mortality and cardiac. Heart Rhythm 2007;4(11):1385–92.

42. Bokma JP, Winter MM, Vehmeijer JT, et al. QRS fragmentation is superior to QRS duration in predicting mortality in adults with tetralogy of Fallot. Heart 2017;103(9):666–71.

43. Vogels RJ, Teuwen CP, Ramdjan TT, et al. Usefulness of fragmented QRS complexes in patients with congenital heart disease to predict ventricular tachyarrhythmias. Am J Cardiol 2017;119(1): 126–31.

44. Conte G, de Asmundis C, Sieira J, et al. Prevalence and clinical impact of early repolarization pattern and QRS-Fragmentation in high-risk patients with Brugada Syndrome. Circ J 2016; 80(10):2109–16.

45. Adler A, Rosso R, Chorin E, et al. Risk stratification in Brugada syndrome: clinical characteristics, electrocardiographic parameters, and auxiliary testing. Heart Rhythm 2016;13(1):299–310.

46. Tokioka K, Kusano KF, Morita H, et al. Electrocardiographic parameters and fatal arrhythmic events in patients with Brugada syndrome: combination of depolarization and repolarization abnormalities. J Am Coll Cardiol 2014;63(20): 2131–8.

47. Wang J, Tang M, Mao KX, et al. Idiopathic ventricular fibrillation with fragmented QRS complex and J wave in resting electrocardiogram. J Geriatr Cardiol 2012;9(2):143–7.

48. Nademanee K, Veerakul G. Overlapping risks of early repolarization and Brugada syndrome. J Am Coll Cardiol 2014;63(20):2139–40.

49. Haraoka K, Morita H, Saito Y, et al. Fragmented QRS is associated with torsades de pointes in patients with acquired long QT syndrome. Heart Rhythm 2010;7(12):1808–14.

50. Konno T, Hayashi K, Fujino N, et al. Electrocardiographic QRS fragmentation as a marker for myocardial fibrosis in hypertrophic cardiomyopathy. J Cardiovasc Electrophysiol 2015;26(10): 1081–7.

51. Baysal E, Yaylak B, Altıntaş B. Fragmented QRS is associated with ventricular tachycardia in patients with apical aneurysm with hypertrophic cardiomyopathy. Indian Heart J 2016;68(2):199.

52. Nomura A, Konno T, Fujita T, et al. Fragmented QRS predicts heart failure progression in patients with hypertrophic cardiomyopathy. Circ J 2015; 79(1):136–43.

53. Zhang L, Mmagu O, Liu L, et al. Hypertrophic cardiomyopathy: can the noninvasive diagnostic testing identify high risk patients. World J Cardiol 2014;6(8):764–70.

54. Kang KW, Janardhan AH, Jung KT, et al. Fragmented QRS as a candidate marker for high-risk assessment in hypertrophic cardiomyopathy. Heart Rhythm 2014;11(8):1433–40.

55. Femenía F, Arce M, Van Grieken J, et al. Fragmented QRS in hypertrophic obstructive cardiomyopathy (FHOCM) Study Investigators. J Interv Card Electrophysiol 2013;38(3):159–65.

56. Canpolat U, Kabakçi G, Aytemir K, et al. Fragmented QRS complex predicts the arrhythmic events in patients with arrhythmogenic right ventricular cardiomyopathy/dysplasia. J Cardiovasc Electrophysiol 2013;24(11):1260–6.

57. Peters S, Trümmel M, Koehler B. QRS fragmentation in standard ECG as a diagnostic marker of arrhythmogenic right ventricular dysplasia-cardiomyopathy. Heart Rhythm 2008;5(10):1417–21.

58. Xu Y, Qiu Z, Xu Y, et al. The role of fQRS in coronary artery disease. A meta-analysis of observational studies. Herz 2015;40(Suppl 1):8–15.

59. Tanriverdi Z, Dursun H, Kaya D. The importance of the number of leads with fQRS for predicting in-hospital mortality in acute STEMI patients treated with primary PCI. Ann Noninvasive Electrocardiol 2016;21(4):413–9.

60. Li M, Wang X, Mi SH, et al. Short-term prognosis of fragmented QRS complex in patients with non-ST elevated acute myocardial infarction. Chin Med J (Engl) 2016;129(5):518–22.

61. Cakmak HA, Aslan S, Gul M, et al. Assessment of the relationship between a narrow fragmented QRS complex and coronary slow flow. Cardiol J 2015;22(4):428–36.

62. Reddy CV, Cheriparambill K, Saul B, et al. Fragmented left sided QRS in absence of bundle branch block: sign of left ventricular aneurysm. Ann Noninvasive Electrocardiol 2006;11(2):132–8.

63. Kadi H, Kevser A, Ozturk A, et al. Fragmented QRS complexes are associated with increased left ventricular mass in patients with essential hypertension. Ann Noninvasive Electrocardiol 2013;18(6):547–54.

64. Bekar L, Katar M, Yetim M, et al. Fragmented QRS complexes are a marker of myocardial fibrosis in hypertensive heart disease. Turk Kardiyol Dern Ars 2016;44(7):554–60.

65. Baranchuk A, Femenia F, López-Diez JC, et al, FECHA Study Investigators. Fragmented surface

ECG was a poor predictor of appropriate therapies in patients with Chagas' cardiomyopathy and ICD implantation (Fragmented ECG in CHAgas' Cardiomyopathy Study). Ann Noninvasive Electrocardiol 2014;19(1):43–9.

66. Bacharova L, Triantafyllou E, Vazaios C, et al. The effect of obstructive sleep apnea on QRS complex morphology. J Electrocardiol 2015;48(2):164–70.

67. Sayin MR, Altuntas M, Aktop Z, et al. Presence of fragmented QRS complexes in patients with obstructive sleep apnea syndrome. Chin Med J (Engl) 2015;128(16):2141–6.

68. Demır K, Avcı A, Yılmaz S, et al. Fragmented QRS in patients with systemic lupus erythematosus. Scand Cardiovasc J 2014;48(4):197–201.

69. Inanir A, Ceyhan K, Okan S, et al. Frequency of fragmented QRS in ankylosing spondylitis: a prospective controlled study. Z Rheumatol 2013;72(5):468–73.

70. Nagao S, Watanabe H, Sobue Y, et al. Electrocardiographic abnormalities and risk of developing cardiac events in extracardiac sarcoidosis. Int J Cardiol 2015;189:1–5.

71. Perlini S, Salinaro F, Cappelli F, et al. Prognostic value of fragmented QRS in cardiac AL amyloidosis. Int J Cardiol 2013;167(5):2156–61.

72. Baş Y, Altunkaş F, Seçkin HY, et al. Frequency of fragmented QRS in patient with psoriasis vulgaris without cardiovascular disease. Arch Dermatol Res 2016;308(5):367–71.

73. Fontaine G, Frank R, Gallais-Hamonno F, et al. Electrocardiography of delayed potentials in post-excitation syndrome. Arch Mal Coeur Vaiss 1978;71(8):854–64.

74. Frank R, Fontaine G, Vedel J, et al. Electrocardiology of 4 cases of right ventricular dysplasia inducing arrhythmia. Arch Mal Coeur Vaiss 1978;71(9):963–72.

75. Marcus FI. Guy Fontaine: a pioneer in electrophysiology. Clin Cardiol 1998;21(2):145–6.

76. Peters S, Trümmel M, Koehler B, et al. The value of different electrocardiographic depolarization criteria in the diagnosis of arrhythmogenic right ventricular dysplasia/cardiomyopathy. J Electrocardiol 2007;40(1):34–7.

77. Maia IG, Sá R, Bassan R, et al. Arrhythmogenic right ventricular dysplasia. Arq Bras Cardiol 1991;57(2):97–102.

78. Okano Y. Electrocardiographic findings in arrhythmogenic right ventricular dysplasia (ARVD) evaluated by body surface mapping. Nihon Rinsho 1995;53(1):230–8.

79. Fontaine G, Guiraudon G, Frank R. Stimulation studies and epicardial mapping in ventricular tachycardia A study of mechanisms and selection for surgery. In: Kulbertus HE, editor. Re-entrant arrhythmias: mechanisms and treatment. Lancaster (PA): MTP Publishers; 1977. p. 334–50.

80. Marcus FI. Epsilon waves aid in the prognosis and risk stratification of patients with ARVC/D. J Cardiovasc Electrophysiol 2015;26(11):1211–2.

81. Protonotarios A, Anastasakis A, Tsatsopoulou A, et al. Clinical significance of epsilon waves in arrhythmogenic cardiomyopathy. J Cardiovasc Electrophysiol 2015;26(11):1204–10.

82. Peters S, Truemmel M, Koehler B. Prognostic value of QRS fragmentation in patients with arrhythmogenic right ventricular cardiomyopathy/dysplasia. J Cardiovasc Med (Hagerstown) 2012;13(5):295–8.

83. Gong B, Li Z. Total Mortality, major adverse cardiac events, and echocardiographic-derived cardiac parameters with fragmented QRS complex. Ann Noninvasive Electrocardiol 2016;21(4):404–12.

84. Morita H, Kusano KF, Miura D, et al. Fragmented QRS as a marker of conduction abnormality and a predictor of prognosis of Brugada syndrome. Circulation 2008;118(17):1697–704.

85. Adler A, Perrin MJ, Spears D, et al. Epsilon wave uncovered by exercise test in a patient with desmoplakin-positive arrhythmogenic right ventricular cardiomyopathy. Can J Cardiol 2015;31(6):819.e1-e2.

86. Saguner AM, Ganahl S, Baldinger SH, et al. Usefulness of electrocardiographic parameters for risk prediction in arrhythmogenic right ventricular dysplasia. Am J Cardiol 2014;113(10):1728–34.

87. Macarie C, Stoian I, Dermengiu D, et al. The electrocardiographic abnormalities in highly trained athletes compared to the genetic study related to causes of unexpected sudden cardiac death. J Med Life 2009;2(4):361–72.

88. Vollmann D, Goette A, Kandolf R, et al. Epsilon waves in giant-cell myocarditis. Eur Heart J 2014;35(1):9.

89. Hurst JW. Naming of the waves in the ECG, with a brief account of their genesis. Circulation 1998;98(18):1937–42.

90. Hoogendijk MG. Diagnostic dilemmas: overlapping features of Brugada syndrome and arrhythmogenic right ventricular cardiomyopathy. Front Physiol 2012;3:144.

91. An HB, Li YY. Epsilon waves seen in a patient with typical electrocardiography pattern of Brugada. Zhonghua Xin Xue Guan Bing Za Zhi 2008;36(2):166.

92. Ozeke O, Cavus UY, Atar I, et al. Epsilon-like electrocardiographic pattern in a patient with Brugada syndrome. Ann Noninvasive Electrocardiol 2009;14(3):305–8.

93. Letsas KP, Efremidis M, Weber R, et al. Epsilon-like waves and ventricular conduction abnormalities in subjects with type 1 ECG pattern of Brugada syndrome. Heart Rhythm 2011;8(6):874–8.

94. Yu J, Hu J, Dai X, et al. SCN5A mutation in Chinese patients with arrhythmogenic right ventricular dysplasia. Herz 2014;39(2):271–5.

95. Valdivia CR, Medeiros-Domingo A, Ye B, et al. Loss-of-function mutation of the SCN3B-encoded sodium channel {beta}3 subunit associated with a case of idiopathic ventricular fibrillation. Cardiovasc Res 2010;86(3):392–400.

96. Perrin MJ, Angaran P, Laksman Z, et al. Exercise testing in asymptomatic gene carriers exposes a latent electrical substrate of arrhythmogenic right ventricular cardiomyopathy. J Am Coll Cardiol 2013;62(19):1772–9.

97. George BA, Ko JM, Lensing FD, et al. "Repaired" tetralogy of Fallot mimicking arrhythmogenic right ventricular cardiomyopathy (another phenocopy). Am J Cardiol 2011;108(2):326–9.

98. Andreou AY. Epsilon waves in right ventricular myocardial infarction. Tex Heart Inst J 2012;39(2): 306.

99. Zorio E, Arnau MA, Rueda J, et al. The presence of epsilon waves in a patient with acute right ventricular infarction. Pacing Clin Electrophysiol 2005; 28(3):245–7.

100. Santucci PA, Morton JB, Picken MM, et al. Electroanatomic mapping of the right ventricle in a patient with a giant epsilon wave, ventricular tachycardia, and cardiac sarcoidosis. J Cardiovasc Electrophysiol 2004;15(9):1091–4.

101. Khaji A, Zhang L, Kowey P, et al. Mega-epsilon waves on 12-lead ECG–just another case of arrhythmogenic right ventricular dysplasia/cardiomyopathy? Electrocardiol 2013;46(6):524–7.

102. McKenna WJ, Thiene G, Nava A, et al. Diagnosis of arrhythmogenic right ventricular dysplasia/cardiomyopathy. Task Force of the Working Group myocardial and Pericardial disease of the European Society of Cardiology and of the Scientific Council on Cardiomyopathies of the International Society and Federation of Cardiology. Br Heart J 1994;71(3):215–8.

103. Chiang BN, Perlman LV, Fulton M, et al. Predisposing factors in sudden cardiac death in Tecumseh, Michigan. A prospective study. Circulation 1970; 41(1):31–7.

104. Shenasa M, Shenasa H. Hypertension, left ventricular hypertrophy, and sudden cardiac death. Int J Cardiol 2017;237:60–3.

105. Corrado D, Basso C, Thiene G. Sudden cardiac death in athletes: what is the role of screening? Curr Opin Cardiol 2012;27(1):41–8.

106. Wheeler MT, Heidenreich PA, Froelicher VF, et al. Cost-effectiveness of preparticipation screening for prevention of sudden cardiac death in young athletes. Ann Intern Med 2010;152(5):276–86.

107. Bottini PB, Carr AA, Prisant LM, et al. Magnetic resonance imaging compared to echocardiography to assess left ventricular mass in the hypertensive patient. Am J Hypertens 1995;8(3):221–8.

108. Chua KC, Teodorescu C, Reinier K, et al. Wide QRS-T angle on the 12-Lead ECG as a predictor of sudden death beyond the LV ejection fraction. J Cardiovasc Electrophysiol 2016;27(7):833–9.

109. Panikkath R, Reinier K, Uy-Evanado A, et al. Electrocardiographic predictors of sudden cardiac death in patients with left ventricular hypertrophy. Ann Noninvasive Electrocardiol 2013;18(3):225–9.

110. Morin DP, Oikarinen L, Viitasalo M, et al. QRS duration predicts sudden cardiac death in hypertensive patients undergoing intensive medical therapy: the LIFE study. Eur Heart J 2009;30(23):2908–14.

111. Nishimura M, Tokoro T, Nishida M, et al. Sympathetic overactivity and sudden cardiac death among hemodialysis patients with left ventricular hypertrophy. Int J Cardiol 2010;142(1):80–6.

112. Stern S. Electrocardiogram: still the cardiologists best friend. Circulation 2006;113:753–6.

Prediction and Prevention of Sudden Cardiac Death

Daniel P. Morin, MD MPH[a],*, Munther K. Homoud, MD[b], N.A. Mark Estes III, MD[b]

KEYWORDS

- Sudden cardiac death • Sudden cardiac arrest • Ischemic heart disease
- Nonischemic cardiomyopathy • Left ventricular ejection fraction

KEY POINTS

- As the most common cause of death worldwide, sudden cardiac death (SCD) has important implications for not only individuals, but for entire populations.
- The most common underlying abnormality associated with SCD is ischemic heart disease, but several other pathophysiological processes (both inherited and acquired) can also predispose to SCD.
- Methods of risk stratification for SCD, and treatments aimed at reducing that risk, have been developed.
- The definitive therapy for most patients at high risk for SCD is the implanted cardioverter-defibrillator (ICD).
- Following the recently published DANISH study, the utility of ICDs in nonischemic cardiomyopathy (NICM) has had renewed interest, and risk stratification in NICM is an area of active investigation.

INTRODUCTION

Sudden cardiac death (SCD), defined as death due to cardiac causes heralded by abrupt loss of consciousness, is the most common cause of death worldwide, accounting for 50% of deaths from cardiovascular disease and approximately 350,000 annual deaths in the United States.[1–6] Although the terms sudden cardiac arrest (SCA) and SCD are commonly used interchangeably, by definition SCA is the sudden cessation of cardiac activity so that the victim becomes unresponsive, with no normal breathing and no signs of circulation.[1] If definitive measures are not taken rapidly, SCA progresses to SCD.[1] Many of these events can be predicted and prevented by implementing evidence-based, guideline-endorsed recommendations for primary or secondary prevention of SCD.[1–6] Risk stratification techniques now allow identification of individuals at risk for SCD because of structural heart disease or inherited channelopathies (**Box 1**).[1–6] Several cardiovascular conditions predisposing to athletic sudden death have been identified.[7–9] Multiple interventions have been identified that can reduce the risk of SCD in these patient populations.[1–9]

Despite contemporary risk stratification techniques, prediction and prevention of SCD represent major challenges, because most SCD events occur in patients who were not previously identified as being at risk for SCD.[1–6] Because most individuals experiencing SCD currently are not identifiable as being at high risk, community-based public access to defibrillation programs is

Speaker's Bureau: Biotronik, Boston Scientific, Medtronic. Research Grants: Boston Scientific, Medtronic (D.P. Morin). No disclosures (M.K. Homoud). Consultant: Boston Scientific, Medtronic, St. Jude (N.A.M. Estes).
[a] Ochsner Medical Center, Ochsner Clinical School, University of Queensland Medical School, 1514 Jefferson Highway, New Orleans, LA 70121, USA; [b] New England Cardiac Arrhythmia Center, Division of Cardiology, Tufts Medical Center, 800 Washington Street, Boston, MA 02111, USA
* Corresponding author.
E-mail address: dmorin@ochsner.org

cardiacEP.theclinics.com

Box 1
Conditions associated with sudden cardiac death

Structural heart disease

Ischemic heart disease

Nonischemic cardiomyopathy

Valvular heart disease

Congenital heart disease

Hypertrophic cardiomyopathy

Arrhythmogenic right ventricular dysplasia

Anomalous coronary artery origin

Primary electrophysiological conditions

Congenital long QT syndromes

Short QT syndrome

Ventricular pre-excitation (Wolff-Parkinson-White syndrome)

Idiopathic ventricular fibrillation

Brugada syndrome

Catecholaminergic polymorphic ventricular tachycardia

essential to save lives and improve outcomes for cardiac arrest victims.

ISCHEMIC HEART DISEASE

Several strategies have evolved to predict and prevent SCD in patients with ischemic heart disease.[1–6] Primary prevention of coronary artery disease (CAD), the most common condition predisposing to SCD, is 1 approach.[1–6] SCD is the first manifestation of CAD in approximately 40% of patients. Risk factors for both CAD and SCD include advanced age, male sex, cigarette smoking, hypertension, diabetes mellitus, hypercholesterolemia, obesity, and a family history of premature CAD.[1,6] These risk factors for SCD are also predictors of myocardial infarction, CAD-related death, and all-cause mortality.[1,6] Lifestyle-based optimization of blood pressure, weight, glucose, cholesterol, smoking, diet, and physical activity is included in this strategy.[1,6] Although this approach is intuitively appealing, evidence showing that it directly prevents SCD does not currently exist.[1,6]

Primary prevention of SCD in patients with CAD, via risk stratification and pharmacologic intervention, revascularization, and/or the implantable cardioverter defibrillator (ICD), represents a strategy supported by multiple clinical trials.[1–6] Impaired left ventricular ejection fraction (LVEF) and other genetic, anatomic, and electrophysiological risk factors for SCD have been identified.[1–6] Pharmacologic interventions that reduce the risk of SCD in patients with impaired LVEF and CAD include beta-blockers, angiotensin-converting enzyme inhibitors, and statins.[6] Antiarrhythmic agents for suppression of ventricular arrhythmias have a neutral or negative effect on mortality based on prospective, randomized trials.[6] Multiple clinical trials randomizing several thousand patients have demonstrated that the ICD reduces SCD and improves overall mortality in selected patient populations, including those with ischemic heart disease and left ventricular dysfunction.[1,6]

Secondary prevention of SCD refers to interventions in patients who have survived a prior cardiac arrest or sustained ventricular tachyarrhythmia.[1–6] Multiple prospective randomized trials have shown the ICD to be superior to antiarrhythmic drug therapy for prolonging survival in such patients.[1–6] All recommendations for ICD therapy apply only to patients who are receiving optimal medical therapy (OMT) and have a reasonable expectation of survival with good functional status for 1 year.[1–6] When indicated for primary or secondary prevention, ICDs have been demonstrated to reduce SCD and improve total mortality, with favorable cost-effectiveness.[1–6] Despite this evidence, many patients who have indications for this therapy are not receiving ICDs.[1–6]

Prevention of SCD immediately after a myocardial infarction (MI) represents a vexing clinical challenge.[6] With advances in the treatment of MI with primary percutaneous coronary intervention and pharmacologic therapy, SCD and total mortality after MI have decreased.[6] Despite optimal therapy with revascularization and drugs, the risk of SCD is highest in the first 30 days.[6] However, clinical trials have demonstrated no mortality improvement from early ICD placement in patients at even extremely high risk for SCD after MI.[6] Autopsy evaluation of patients experiencing SCD in the immediate post-MI period has demonstrated that there is a high frequency of cardiac rupture or recurrent MI in the first month after the index MI, whereas arrhythmic death becomes more likely subsequently.[6] These observations may help to explain the lack of benefit of early ICD therapy after MI.[6]

Contemporary clinical guidelines restrict ICD implants to patients at least 40 days after MI with continued impairment of LVEF despite OMT.[1–6] The home automated external defibrillator in high-risk post-MI patients does not improve survival compared with conventional resuscitation methods.[1–6] Based on these considerations, clinicians commonly employ the wearable cardioverter defibrillator (WCD).[5] Although the short-term use of the WCD is a reasonable approach for high-risk post-MI patients, it remains to be evaluated in appropriately designed prospective trials.[5] Additional research is needed to identify risk stratification and intervention strategies to prevent SCD immediately after MI. In the meantime, clinicians should optimize and individualize therapy in the immediate post-MI period while carefully considering the risks of sudden death and mortality from other causes.[1–6]

NONISCHEMIC CARDIOMYOPATHY

Although most systolic cardiomyopathy is caused by CAD, a significant minority of cases have no associated CAD. Nonischemic cardiomyopathy (NICM) is the second most common cause of systolic heart failure, accounting for approximately 10% of cases.[10,11] Although the prognosis of patients with idiopathic NICM is better than that of those with ICM, NICM still carries a substantial risk of death, with 5-year mortality in the 25% to 50% range.[10,12,13] As many as 35% of these deaths are sudden, with much of the remainder resulting from progressive congestive heart failure or noncardiac causes.[13,14]

Several randomized controlled trials have examined the utility of the ICD for mortality reduction in NICM.[15,16] Based on this evidence, societal guidelines include ICD implantation as a Class I indication in patients with NICM, LVEF of no more than 35%, and New York Heart Association (NYHA) Class II or III, and a Class IIb indication for such patients in NYHA Class I.[17] In 2004, the Defibrillators in Non-Ischemic Cardiomyopathy Treatment Evaluation (DEFINITE) investigators reported that in patients with OMT-treated NICM and LVEF of no more than 35%, ICD implantation reduced the risk of SCD and trended strongly toward a reduction in all-cause mortality.[13] During that same era, the Comparison of Medical Therapy, Pacing, and Defibrillation in Heart Failure (COMPANION) trial showed that in patients with cardiomyopathy (~45% nonischemic) and QRS duration of at least 120 milliseconds, CRT-*P* alone (ie, no ICD) reduced the combined risk of mortality and heart failure hospitalization, and CRT-*D* implantation significantly reduced mortality.[18] Subsequently, the Sudden Cardiac Death in Heart Failure Trial (SCD-HeFT) showed that ICD-treated patients had 23% lower overall mortality, although this benefit was limited to those with milder heart failure symptoms.[12] The nonischemic subset with NYHA III symptoms showed no mortality benefit.

Perhaps because of the statistically nonsignificant mortality result in DEFINITE, the disparate subgroup results in SCD-HeFT, and the possible confounding of ICD benefit due to universal CRT use in COMPANION, the Netherlands did not adopt widespread ICD implantation for patients with NICM. This allowed the conduct of the recently reported Danish Study to Assess the Efficacy of ICDs in Patients with Non-ischemic Systolic Heart Failure on Mortality (DANISH), which randomized patients with symptomatic NICM (LVEF ≤35%) to ICD versus no ICD.[14] A similar proportion of patients in each arm (58%) received cardiac resynchronization therapy (CRT). Although the incidence of SCD in patients who received ICDs was 50% lower than in those who did not, the primary outcome of all-cause mortality occurred at similar rates. Importantly, subgroup analysis showed that ICDs were beneficial in younger patients (<68 years) but not in older patients. Some authors have reconciled this age-based difference by correlating older age with the accumulation of comorbidities, and thereby with risk for nonarrhythmic death that is not lessened by the presence of an ICD.[19]

Beyond Left Ventricular Ejection Fraction: Further Risk Stratification for Sudden Cardiac Death in Nonischemic Cardiomyopathy

Especially in light of the DANISH trial's recent challenge to ICD use in NICM, further risk stratification of the NICM population has become a priority. Several modalities have been evaluated. Although it may be that none is strong enough to be used as a sole marker of risk, it seems likely that a combination of electrocardiogram (ECG) parameters, imaging studies, and perhaps genetics, may be able to risk-stratify patients with NICM.[11,20]

A significant body of evidence supports contrast-enhanced cardiac MRI (CMR/MRI) as a powerful risk stratifier in NICM. Myocardial scar promotes ventricular arrhythmia via heterogeneous conduction and electrical reentry.[16,21] As illustrated in **Fig. 1**, in a review of 29 observational studies

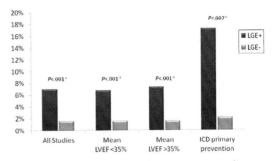

Fig. 1. Annual rate of VF/VF or SCD according to LGE status. [a]p values for weighted difference. ICD, implantable cardioverter defibrillator; LGE, late gadolinium enhancement on MRI; LVEF, left ventricular ejection fraction. (*Adapted from* Di Marco A, Anguera I, Schmitt M, et al. Late gadolinium enhancement and the risk for ventricular arrhythmias or sudden death in dilated cardiomyopathy. JACC Heart Fail 2017;5(1):36; with permission.)

including 2948 patients with NICM, there was much more SCA among LGE-positive patients than among LGE-negative patients, with no correlation between studies' mean LVEF and event rates.[16] In fact, the higher risk implied by LGE persisted among studies with mean LVEF greater than 35%, and was especially pronounced in the primary prevention population. The ongoing randomized CMR Guide trial (NCT01918215) is further evaluating SCA risk, and the utility of ICD therapy, in LGE-positive patients with only mildly depressed LVEF (36%–50%).

Several other candidate risk factors have been evaluated in the NICM population.[11] On meta-analysis, some ECG-based measures of abnormal depolarization can improve risk stratification.[11] Similarly, the repolarization indices T-wave alternans, QRS-T angle, and the duration between the T wave's peak and end have proven useful.[11,22,23] Trials evaluating the significance of nonsustained ventricular tachycardia (NSVT) have come to conflicting conclusions, but their combination via meta-analysis indicates a net higher risk when NSVT is present. The same is true for inducibility of ventricular tachyarrhythmia at invasive electrophysiology study.[11] In contrast, several measures of autonomic function have not demonstrated a net improvement in risk stratification.[11] Although recent discoveries in genetic analysis have great potential, the present knowledge base is not sufficient to warrant widespread genetic screening.[1]

Prevention of Sudden Cardiac Death in Nonischemic Cardiomyopathy

As SCD most often results from ventricular tachyarrhythmia, the most effective available therapy is the ICD.[1,24] In survivors of SCA with no reversible cause, ICD implantation is indicated. Following the application of OMT for NICM, there can be significant improvement in HF symptoms and an increase in the initially depressed LVEF.[25] As shown in **Fig. 2**, Broch and colleagues[10] recently found an average 1-year improvement from 26% +/− 10% to 41% +/− 11%, and significant favorable change in NYHA class, despite only 14% being treated with cardiac resynchronization therapy (CRT). Although not specifically included in guidelines, most payors require 3 months of OMT for newly diagnosed NICM, followed by reassessment of LVEF, prior to ICD implantation. During this time, reversible causes of NICM should be sought, and the use of a wearable defibrillator vest may be considered.[5,20,26]

If the LVEF remains depressed despite OMT (and other therapy as needed), device therapy should be considered. Even potent antiarrhythmic therapy, most often amiodarone, cannot sufficiently reduce SCA risk.[12] The evidence supports ICD implantation for those with NICM and LVEF of no more than 35% who have a life expectancy at least 12 months, and/or cardiac resynchronization therapy in those with LVEF of no more than 35%, significant symptoms, and a wide QRS.[12,24] As seen in **Fig. 3**, this therapeutic strategy is further endorsed by recent meta-analyses of ICD use in nonischemics, despite the negative results of the DANISH trial.[15] Because of patients' variable relative risk of arrhythmic versus nonarrhythmic death, ICDs may be particularly attractive for younger patients, those with less symptomatic heart failure, and/or those with fewer comorbidities.[19] In older or sicker patients, ICDs are less likely to prolong life, but still impose risk in terms of complications (procedural or otherwise).

RISK STRATIFICATION OF SUDDEN CARDIAC DEATH IN INHERITED CHANNELOPATHIES

Some rare hereditary diseases cause SCD in the young through mutation(s) in the channels that regulate the flow of electrolytes across cardiac

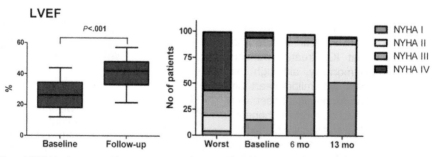

Fig. 2. LVEF and NYHA class over time among patients with NYHA, showing highly significant improvement in both measures of cardiovascular function. (*Adapted from* Broch K, Murbraech K, Andreassen AK, et al. Contemporary outcome in patients with idiopathic dilated cardiomyopathy. Am J Cardiol 2015;116:955–7; with permission.)

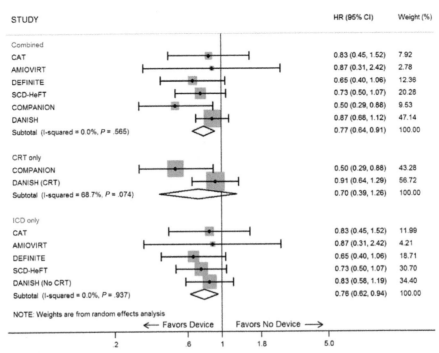

Fig. 3. Meta-analysis of studies examining ICDs and CRT for primary prevention of SCD in NICM. CRT, cardiac resynchronization therapy; ICD, implantable cardioverter defibrillator. (*Adapted from* Golwala H, Bajaj NS, Arora G, et al. Implantable cardioverter-defibrillator for nonischemic cardiomyopathy: an updated analysis. Circulation 2017;135:202; with permission.)

cell membranes.[27] Risk stratification can be challenging, largely because the natural history of these rare diseases is not fully understood.

The Long QT Syndrome

The incidence of the long QT syndrome (LQTS) is estimated at 1 case per 2500 live, otherwise healthy white births.[28] Thirteen different genetic forms of LQTS have been identified, with mutations involving KCNQ1 (LQT1), KCNH2 (LQT2), and SCN5A (LQT3) accounting for more than 90% of genotyped patients.[29] Fifteen percent to 20% of LQTS cases have no identified genetic mutation.[29] The most important determinants of risk are the extent of QT prolongation (especially ≥500 milliseconds), age of first arrhythmic event of no more than 7 years, and whether syncope occurs despite beta blocker use.[30–32] A correlation between genotype and the risk of SCD has been established. Patients with LQT2 (especially females) and LQT3 (especially young males) carry particularly high risk.[30,31] The type of mutation and its location within the causative gene can modify the risk.[32] The association of LQTS with extracardiac abnormalities, such as in the Jervell and Lange-Nielsen syndrome, the Timothy syndrome, and the Andersen-Tawil syndrome, signify higher risk.[32]

Brugada Syndrome

Brugada syndrome (BrS), a hereditary channelopathy presenting predominantly in men, accounts for up to 20% of SCDs in the absence of structural heart disease.[33] The classical Type 1 pattern displays ST-segment elevation of at least 2 mm with a coved morphology, followed by an inverted T wave, in lead V_1 or V_2.[34] The prevalence of this electrocardiographic pattern (and of the disease) varies geographically, with a much higher prevalence in Southeast Asia and Japan compared with the Americas and Europe.[33] Ten genetic variants leading to BrS have been identified, predominantly involving the sodium channel, and, less commonly, the calcium and potassium channel genes.[32] Although patients with other Brugada-related ECG patterns (ie, Type II and Type III, which importantly do not indicate BrS) do not have elevated risk, those with true BrS may display dynamic electrocardiographic changes; the Type 1 pattern may be induced by pyrexia, vagotonia, or the administration of sodium channel-blocking agents.[34] Compared with the LQTS, there is no reliable medical treatment. The ICD is the only effective intervention to prevent SCD. Patients at highest risk are survivors of SCD, as are men and patients with ventricular arrhythmias, syncope, and spontaneous Type 1 pattern.[34–36] Risk stratification of asymptomatic patients is challenging. Some studies have indicated a value to programmed electrical stimulation in determining the risk of future events, but this has not been uniformly demonstrated.[35,36] Neither a family history of SCD nor the type of genetic mutation has any bearing on prognosis.[36]

Catecholaminergic Polymorphic Ventricular Tachycardia

Catecholaminergic polymorphic ventricular tachycardia is a rare but highly lethal channelopathy characterized by an absence of resting electrocardiographic abnormalities but polymorphic ventricular tachyarrhythmias precipitated by exercise or emotion.[37] Altered handling of calcium homeostasis across the sarcoplasmic reticulum caused by mutations in the RyR2 and the CASQ1 receptors has been implicated.[27] Young age at presentation, survival from SCA, and the absence of therapy with beta blockers are identified high risk factors.[38] With a 20-year mortality rate of up to 50%, no identified low risk features have been identified.[37]

Short QT Syndrome

The short QT syndrome (SQTS) is a rare inherited channelopathy characterized by QTc interval less than 330 milliseconds, carrying elevated risk of ventricular and atrial fibrillation.[34] Six forms of SQTS have been identified involving gain-of-function mutations in some of the same potassium channel genes involved in LQTS, and loss-of-function mutations of L-type calcium channels.[32] The most common presentation is SCD, with incidence peaks during the first year of life and later between ages 20 and 40.[39] Most arrhythmic events occur at rest.[39] The limited number of patients has made risk stratification difficult, with SCA being the only predictor of future adverse events.[39]

Early Repolarization Syndrome

Although electrocardiographic early repolarization (ER) has long been associated with a benign prognosis, ER syndrome (ERS) has been demonstrated with greater frequency in individuals with idiopathic VF.[34] Findings distinguishing ERS from the benign variety are notching or slurring of the J point elevation, and a horizontal or downsloping ST segment, particularly in the inferolateral leads. J point elevation of at least 2 mV and ER in the inferior leads have been associated with a higher risk of SCA.[34] No genetic marker has been identified.

SUDDEN CARDIAC DEATH IN THE ATHLETE

SCD in athletes commonly brings to the forefront the lack of evidence-based strategies that predict and prevent these tragic events.[7–9] The frequency of SCD in young athletes is relatively low, with 100 to 150 SCDs during sports in the United States annually.[7–9] Although SCD is a rare occurrence among athletes, specific underlying conditions may dramatically increase the risk.[7–9] It is important for the clinician to recognize conditions predisposing to athletic SCD, as lifestyle restrictions and treatments with proven efficacy exist.[7–9] These conditions include hypertrophic cardiomyopathy (HCM), arrhythmogenic right ventricular dysplasia (ARVD), LQTS, Wolff-Parkinson-White syndrome, and anomalous origin of a coronary artery.[7–9] In North America, HCM has been implicated in as many as 50% of cases of SCD in athletes younger than 35 years. Interestingly, in Italy, ARVD has been implicated in the majority of SCDs. In patients over age 35, CAD predominates as the underlying cause, occurring in over 75% of patients.[7–9] Importantly, risk stratification for SCD is possible for all of the cardiovascular conditions that predispose to athletic SCD, independent of athletic participation.[7–9] In selected patients with these conditions, ICD implantation is commonly recommended to reduce the risk of SCD.

Despite identification of conditions that predispose to SCD, considerable uncertainty remains related to many fundamental issues regarding athletic SCD.[7–9] Due to the absence of athletic death registries with mandatory reporting requirements, data related to the frequency with which these events occur remain unavailable.[7–9] Fundamental gaps in evidence persist regarding the utility of preparticipation screening strategies for preventing SCD in the athlete.[7–9] Restriction from athletics is not supported by robust evidence. Despite these limitations, a recent interassociation consensus statement related to cardiovascular care of the athlete has highlighted the importance of preparticipation cardiovascular screening, including a comprehensive personal and family history and physical examination.[7] Although the consensus statement mentions that electrocardiographic screening can increase the sensitivity to detect potentially lethal cardiac conditions if cardiology expertise is available, it offers no firm recommendation about whether a screening ECG should be performed in all athletes.[7–9]

Another recent consensus statement offers multiple specific recommendations related to public access to defibrillation, a measure that has been demonstrated to improve outcomes of athletes and spectators at athletic events.[9] Schools and other organizations hosting athletic events or providing training facilities for competitive athletic programs should have an emergency action plan that incorporates basic life support and automated external defibrillator (AED) use within a broader plan to activate emergency medical services (EMS).[9] Additionally, coaches and athletic trainers should be trained to recognize SCA and to implement timely cardiopulmonary resuscitation along with AED deployment.[9] AEDs should be available to all SCA victims within 5 minutes, in all settings, including competition, training, and practice. Finally, advanced post–SCA care, including targeted temperature management, should be available at sites where patients are transferred by EMS.[9]

SUMMARY

Sudden death remains a major problem, with significant impact on public health. Many conditions predispose to SCA/SCD, foremost among them CAD, and an effective therapy exists in the form of the ICD. Risk stratification for SCA remains imperfect, especially for patients with nonischemic cardiomyopathy. Ongoing trials may improve the ability to identify those at high risk, and potentially those at very low risk, in the future.

REFERENCES

1. Al-Khatib SM, Yancy CW, Solis P, et al. 2016 AHA/ACC clinical performance and quality measures for prevention of sudden cardiac death. J Am Coll Cardiol 2017;69(6):712–44.
2. Priori SG, Blomström-Lundqvist C, Mazzanti A, et al. 2015 ESC Guidelines for the management of patients with ventricular arrhythmias and the prevention of sudden cardiac death. Eur Heart J 2015;36(41):2793–867.
3. Bennett M, Parkash R, Nery P, et al. Canadian Cardiovascular Society/Canadian Heart Rhythm Society 2016 implantable cardioverter-defibrillator guidelines. Can J Cardiol 2017;33(2):174–88.
4. Neumar RW, Eigel B, Callaway CW, et al. American Heart Association response to the 2015 Institute of Medicine report on strategies to improve cardiac arrest survival. Circulation 2015;132(11):1049–70.
5. Piccini JP, Allen LA, Kudenchuk PJ, et al. Wearable cardioverter-defibrillator therapy for the prevention of sudden cardiac death: a science advisory from the American Heart Association. Circulation 2016;133(17):1715–27.
6. Estes NAM. Predicting and preventing sudden cardiac death. Circulation 2011;124(5):651–6.
7. Hainline B, Drezner JA, Baggish A, et al. Interassociation consensus statement on cardiovascular care of college student-athletes. J Am Coll Cardiol 2016;67(25):2981–95.
8. Maron BJ, Zipes DP, Kovacs RJ. Eligibility and disqualification recommendations for competitive athletes with cardiovascular abnormalities: preamble, principles, and general considerations. J Am Coll Cardiol 2015;66(21):2343–9.
9. Link MS, Myerburg RJ, Estes NAM. Eligibility and disqualification recommendations for competitive athletes with cardiovascular abnormalities: Task Force 12: emergency action plans, resuscitation, cardiopulmonary resuscitation, and automated external defibrillators. J Am Coll Cardiol 2015;66(21):2434–8.
10. Broch K, Murbræch K, Andreassen AK, et al. Contemporary outcome in patients with idiopathic dilated cardiomyopathy. Am J Cardiol 2015;116(6):952–9.
11. Goldberger JJ, Subačius H, Patel T, et al. Sudden cardiac death risk stratification in patients with non-ischemic dilated cardiomyopathy. J Am Coll Cardiol 2014;63(18):1879–89.
12. Bardy GH, Lee KL, Mark DB, et al. Amiodarone or an implantable cardioverter-defibrillator for congestive heart failure. N Engl J Med 2005;352(3):225–37.
13. Kadish A, Dyer A, Daubert JP, et al. Prophylactic defibrillator implantation in patients with nonischemic dilated cardiomyopathy. N Engl J Med 2004;350(21):2151–8.
14. Køber L, Thune JJ, Nielsen JC, et al. Defibrillator implantation in patients with nonischemic systolic heart failure. N Engl J Med 2016;375(13):1221–30.
15. Golwala H, Bajaj NS, Arora G, et al. Implantable cardioverter-defibrillator for nonischemic cardiomyopathy: an updated meta-analysis. Circulation 2017;135(2):201–3.
16. Di Marco A, Anguera I, Schmitt M, et al. Late gadolinium enhancement and the risk for ventricular arrhythmias or sudden death in dilated cardiomyopathy. JACC Heart Fail 2017;5(1):28–38.
17. Epstein AE, DiMarco JP, Ellenbogen KA, et al. 2012 ACCF/AHA/HRS focused update incorporated into the ACCF/AHA/HRS 2008 guidelines for device-based therapy of cardiac rhythm abnormalities: a report of the American College of Cardiology Foundation/American Heart Association Task Force on Practice Guide. J Am Coll Cardiol 2013;61(3):e6–75.
18. Bristow MR, Saxon LA, Boehmer J, et al. Cardiac-resynchronization therapy with or without an implantable defibrillator in advanced chronic heart failure. N Engl J Med 2004;350(21):2140–50.
19. Berger RE, Ellenbogen KA, Stevenson WG. Implantable cardioverter–defibrillators in nonischemic cardiomyopathy. N Engl J Med 2016;375(23):2290–2.

20. Japp AG, Gulati A, Cook SA, et al. The diagnosis and evaluation of dilated cardiomyopathy. J Am Coll Cardiol 2016;67(25):2996–3010.

21. Arbustini E, Disertori M, Narula J. Primary prevention of sudden arrhythmic death in dilated cardiomyopathy. JACC Heart Fail 2017;5(1):39–43.

22. Cantillon DJ, Stein KM, Markowitz SM, et al. Predictive value of microvolt T-wave alternans in patients with left ventricular dysfunction. J Am Coll Cardiol 2007;50(2):166–73.

23. Rosenthal TM, Stahls PF, Abi Samra FM, et al. T-peak to T-end interval for prediction of ventricular tachyarrhythmia and mortality in a primary prevention population with systolic cardiomyopathy. Heart Rhythm 2015;12(8):1789–97.

24. Tracy CM, Epstein AE, Darbar D, et al. 2012 ACCF/AHA/HRS focused update of the 2008 guidelines for device-based therapy of cardiac rhythm abnormalities: a report of the American College of Cardiology Foundation/American Heart Association Task Force on practice guidelines and the Heart Rhythm Society. Circulation 2012;126(14):1784–800.

25. Merlo M, Pyxaras SA, Pinamonti B, et al. Prevalence and prognostic significance of left ventricular reverse remodeling in dilated cardiomyopathy receiving tailored medical treatment. J Am Coll Cardiol 2011;57(13):1468–76.

26. Adler A, Halkin A, Viskin S. Wearable cardioverter-defibrillators. Circulation 2013;127(7):854–60.

27. Cerrone M, Priori SG. Genetics of sudden death: focus on inherited channelopathies. Eur Heart J 2011;32(17):2109–18.

28. Schwartz PJ, Stramba-Badiale M, Crotti L, et al. Prevalence of the congenital long-QT syndrome. Circulation 2009;120(18):1761–7.

29. Ackerman MJ, Priori SG, Willems S, et al. HRS/EHRA expert consensus statement on the state of genetic testing for the channelopathies and cardiomyopathies. Heart Rhythm 2011;8(8):1308.

30. Priori SG, Napolitano C, Schwartz PJ, et al. Association of long QT syndrome loci and cardiac events among patients treated with beta-blockers. JAMA 2004;292(11):1341–4.

31. Priori SG, Schwartz PJ, Napolitano C, et al. Risk stratification in the long-QT syndrome. N Engl J Med 2003;348(19):1866–74.

32. Napolitano C, Bloise R, Monteforte N, et al. Sudden cardiac death and genetic ion channelopathies: long QT, Brugada, short QT, catecholaminergic polymorphic ventricular tachycardia, and idiopathic ventricular fibrillation. Circulation 2012;125(16):2027–34.

33. Antzelevitch C, Brugada P, Borggrefe M, et al. Brugada syndrome: report of the second consensus conference. Heart Rhythm 2005;2(4):429–40.

34. Priori SG, Wilde AA, Horie M, et al. HRS/EHRA/APHRS expert consensus statement on the diagnosis and management of patients with inherited primary arrhythmia syndromes. Heart Rhythm 2013;10(12):1932–63.

35. Priori SG, Gasparini M, Napolitano C, et al. Risk stratification in Brugada syndrome: results of the PRELUDE (PRogrammed ELectrical stimUlation preDictive valuE) registry. J Am Coll Cardiol 2012;59(1):37–45.

36. Gehi AK, Duong TD, Metz LD, et al. Risk stratification of individuals with the Brugada electrocardiogram: a meta-analysis. J Cardiovasc Electrophysiol 2006;17(6):577–83.

37. van der Werf C, Wilde AAM. Catecholaminergic polymorphic ventricular tachycardia: from bench to bedside. Heart 2013;99(7):497–504.

38. Hayashi M, Denjoy I, Extramiana F, et al. Incidence and risk factors of arrhythmic events in catecholaminergic polymorphic ventricular tachycardia. Circulation 2009;119(18):2426–34.

39. Mazzanti A, Kanthan A, Monteforte N, et al. Novel insight into the natural history of short QT syndrome. J Am Coll Cardiol 2014;63(13):1300–8.

Role of Cardiac Imaging in Evaluating Risk for Sudden Cardiac Death

Constancia Macatangay, MD, Juan F. Viles-Gonzalez, MD,
Jeffrey J. Goldberger, MD*

KEYWORDS

- Sudden cardiac death • Risk stratification • Cardiac imaging • Ventricular tachycardia
- Ventricular fibrillation

KEY POINTS

- Sudden cardiac death (SCD) continues to be a major cause of death from cardiovascular disease.
- Our ability to predict patients at the highest risk of developing lethal ventricular arrhythmias remains limited.
- Despite all the recent studies evaluating different risk stratification tools, there is no single optimal strategy for risk stratification.
- Cardiac imaging provides the opportunity to assess left ventricular ejection fraction, strain, fibrosis, and sympathetic innervation, all of which are pathophysiologically related to risk for SCD.
- Further studies are required to identify the optimal imaging platform for risk assessment for SCD.

INTRODUCTION

Sudden cardiac death (SCD) is defined as death from an unexpected circulatory arrest occurring within an hour of the onset of symptoms.[1] It is a major public health concern that accounts for 18.5% of all natural deaths and 50% of all cardiovascular deaths in the United States.[2,3] This proportion has remained unchanged despite the overall decreasing cardiovascular mortality in recent decades. In 2011, the incidence of emergency medical services–assessed out-of-hospital cardiac arrests (OHCA) in the United States is approximately 326,200. Twenty-five percent of the emergency medical services–treated OHCA have no symptoms before the onset of cardiac arrest.[4,5]

Certain patient groups are known to be at a particularly increased risk for SCD. The annual incidence of SCD increases with advancing age, with it being 100-fold less frequent in people less than 30 years of age (0.001%) compared with those older than 35 years.[6,7] According to the Department of Defense Cardiovascular Death Registry, the US incidence of sudden unexplained death per 100,000 person-years is 1.2 for persons aged 18 to 35 years and 2.0 for persons greater than 35 years of age.[8] SCD risk is higher in men. In the Framingham Heart Study, at 45 years of age, lifetime risks were 10.9% for men (95% CI, 9.4%–12.5%) and 2.8% for women (95% CI, 2.1%–3.5%).[9] In the Oregon Sudden Unexpected Death Study, the annual incidence of sudden cardiac arrest (SCA) among blacks was more than 2-fold higher than in whites for both men and women.[10] Finally, a family history of cardiac arrest in a first-degree relative (parents, offspring, siblings) is associated with a 2-fold increase in risk of cardiac arrest.[5]

CONCEPTS IN RISK STRATIFICATION

SCD includes arrhythmic and nonarrhythmic causes. Arrhythmic SCD may be due to ventricular

Cardiovascular Division, Department of Medicine, Miller School of Medicine, University of Miami, 1120 NW 14th Street, Miami, FL 33136, USA
* Corresponding author.
E-mail address: j-goldberger@miami.edu

fibrillation (VF), ventricular tachycardia (VT) or pulseless electric activity/asystole. Among emergency medical services–treated OHCA, 23% have an initial rhythm of VF or VT.[5] Epidemiologic studies show that there has been a decline in cardiac arrest caused by VT/VF and an increasing trend in the occurrence of pulseless electric activity/asystole.[11] The cause of this trend is unclear; however, possible explanations include improved therapies to prevent and treat coronary artery disease, increased use of beta-blockers and implantable cardioverter-defibrillators (ICDs) in high-risk patients, aging population, increased prevalence of end-stage cardiovascular disease with severe comorbidities, and a majority of OHCAs occurring at home.[12–17] Recent data demonstrated a pulseless electric activity incidence of 19% to 23%, with approximately 50% of patients initially having asystole.[18]

Current risk stratification is focused on SCD due to VT/VF (SCD-VT-VF) because the pathophysiologic understanding, outcomes, and available treatments for this are superior to those for pulseless electric activity/asystole.[15] There are several key concepts in the risk stratification of SCD that must be highlighted to understand the importance and use of the different modalities being used to evaluate patients.

First, SCD is a complex state that it is multifactorial and is associated with a continuous risk function.[19] Therefore, ideal SCD risk stratification should minimize dichotomization into high or low risk. Second, risk functions are dynamic. The quantitative and qualitative durability of a risk marker changes over time. Thus, it is likely that repeated measures need to be made over time. The timing of risk assessment is an important variable in risk stratification.[20] This is exemplified by the VALIANT study (Valsartan in Acute Myocardial Infarction), which reported the SCD risk after a myocardial infarction (MI). The monthly risk of SCD declined from 1.4% the first month to 0.14% after 2 years.[21] Third, is the important concept of competing risks for nonsudden death. Many risk factors for SCD are also significantly associated with death owing to other cardiovascular or noncardiovascular causes.[22] Thus, the risk for nonsudden death can modify the relationship between arrhythmia risk and mortality.[23]

CARDIAC IMAGING AND SUDDEN CARDIAC DEATH PATHOPHYSIOLOGY

The majority of SCD victims either have no known heart disease or heart disease with normal or mildly impaired cardiac function. Between 45% and 50% of those who experience SCD are not previously diagnosed with cardiovascular disease,

and therefore SCD is the first manifestation of heart disease.[24–26] The data on the different pathologies underlying SCD is based on autopsy series and cardiac evaluations in cardiac arrest survivors. The epidemiology of SCD directly relates to its underlying pathophysiology. Coronary artery disease is the most common underlying cause of SCD in the Western world, comprising 75% to 80% of the cases.[27,28] In the Framingham Study, preexisting coronary artery disease was associated with 2.8- to 5.3-fold increases in SCD risk,[29] and women and men had a 4- to 10-fold higher risk of SCD, respectively, after experiencing an MI.[30,31] Cardiomyopathies and ion channelopathies account for most of the remaining causes.[27,28] Despite evaluation, no cardiac abnormality is found in 5% of SCD cases.

The pathophysiology of SCD is complex and involves an interaction between an underlying substrate and a transient trigger. Myocardial cell death owing to toxins, ischemia, infectious agents, or chronic volume/pressure overload leads to scar formation, alterations in chamber geometry, and anatomic and electrical remodeling. The electrophysiologic alterations in this vulnerable substrate initiate and maintain VT/VF likely via a reentrant mechanism, although abnormal automaticity, triggered activity, or a combination of these mechanisms may occur. Factors that are known to trigger or modulate VT/VF include sympathetic activation, ischemia, metabolic disturbance, ion channel abnormalities, and/or acute hemodynamic stress. The interaction between the various substrates and triggering events induces electric instability and lethal ventricular arrhythmias, followed by hemodynamic collapse.[27,32]

The role of cardiac imaging in the risk stratification for SCD lies in its ability to assess the presence of structural arrhythmogenic factors that initiate or maintain VT/VF. This review article focuses on cardiac imaging for risk stratification to identify patients susceptible to SCD-VT/VF.

EVALUATION OF ARRHYTHMIC SUBSTRATES

Ventricular arrhythmias are felt to originate in diseased myocardium, particularly regions of myocardial scar and surrounding border regions.[33–35] The slow and heterogeneous electrical conduction that may occur within or adjacent to the scar are central to the development of VT and VF. Thus, the evaluation and quantification of myocardial scar provide useful tools for risk stratification. There are, however, limitations to the use of scar as a risk measure of SCD-VT/VF: not all scar is arrhythmogenic and electric properties of scar may evolve over time.[36]

Left Ventricular Systolic Function

Global left ventricular (LV) systolic function is a crude marker for overall scar burden. LV ejection fraction (LVEF) is the most widely used measure of LV systolic function with a long history.[37,38] Since the 1980s, the link between SCD-VT/VF and LVEF in patients with LV dysfunction after an MI has been established.[37,38] Large clinical trials have established mortality reduction with ICD use in patients with a reduced LVEF.[39–43] Thus, despite its limited sensitivity and specificity, LVEF has been a mainstay of current clinical guidelines in the determination of patients who are at high risk for SCD.[44,45] Although LVEF is related to scar burden, the strength of the relationship is weak.[46]

LVEF has several advantages as a risk stratification tool for SCD-VT/VF, such as ease of measurement and interpretation by physicians, and availability in a large number of patients. Different cardiac imaging modalities have been used for the assessment of LVEF.

Echocardiographic LVEF measurement has been the most commonly used tool in clinical practice because it does not involve the use of ionizing radiation and is highly accessible and portable. Many methods to measure LVEF using echocardiography have been developed. Methods differ based on the type of image used (M-mode, 2-dimensional, 3-dimensional), the measurements needed, and geometric assumptions. The American Society of Echocardiography recommends the biplane method of disks (modified Simpson method) for measuring LVEF.[47] Limitations of this technique include the need for adequate visualization of the blood–endocardial border and good apical windows to allow accurate measurement. Three-dimensional echocardiography is now being more commonly used for LVEF assessment. In this technique, data are acquired over several heartbeats and minimal assumptions of the LV cavity shape are made. It has been shown to be less variable and more accurate than the other echocardiographic methods, when compared with MRI as a reference standard.[48]

The 2 most common methods in nuclear cardiac imaging used to calculate LVEF are radionuclide angiography (blood pool imaging) and gated myocardial perfusion imaging with either single photon emission computed tomography (SPECT) or PET. The accuracy of LVEF assessment is approximately ±2% to 6% for radionuclide angiography versus in excess of ± 10% for both visual estimation and calculation by Simpson's method with echocardiography.[49,50] LVEF assessment in the patients enrolled in the SCD-HEFT trial (Sudden Cardiac Death in Heart Failure Trial) showed that LVEF measurement tended to be skewed toward higher values among patients who underwent radionuclide scan, whereas echocardiography and contrast angiography seemed to be more symmetric. Despite such trend, there were no differences in survival between patients enrolled based on radionuclide angiography versus echocardiography (hazard ratio [HR], 1.06; 95% CI, 0.88–1.28), radionuclide angiography versus contrast angiography (HR 1.25; 95% CI, 0.97–1.62), or echocardiography versus contrast angiography (HR 1.18; 95% CI, 0.94–1.48).[41,51]

MRI and computed tomography scan are also currently used for LVEF measurement. Both offer high-contrast resolution and high signal to noise ratio, and the endocardial border is more well-defined. However, owing to the limited availability and use of contrast or radiation, these modalities are not commonly used.

Despite the advantages of LVEF as a risk stratification tool for SCD, it has a number of limitations. Large population-based studies and postinfarction trials provide information on the sensitivity of the LVEF to predict SCD.[52] The Maastricht Circulatory Arrest Registry reported that for patients in whom LVEF had been determined before cardiac arrest, 52% had an LVEF of greater than 30% and 32% had an LVEF of greater than 40%. Of those patients with a cardiac history, overt heart failure was present in only 26% of cases.[53] The Oregon Sudden Unexpected Death study had similar results, wherein an LVEF of greater than 35% was found in 70% of sudden death victims who had LVEF measured before their cardiac arrest.[26] The sensitivity of LVEF for the prediction of sudden death in several studies of acute MI patients show a median sensitivity of approximately 45%.[54–59]

Because the LVEF is also a powerful predictor of overall mortality and non-SCD, its specificity as a predictor for SCD-VT/VF is limited.[60] In fact, the majority of the post-MI trials show that LVEF is not associated with incremental relative risk for sudden death versus nonsudden death.[52,55,57–63] This concept is exhibited by the recent studies showing that only 11% to 35% of post-MI patients with ICDs implanted for primary prevention of SCD, that is, LVEF as the main criterion for ICD implantation, actually receive appropriate ICD therapy in the succeeding years. A recent meta-analysis of 6088 patients with nonischemic dilated cardiomyopathy (LVEF range, 17%–45%) showed that the LVEF association to arrhythmic events had an odds ratio of 2.86, a sensitivity of 71.1%, and specificity of 50.5%.[64]

Finally, LVEF can vary with different loading conditions owing to changes in adrenergic drive or intravascular volumes.[65,66] Like all other risk factors, LVEF changes over time in response to medical therapy or lack thereof.[67]

In summary, impaired LVEF is a significant component underlying SCD risk; however, it should not be used as a sole criterion to stratify patient risk for SCD.

Left Ventricular Size

Because patients with a very low LVEF comprise a minority of the cases of SCD in the general population,[25,26] clinical markers are needed that can help to address the heterogeneity of risk in relation to LV function. The LV diameter is easily obtained during echocardiography at the time of LVEF measurement. Previous studies have established the importance of LV size with regard to cardiac mortality. In fact, the MADIT-CRT trial (Multicenter Automatic Defibrillator Implantation Trial with Cardiac Resynchronization Therapy) showed a graded reduction in risk of death or heart failure with decreasing LV diastolic volumes.[68] From a large community-based study of SCD (The Oregon Sudden Unexpected Death Study), the LV diameter was jointly evaluated with LVEF for risk stratification of SCD.[69] LV dilatation was classified as mild if the LV internal dimension in diastole was 60 to 63 mm in men and 54 to 57 mm in women; moderate if 64 to 68 mm in men and 58 to 61 mm in women; and severe if 69 mm or greater in men and 62 mm or greater in women. Multivariate analysis showed that severe LV dilatation was an independent predictor of SCD with an odds ratio of 2.5 (95% CI, 1.03–5.9; $P = .04$). In addition, people with both an LVEF of 35% or less and severe LV dilatation had higher odds for SCD compared with those with low LVEF only (odds ratio, 3.8 [95% CI, 1.5–10.2] for both vs 1.7 [95% CI, 1.2–2.5] for low LVEF only), suggesting that severe LV dilatation independently increases SCD risk.[69]

Strain Echocardiography

Two-dimensional speckle-tracking analysis is based on the detection and the motion tracking of natural acoustic myocardial reflections and interference patterns. The tracking system permits the measurement of myocardial deformation or strain. Strain parameters may be specific or individualized for each myocardial segment or averaged and expressed as global strain. The global longitudinal strain (GLS) is the mean value of segmental myocardial deformation.[70] Strain imaging is readily measured during routine echocardiography and is used to reflect myocardial heterogeneity. Strain imaging is a promising marker of SCD risk in patients with normal or mildly impaired LV function. Its value lies in its ability to detect subclinical ventricular dysfunction and identification of scar beyond wall motion abnormalities.

In a prospective, multicenter study of 569 patients more than 40 days after MI, strain echocardiography predicted arrhythmic events independently of LVEF (HR, 1.7; 95% CI, 1.2–2.5; $P<.01$). A combination of mechanical dispersion of greater than 75 ms and GLS worse than -16%, showed the best positive predictive value for arrhythmic events compared with LVEF alone (21% vs 11%), particularly in patients with an LVEF of greater than 35%.[71] In another study with 308 patients with heart failure, receiving operating characteristic analysis identified an optimal GLS cutoff value of -10%, with a 73% sensitivity and 61% specificity (area under the curve, 0.76) for 1-year occurrence of arrhythmic events. Furthermore, when GLS was added to LVEF, there was a significant increase in χ^2 values for the association with ventricular arrhythmic events (17–21; $P = .04$).[70]

In a study of 569 post-MI patients,[72] echocardiography was performed a median of 4 months after MI. Sustained VT or SCD occurred in 15 patients at median follow-up of 30 months. These patients had lower LVEF (48 ± 17% vs 55 ± 11%; $P<.001$), reduced global strain ($-14.8 ± 4.7\%$ vs $-18.2 ± 3.7\%$; $P = .001$), and increased mechanical dispersion (63 ± 25 ms vs 42 ± 17 ms; $P<.001$). Mechanical dispersion and the postsystolic strain index discriminated those with versus without an arrhythmic event with a C-statistic of 0.75.

Radionuclide Imaging

Nuclear imaging has the ability to detect different pathophysiological aspects of the arrhythmic substrate. SPECT and PET allow the evaluation of perfusion, scar, metabolism, and sympathetic innervation. The relative tracer myocardial uptake during rest and stress provides information on the size of resting perfusion defects (scar or hibernating myocardium), stress perfusion defects (scar, hibernating myocardium, and/or ischemia), and their reversibility (ischemia).[73,74]

The presence and size of resting perfusion defects in patients with ischemic cardiomyopathy (ICM) have been shown to correlate with the inducibility of ventricular arrhythmias during an electrophysiologic study.[75,76] VTs were found to originate close to the border of the resting perfusion defects.[77] Moreover, it was demonstrated that impairment of thallium uptake, signifying zone of infarct, accurately predicted endocardial voltage-defined scar, which was the site of successful ablation in all patients.[78]

With the ability of nuclear imaging to identify areas of scar, a vulnerable substrate integral to the pathophysiology of ventricular arrhythmias, several studies have correlated nuclear imaging with VT/VF and SCD.[79,80] In a study of 51 patients who had received cardiac resynchronization therapy for at least 6 months and underwent resting gated myocardial perfusion SPECT, survival analysis showed that the survival probability for VT/VF in those with an LVEF of greater than 29%, scar areas of less than 23%, and LV dyssynchrony phase standard deviation of less than 50° was significantly better than others (HR, 5.16; 95% CI, 1.20–22.16).[80] In a secondary prevention population study that included survivors of SCA with ICM the relationship among ischemia, viability, scar, and recurrent arrhythmic events was studied.[81] Patients with SPECT-detected scar involving more than 1 vascular territory had significantly higher recurrent event rates when compared with those with less extensive or no scar (54% vs 16%; P<.05). Multivariate analysis showed that an LVEF of 30% or less and the presence of extensive scar were the only independent predictors of death and recurrent ventricular arrhythmias. In patients with non ischemic cardiomyopathy (NICM), it was shown that the presence of myocardial scar on SPECT further risk stratifies patients with low heart-mediastinal ratio (HMR) of less than 1.6 detected with ^{123}I-meta-iodobenzyl-guanidine (^{123}I-mIBG) imaging.[82,83] Among the 317 patients from the ADMIRE-HF cohort (AdreView Myocardial Imaging for Risk Evaluation in Heart Failure), those with a late HMR of less than 1.6 but a summed rest score of 8 or less had fewer episodes of sustained VT, resuscitated SCA, and appropriate ICD therapies when compared with those with a summed rest score of greater than 8 (3.9% vs 11.9%; P = .001).

Cardiac Magnetic Resonance

Cardiac magnetic resonance (CMR) provides good myocardial tissue characterization and has greater spatial and temporal resolution than nuclear imaging, thus an excellent tool in quantifying LVEF, mass, structure, and fibrosis.[84] CMR late gadolinium enhancement (LGE) imaging allows detection of contrast accumulation in areas of infarction or fibrosis owing to slower contrast kinetics and a greater volume of distribution in the extracellular matrix. Fibrosis extent is then quantified as a percentage of total LV mass using dedicated software.[85]

Heterogeneity in scar tissue is thought to create electrical dispersion and areas of slow conduction that form the substrate for electrical reentry and malignant arrhythmia.[86] The presence and extent of fibrosis on LGE imaging has been shown to correlate with a greater probability of inducible VT, increased arrhythmic risk, and composite cardiovascular outcomes both in ICM and other cardiomyopathies.[46,87–96]

Using CMR, the infarcted myocardial region can be divided into a central core infarct zone and a periinfarct gray zone extending both circumferentially to the viable remote region as well as transmurally to the viable subepicardium. This gray zone is suggested to be heterogeneous islands of viable myocardium and fibrotic tissue, and has been found to be related to arrhythmogenic substrates in electrophysiologic studies. Although there is a consensus about the prognostic value of scar among all the studies involving CMR in ICM, there is a disagreement with regard to the pathologic correlate of the gray zone and which type of scar—total scar, core infarct, or periinfarct—is the most predictive of endpoints. Various approaches have been used.[97] Nevertheless, this characterization has been used to identify conduction gaps[98] that may provide substrate for VT, as well as direct identification of VT circuits using computer modeling of the imaging data.[99,100]

The role of LGE for risk stratification was evaluated in a prospective cohort of 137 patients undergoing evaluation for possible ICD placement. Adverse events were reported as death or ICD discharge. In patients with an LVEF of greater than 30%, significant scarring (>5% LV) identified a high-risk cohort similar in risk to those with an LVEF of 30% or less. Conversely an LVEF of 30% or less and minimal or no scarring identified a low-risk cohort similar in risk to those with an LVEF of greater than 30%.[101]

NICM includes various etiologies, namely, idiopathic dilated, hypertrophic (HCM), infectious, neuromuscular, infiltrative, postpartum. In patients with dilated cardiomyopathy, it is not uncommon to have LGE on CMR imaging.[102] In fact, it was shown that up to 71% of patients have scar with midwall pattern hyperenhancement and, less commonly, an epicardial pattern. Subendocardial injury was seen in 17% of patients and attributed to embolic events.[87] Several studies showed that aside from scar, the extent of scar (transmurality or percentage of LV mass) was most predictive of outcomes.[87–89,101–105]

Although LGE has been an established method for CMR assessment of scar, it relies on regional segregation of tissue characteristics to generate imaging contrast. Thus, in cardiomyopathies with diffuse and global inflammation, fibrosis, hypertrophy, and infiltration, LGE might be of limited value. T1 mapping is a CMR technique, which allows the detection of diffuse myocardial conditions by measurement of T1 values, which directly correspond with variations in intrinsic myocardial tissue properties and extracellular volume. Aside from its ability to detect diffuse myocardial disease, it also complements LGE in visualization of the regional changes in early and advanced myocardial disease.[105] The role of T1 mapping in the assessment of ventricular arrhythmia risk has been recently studied. In a prospective longitudinal study, 130 patients with either ICM or NICM receiving ICD underwent myocardial tissue characterization using T1 mapping and conventional LGE.[104] T1 mapping showed independent prediction of ventricular arrhythmia in both ICM and NICM cardiomyopathies (HR, 1.10; 95% CI, 1.04–1.16). Other factors that were significantly associated with the primary endpoint of ICD therapy or documented sustained ventricular arrhythmia were ICD implantation for secondary prevention (HR, 1.7; 95% CI, 1.01–1.91) and gray zone LGE index (HR, 1.36; 95% CI, 1.15–1.61).

SCD is a common cause of death in patients with HCM. Established risk factors associated with SCD include unexplained syncope, a family history of SCD, an interventricular septum thickness of greater than 3 cm, abnormal blood pressure response to exercise, and nonsustained VT. Recently, it has been shown that LV mass index, maximal LV wall thickness, and myocardial fibrosis are also predictive of SCD.[106] A pooled number of 1915 HCM patients (30 with SCD and 36 cardiac deaths) showed that LV scar is an independent predictor of inducible VT,[93] SCD,[94,95] or cardiac death.[94,96] The most current study with 594 HCM patients showed that the extent of LGE was independently associated with increased risk for SCD even after the traditional clinical risk factors are controlled (adjusted OR, 1.25/5% LGE increase; $P = .002$).[95] Furthermore, the absence of LGE was associated with a low likelihood of adverse events (adjusted odds ratio, 0.59; 95% CI:0.34–0.99). CMR may also provide incremental diagnostic information in patients with unusual forms of HCM (**Fig. 1**).

Myocarditis is an acute or chronic inflammatory myocardial disease that may be triggered by toxins, chemotherapy, or infectious diseases. CMR has played a major role in the diagnosis and prognostication of patients with myocarditis. It can visualize scar on LGE and tissue edema (T1 mapping) in the acute phase of inflammation. Grun and colleagues[107] enrolled 222 patients with biopsy-proven viral myocarditis and CMR in their study. These investigators showed that none of the patients without LGE had SCD (negative predictive value, 100%), irrespective of LVEF or LV volumes. Hence, the absence of LGE might identify patients at particularly low risk for SCD.

CMR has had an increasing role in the diagnosis, and possibly prognostication, of other types of cardiomyopathies, such as arrhythmogenic right ventricular dysplasia, cardiac sarcoidosis, amyloidosis, cardiomyopathies associated with neuromuscular disease, and cardiac siderosis. Currently, there is limited evidence with regard to risk stratification for SCD.

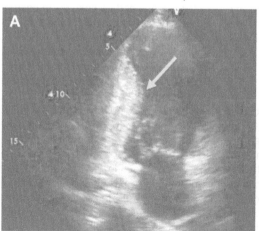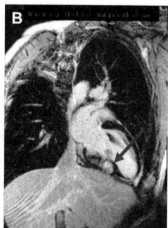

Fig. 1. (*A*) An echocardiographic 2-chamber view with poor visualization of the endocardial borders, but slight thickening of the midinferior wall (*yellow arrow*). (*B*) An MRI demonstrating focal thickening of the midinferior wall with a focal area of hyperenhancement at that site (*red arrow*).

MYOCARDIAL SYMPATHETIC DENERVATION AND THE RISK OF SUDDEN CARDIAC DEATH

Both cardiac mechanical and electrical function are influenced by the balance between sympathetic and parasympathetic inputs.[108] Alterations in the cardiac sympathetic activity have been linked to disease progression and increased mortality in cardiovascular disease. Furthermore, the autonomic nervous system plays an integral role in the development of ventricular arrhythmias, particularly in patients with MI or LV dysfunction.[109] Therefore, measures of autonomic tone have been considered prime targets for risk stratification tools.[36]

Radiolabeled norepinephrine analogs have been developed to quantify myocardial sympathetic innervation in vivo. The principle of innervation imaging is based on the uptake, storage, and release of norepinephrine, which is mediated by presynaptic sympathetic nerve terminals in response to variations of sympathetic drive. To date, most commonly used tracers are norepinephrine analogues [123]I-*m*IBG for SPECT and [^{11}C]hydroxyephedrine for PET. The [123]I-*m*IBG studies on prognostic significance of cardiac sympathetic denervation examined predominantly the global HMR of [123]I-*m*IBG.[84]

In a cohort study of 90 patients with ICM and NICM, HMR was found to be the strongest predictor of survival over short-term follow-up.[110] Subsequent to this finding, [123]I-*m*IBG HMR was found to be the most significant clinical predictor of cardiac mortality in ICM and NICM over a mean follow-up of approximately 4.5 years.[111] This predictive capacity of global [123]I-*m*IBG was independent of the etiology of LV dysfunction, and also provided prognostic value among those with only mildly reduced LVEF (40%–50%).

The ADMIRE-HF study is the largest prospective study evaluating global [123]I-*m*IBG uptake and clinical outcomes. [123]I-*m*IBG and SPECT perfusion were done in 961 patients with New York Heart Association functional class II or III heart failure and an LVEF of 35% or less.[82] The median follow-up was 17 months and the majority of patients (66%) had ICM. The primary composite endpoints of heart failure progression, all arrhythmic events, and cardiac death occurred more frequently among those with a global reduction in myocardial [123]I-*m*IBG uptake, defined as a late HMR of less than 1.6. The 2-year event rate was 15% for an HMR of 1.60 or greater and 37% for an HMR less than 1.60. Sudden death, resuscitated SCA, and appropriate ICD discharges (including shock and antitachycardia pacing) were a small portion of the total composite endpoints. The frequency of arrhythmic events, the majority of which were nonsustained VT, was significantly

higher among those with an HMR less than 1.6 (HR for arrhythmic events, 0.37; $P = .02$). In the PARAPET prospective study (Prediction of ARrhythmic Events with Positron Emission Tomography), 204 patients with ICM and an LVEF of 35% or less had PET imaging with [^{11}C]hydroxyephedrine. With 4 years of follow-up, the amount of viable but denervated myocardium was independently predictive of the development of VT or arrhythmic death.[112]

A subanalysis of the ADMIRE-HF demonstrated improved risk stratification of [123]I-*m*IBG over LVEF.[83] A late HMR less than 1.6 conferred a greater risk of death and arrhythmic events across all LVEF subgroups. Among subjects with a relatively preserved LVEF of greater than 40%, an HMR greater than 1.6 was associated with excellent prognosis and no mortality or arrhythmic events in the follow-up period. In contrast, individuals having an LVEF greater than 40% and a late HMR less than 1.6 had a 7.5% per 100 person-years risk of death and composite arrhythmic events. Another post hoc analysis of the ADMIRE-HF study showed a relationship between HMR on planar imaging and arrhythmic events (defined as composite of SCA, appropriate ICD therapy, resuscitated cardiac arrest, or sustained VT).[113] The composite arrhythmic event rate was 6.9% in 1 year and 9.4% in 2 years. An HMR less than 1.6 (HR, 3.5; 95% CI, 1.5–8), an LVEF less than 25% (HR, 1.9; 95% CI, 1.2–3.0), and a systolic blood pressure less than 120 mm Hg (HR, 1.2; 95% CI, 1.0–1.4) were independent predictors of arrhythmic events.

SUMMARY

SCD continues to be a major cause of death from cardiovascular disease. Our ability to predict patients at the greatest risk of developing lethal ventricular arrhythmias remains limited. Despite all the recent studies evaluating different risk stratification tools, there is no single optimal strategy for risk stratification. Cardiac imaging provides the opportunity to assess LVEF, strain, fibrosis, and sympathetic innervation, all of which are pathophysiologically related to risk for SCD. These modalities may play a role in the identification of vulnerable anatomic substrates that provide the pathophysiologic basis for SCD. Further studies are required to identify the optimal imaging platform for risk assessment for SCD.

REFERENCES

1. Zipes DP, Camm AJ, Borggrefe M, et al. ACC/AHA/ESC 2006 guidelines for management of patients

with ventricular arrhythmias and the prevention of sudden cardiac death: a report of the American College of Cardiology/American Heart Association Task Force and the European Society of Cardiology Committee for Practice Guidelines (Writing Committee to Develop Guidelines for Management of Patients With Ventricular Arrhythmias and the Prevention of Sudden Cardiac Death). J Am Coll Cardiol 2006;48:e247–346.

2. Myerburg RJ, Junttila MJ. Sudden cardiac death caused by coronary heart disease. Circulation 2012;125:1043–52.

3. Go AS, Mozaffarian D, Roger VL, et al. Heart disease and stroke statistics–2014 update: a report from the American Heart Association. Circulation 2014;129:e28–292.

4. Fishman GI, Chugh SS, Dimarco JP, et al. Sudden cardiac death prediction and prevention: report from a National Heart, Lung, and Blood Institute and Heart Rhythm Society Workshop. Circulation 2010;122:2335–48.

5. Mozaffarian D, Benjamin EJ, Go AS, et al. Heart disease and stroke Statistics—2015 update: a report from the American Heart Association. Circulation 2015;131:e29–322.

6. Stecker EC, Reinier K, Marijon E, et al. Public health burden of sudden cardiac death in the United States. Circ Arrhythm Electrophysiol 2014; 7:212–7.

7. Kong MH, Fonarow GC, Peterson ED, et al. Systematic review of the incidence of sudden cardiac death in the United States. J Am Coll Cardiol 2011; 57:794–801.

8. Eckart RE, Shry EA, Burke AP, et al. Sudden death in young adults: an autopsy-based series of a population undergoing active surveillance. J Am Coll Cardiol 2011;58:1254–61.

9. Bogle BM, Ning H, Mehrotra S, et al. Lifetime risk for sudden cardiac death in the community. J Am Heart Assoc 2016;5(7) [pii:e002398].

10. Reinier K, Nichols GA, Huertas-Vazquez A, et al. Distinctive clinical profile of blacks versus whites presenting with sudden cardiac arrest. Circulation 2015;132:380–7.

11. Hulleman M, Berdowski J, de Groot JR, et al. Implantable cardioverter-defibrillators have reduced the incidence of resuscitation for out-of-hospital cardiac arrest caused by lethal arrhythmias. Circulation 2012;126:815–21.

12. Bloch Thomsen PE, Jons C, Raatikainen MJ, et al. Long-term recording of cardiac arrhythmias with an implantable cardiac monitor in patients with reduced ejection fraction after acute myocardial infarction: the Cardiac Arrhythmias and Risk Stratification after Acute Myocardial Infarction (CARISMA) study. Circulation 2010; 122:1258–64.

13. Youngquist ST, Kaji AH, Niemann JT. Beta-blocker use and the changing epidemiology of out-of-hospital cardiac arrest rhythms. Resuscitation 2008;76:376–80.

14. Levantesi G, Scarano M, Marfisi R, et al. Meta-analysis of effect of statin treatment on risk of sudden death. Am J Cardiol 2007;100:1644–50.

15. Engdahl J, Bång A, Lindqvist J, et al. Factors affecting short- and long-term prognosis among 1069 patients with out-of-hospital cardiac arrest and pulseless electrical activity. Resuscitation 2001;51:17–25.

16. Hansen SM, Hansen CM, Folke F, et al. Bystander defibrillation for out-of-hospital cardiac arrest in public vs residential locations. JAMA Cardiol 2017;2(5):507–14.

17. Chan PS, McNally B, Tang F, et al. Recent trends in survival from out-of-hospital cardiac arrest in the United States. Circulation 2014;130:1876–82.

18. Myerburg RJ, Halperin H, Egan DA, et al. Pulseless electric activity: definition, causes, mechanisms, management, and research priorities for the next decade: report from a National Heart, Lung, and Blood Institute workshop. Circulation 2013;128: 2532–41.

19. Buxton AE, Lee KL, Hafley GE, et al. Limitations of ejection fraction for prediction of sudden death risk in patients with coronary artery disease: lessons from the MUSTT study. J Am Coll Cardiol 2007; 50:1150–7.

20. Myerburg RJ, Reddy V, Castellanos A. Indications for implantable cardioverter-defibrillators based on evidence and judgment. J Am Coll Cardiol 2009;54:747–63.

21. Solomon SD, Zelenkofske S, McMurray JJ, et al. Sudden death in patients with myocardial infarction and left ventricular dysfunction, heart failure, or both. N Engl J Med 2005;352:2581–8.

22. Lloyd-Jones DM, Dyer AR, Wang R, et al. Risk factor burden in middle age and lifetime risks for cardiovascular and non-cardiovascular death (Chicago Heart Association Detection Project in Industry). Am J Cardiol 2007;99:535–40.

23. Goldberger JJ, Buxton AE, Cain M, et al. Risk stratification for arrhythmic sudden cardiac death: identifying the roadblocks. Circulation 2011;123: 2423–30.

24. Myerburg RJ, Kessler KM, Castellanos A. Sudden cardiac death. Structure, function, and time-dependence of risk. Circulation 1992;85:I2–10.

25. de Vreede-Swagemakers JJM, Gorgels APM, Dubois-Arbouw WI, et al. Out-of-hospital cardiac arrest in the 1990s: a population-based study in the Maastricht area on incidence, characteristics and survival. J Am Coll Cardiol 1997;30:1500–5.

26. Stecker EC, Vickers C, Waltz J, et al. Population-based analysis of sudden cardiac death with and

without left ventricular systolic dysfunction. J Am Coll Cardiol 2006;47:1161–6.

27. Deo R, Albert CM. Epidemiology and genetics of sudden cardiac death. Circulation 2012;125: 620–37.

28. Risgaard B, Winkel BG, Jabbari R, et al. Burden of sudden cardiac death in persons aged 1 to 49 years: nationwide study in Denmark. Circ Arrhythm Electrophysiol 2014;7:205–11.

29. Cupples LA, Gagnon DR, Kannel WB. Long- and short-term risk of sudden coronary death. Circulation 1992;85:I11–8.

30. Albert CM, Chae CU, Grodstein F, et al. Prospective study of sudden cardiac death among women in the United States. Circulation 2003;107: 2096–101.

31. Kannel WB, Wilson PW, D'Agostino RB, et al. Sudden coronary death in women. Am Heart J 1998; 136:205–12.

32. Goldberger JJ, Cain ME, Hohnloser SH, et al. American Heart Association/American College of Cardiology Foundation/Heart Rhythm Society Scientific Statement on Noninvasive Risk Stratification Techniques for identifying patients at risk for sudden cardiac death. J Am Coll Cardiol 2008;52: 1179–99.

33. Hsia HH, Marchlinski FE. Characterization of the electroanatomic substrate for monomorphic ventricular tachycardia in patients with nonischemic cardiomyopathy. Pacing Clin Electrophysiol 2002; 25:1114–27.

34. Stevenson WG, Brugada P, Waldecker B, et al. Clinical, angiographic, and electrophysiologic findings in patients with aborted sudden death as compared with patients with sustained ventricular tachycardia after myocardial infarction. Circulation 1985;71:1146–52.

35. Vassallo JA, Cassidy D, Simson MB, et al. Relation of late potentials to site of origin of ventricular tachycardia associated with coronary heart disease. Am J Cardiol 1985;55:985–9.

36. Deyell MW, Krahn AD, Goldberger JJ. Sudden cardiac death risk stratification. Circ Res 2015;116: 1907–18.

37. Bigger JT Jr, Fleiss JL, Kleiger R, et al. The relationships among ventricular arrhythmias, left ventricular dysfunction, and mortality in the 2 years after myocardial infarction. Circulation 1984;69:250–8.

38. Gradman A, Deedwania P, Cody R, et al. Predictors of total mortality and sudden death in mild to moderate heart failure. J Am Coll Cardiol 1989; 14:564–70.

39. Buxton AE, Lee KL, Fisher JD, et al. A randomized study of the prevention of sudden death in patients with coronary artery disease. Multicenter Unsustained Tachycardia Trial Investigators. N Engl J Med 1999;341:1882–90.

40. Moss AJ, Zareba W, Hall WJ, et al. Prophylactic implantation of a defibrillator in patients with myocardial infarction and reduced ejection fraction. N Engl J Med 2002;346:877–83.

41. Bardy GH, Lee KL, Mark DB, et al. Amiodarone or an implantable cardioverter-defibrillator for congestive heart failure. N Engl J Med 2005;352: 225–37.

42. Kadish A, Dyer A, Daubert JP, et al, for the Defibrillators in Non-ischemic Cardiomyopathy Treatment Evaluation (DEFINITE) Investigators. Prophylactic defibrillator implantation in patients with nonischemic dilated cardiomyopathy. N Engl J Med 2004; 350:2151–8.

43. Moss AM, Hall WJ, Cannom DS, et al. Improved survival with an implanted defibrillator in patients with coronary disease at high risk for ventricular arrhythmia. N Engl J Med 1996;335:1933–40.

44. Epstein AE, DiMarco JP, Ellenbogen KA, et al. 2012 ACCF/AHA/HRS focused update incorporated into the ACCF/AHA/HRS 2008 guidelines for device-based therapy of cardiac rhythm abnormalities: a report of the American College of Cardiology Foundation/American Heart Association Task Force on Practice Guidelines and the Heart Rhythm Society. J Am Coll Cardiol 2013;61:e6–75.

45. Tang AS, Ross H, Simpson CS, et al. Canadian Cardiovascular Society/Canadian Heart Rhythm Society position paper on implantable cardioverter defibrillator use in Canada. Can J Cardiol 2005; 21(Suppl A):11a–8a.

46. Bello D, Fieno DS, Kim RJ, et al. Infarct morphology identifies patients with substrate for sustained ventricular tachycardia. J Am Coll Cardiol 2005;45: 1104–8.

47. Lang RM, Bierig M, Devereux RB, et al. Recommendations for chamber quantification: a report from the American Society of Echocardiography's Guidelines and Standards Committee and The Chamber Quantification Writing Group, developed in conjunction with the European Association of Echocardiography, a branch of the European Society of Cardiology. J Am Soc Echocardiogr 2005;18: 1440–63.

48. Jenkins C, Bricknell K, Chan J, et al. Comparison of two- and three-dimensional echocardiography with sequential magnetic resonance imaging for evaluating left ventricular volume and ejection fraction over time in patients with healed myocardial infarction. Am J Cardiol 2007;99:300–6.

49. Wackers FJ, Berger HJ, Johnstone DE, et al. Multiple gated cardiac blood pool imaging for left ventricular ejection fraction: validation of the technique and assessment of variability. Am J Cardiol 1979;43:1159–66.

50. McGowan JH, Cleland JG. Reliability of reporting left ventricular systolic function by echocardiography: a

systematic review of 3 methods. Am Heart J 2003; 146:388–97.

51. Gula LJ, Klein GJ, Hellkamp AS, et al. Ejection fraction assessment and survival: an analysis of the sudden cardiac death in heart failure trial (SCD-HeFT). Am Heart J 2008;156:1196–200.

52. Buxton AE, Ellison KE, Lorvidhaya P, et al. Left ventricular ejection fraction for sudden death risk stratification and guiding implantable cardioverter-defibrillators implantation. J Cardiovasc Pharmacol 2010;55:450–5.

53. Gorgels AP, Gijsbers C, de Vreede-Swagemakers J, et al. Out-of-hospital cardiac arrest–the relevance of heart failure. The Maastricht Circulatory Arrest Registry. Eur Heart J 2003;24:1204–9.

54. Bailey JJ, Berson AS, Handelsman H, et al. Utility of current risk stratification tests for predicting major arrhythmic events after myocardial infarction. J Am Coll Cardiol 2001;38:1902–11.

55. Bauer A, Guzik P, Barthel P, et al. Reduced prognostic power of ventricular late potentials in post-infarction patients of the reperfusion era. Eur Heart J 2005;26:755–61.

56. Huikuri HV, Raatikainen MJ, Moerch-Joergensen R, et al. Prediction of fatal or near-fatal cardiac arrhythmia events in patients with depressed left ventricular function after an acute myocardial infarction. Eur Heart J 2009;30:689–98.

57. Huikuri HV, Tapanainen JM, Lindgren K, et al. Prediction of sudden cardiac death after myocardial infarction in the beta-blocking era. J Am Coll Cardiol 2003;42:652–8.

58. Makikallio TH, Barthel P, Schneider R, et al. Prediction of sudden cardiac death after acute myocardial infarction: role of Holter monitoring in the modern treatment era. Eur Heart J 2005;26:762–9.

59. Hohnloser SH, Klingenheben T, Zabel M, et al. Prevalence, characteristics and prognostic value during long-term follow-up of nonsustained ventricular tachycardia after myocardial infarction in the thrombolytic era. J Am Coll Cardiol 1999;33:1895–902.

60. Mukharji J, Rude RE, Poole WK, et al. Risk factors for sudden death after acute myocardial infarction: two-year follow-up. Am J Cardiol 1984;54:31–6.

61. Richards DA, Byth K, Ross DL, et al. What is the best predictor of spontaneous ventricular tachycardia and sudden death after myocardial infarction? Circulation 1991;83:756–63.

62. Copie X, Hnatkova K, Staunton A, et al. Predictive power of increased heart rate versus depressed left ventricular ejection fraction and heart rate variability for risk stratification after myocardial infarction. J Am Coll Cardiol 1996;27:270–6.

63. Farrell TG, Bashir Y, Cripps T, et al. Risk stratification for arrhythmic events in postinfarction patients based on heart rate variability, ambulatory electrocardiographic variables and the signal-averaged electrocardiogram. J Am Coll Cardiol 1991;18:687–97.

64. Goldberger JJ, Subacius H, Patel T, et al. Sudden cardiac death risk stratification in patients with non-ischemic dilated cardiomyopathy. J Am Coll Cardiol 2014;63:1879–89.

65. Carabello BA, Spann JF. The uses and limitations of end-systolic indexes of left ventricular function. Circulation 1984;69(5):1058–64.

66. Thomas JD, Popovic ZB. Assessment of left ventricular function by cardiac ultrasound. J Am Coll Cardiol 2006;48:2012–25.

67. Zecchin M, Merlo M, Pivetta A, et al. How can optimization of medical treatment avoid unnecessary implantable cardioverter-defibrillator implantations in patients with idiopathic dilated cardiomyopathy presenting with "SCD-HeFT criteria?". Am J Cardiol 2012;109:729–35.

68. Solomon SD, Foster E, Bourgoun M, et al. Effect of cardiac resynchronization therapy on reverse remodeling and relation to outcome: multicenter automatic defibrillator implantation trial: cardiac resynchronization therapy. Circulation 2010;122:985–92.

69. Narayanan K, Reinier K, Teodorescu C, et al. Left ventricular diameter and risk stratification for sudden cardiac death. J Am Heart Assoc 2014;3:e001193.

70. Iacoviello M, Puzzovivo A, Guida P, et al. Independent role of left ventricular global longitudinal strain in predicting prognosis of chronic heart failure patients. Echocardiography 2013;30:803–11.

71. Haugaa KH, Grenne BL, Eek CH, et al. Strain echocardiography improves risk prediction of ventricular arrhythmias after myocardial infarction. JACC Cardiovasc Imaging 2013;6:841–50.

72. Haugaa KH, Smedsrud MK, Steen T, et al. Mechanical dispersion assessed by myocardial strain in patients after myocardial infarction for risk prediction of ventricular arrhythmia. JACC Cardiovasc Imaging 2010;3:247–56.

73. Partington SL, Kwong RY, Dorbala S. Multimodality imaging in the assessment of myocardial viability. Heart Fail Rev 2011;16:381–95.

74. Roes SD, Kaandorp TA, Marsan NA, et al. Agreement and disagreement between contrast-enhanced magnetic resonance imaging and nuclear imaging for assessment of myocardial viability. Eur J Nucl Med Mol Imaging 2009;36:594–601.

75. Gradel C, Jain D, Batsford WP, et al. Relationship of scar and ischemia to the results of programmed electrophysiological stimulation in patients with coronary artery disease. J Nucl Cardiol 1997;4:379–86.

76. Sellers TD, Beller GA, Gibson RS, et al. Prevalence of ischemia by quantitative thallium-201 scintigraphy in patients with ventricular tachycardia or fibrillation inducible by programmed stimulation. Am J Cardiol 1987;59:828–32.

77. McFarland TM, McCarthy DM, Makler PT Jr, et al. Relation between site of origin of ventricular tachycardia and relative left ventricular myocardial perfusion and wall motion. Am J Cardiol 1983;51:1329–33.

78. Tian J, Smith MF, Ahmad G, et al. Integration of 3-dimensional scar models from SPECT to guide ventricular tachycardia ablation. J Nucl Med 2012;53:894–901.

79. Hung G-U, Huang W-S, Chen J. The prognostic value of myocardial perfusion imaging in predicting ventricular arrhythmia in patients with CRT. J Nucl Med 2015;56:240.

80. Hou P-N, Tsai S-C, Lin W-Y, et al. Relationship of quantitative parameters of myocardial perfusion SPECT and ventricular arrhythmia in patients receiving cardiac resynchronization therapy. Ann Nucl Med 2015;29:772–8.

81. van der Burg AE, Bax JJ, Boersma E, et al. Impact of viability, ischemia, scar tissue, and revascularization on outcome after aborted sudden death. Circulation 2003;108:1954–9.

82. Jacobson AF, Senior R, Cerqueira MD, et al. Myocardial iodine-123 meta-iodobenzylguanidine imaging and cardiac events in heart failure. Results of the prospective ADMIRE-HF (AdreView Myocardial Imaging for Risk Evaluation in Heart Failure) study. J Am Coll Cardiol 2010;55:2212–21.

83. Sood N, Al Badarin F, Parker M, et al. Resting perfusion MPI-SPECT combined with cardiac 123I-mIBG sympathetic innervation imaging improves prediction of arrhythmic events in non-ischemic cardiomyopathy patients: sub-study from the ADMIRE-HF trial. J Nucl Cardiol 2013;20:813–20.

84. Malhotra S, Canty JM Jr. Life-threatening ventricular arrhythmias: current role of imaging in diagnosis and risk assessment. J Nucl Cardiol 2016;23:1322–34.

85. Iacoviello M, Monitillo F. Non-invasive evaluation of arrhythmic risk in dilated cardiomyopathy: from imaging to electrocardiographic measures. World J Cardiol 2014;6:562–76.

86. Arenal A, Hernández J, Pérez-David E, et al. Do the spatial characteristics of myocardial scar tissue determine the risk of ventricular arrhythmias? Cardiovasc Res 2012;94:324–32.

87. Gao P, Yee R, Gula L, et al. Prediction of arrhythmic events in ischemic and dilated cardiomyopathy patients referred for implantable cardiac defibrillator: evaluation of multiple scar quantification measures for late gadolinium enhancement magnetic resonance imaging. Circ Cardiovasc Imaging 2012;5:448–56.

88. Nazarian S, Bluemke DA, Lardo AC, et al. Magnetic resonance assessment of the substrate for inducible ventricular tachycardia in nonischemic cardiomyopathy. Circulation 2005;112:2821–5.

89. Wu KC, Gerstenblith G, Guallar E, et al. Combined cardiac MRI and c-reactive protein levels identify a cohort at low risk for defibrillator firings and death. Circ Cardiovasc Imaging 2012;5:178–86.

90. Schmidt A, Azevedo CF, Cheng A, et al. Infarct tissue heterogeneity by magnetic resonance imaging identifies enhanced cardiac arrhythmia susceptibility in patients with left ventricular dysfunction. Circulation 2007;115:2006–14.

91. de Haan S, Meijers TA, Knaapen P, et al. Scar size and characteristics assessed by CMR predict ventricular arrhythmias in ischaemic cardiomyopathy: comparison of previously validated models. Heart 2011;97:1951–6.

92. Roes SD, Borleffs CJ, van der Geest RJ, et al. Infarct tissue heterogeneity assessed with contrast-enhanced MRI predicts spontaneous ventricular arrhythmia in patients with ischemic cardiomyopathy and implantable cardioverter-defibrillator. Circ Cardiovasc Imaging 2009;2:183–90.

93. Fluechter S, Kuschyk J, Wolpert C, et al. Extent of late gadolinium enhancement detected by cardiovascular magnetic resonance correlates with the inducibility of ventricular tachyarrhythmia in hypertrophic cardiomyopathy. J Cardiovasc Magn Reson 2010;12:30.

94. Green JJ, Berger JS, Kramer CM, et al. Prognostic value of late gadolinium enhancement in clinical outcomes for hypertrophic cardiomyopathy. JACC Cardiovasc Imaging 2012;5:370–7.

95. Chan RH, Maron BJ, Olivotto I, et al. Prognostic utility of contrast-enhanced cardiovascular magnetic resonance imaging in hypertrophic cardiomyopathy: an international multicenter study. Circulation 2012;126:A552.

96. Bruder O, Wagner A, Jensen CJ, et al. Myocardial scar visualized by cardiovascular magnetic resonance imaging predicts major adverse events in patients with hypertrophic cardiomyopathy. J Am Coll Cardiol 2010;56:875–87.

97. Lee DC, Goldberger JJ. CMR for sudden cardiac death risk stratification: are we there yet? JACC Cardiovasc Imaging 2013;6:345–8.

98. Perez-David E, Arenal Á, Rubio-Guivernau JL, et al. Noninvasive identification of ventricular tachycardia-related conducting channels using contrast-enhanced magnetic resonance imaging in patients with chronic myocardial infarction. J Am Coll Cardiol 2011;57:184–94.

99. Ng J, Jacobson JT, Ng JK, et al. Virtual electrophysiological study in a 3-dimensional cardiac

magnetic resonance imaging model of porcine myocardial infarction. J Am Coll Cardiol 2012;60: 423–30.

100. Deng D, Arevalo H, Pashakhanloo F, et al. Accuracy of prediction of infarct-related arrhythmic circuits from image-based models reconstructed from low and high resolution MRI. Front Physiol 2015;6:282.

101. Aljaroudi WA, Flamm SD, Saliba W, et al. Role of CMR imaging in risk stratification for sudden cardiac death. JACC Cardiovasc Imaging 2013;6: 392–406.

102. Klem I, Weinsaft JW, Bahnson TD, et al. Assessment of myocardial scarring improves risk stratification in patients evaluated for cardiac defibrillator implantation. J Am Coll Cardiol 2012;60: 408–20.

103. Iles L, Pfluger H, Phrommintikul A, et al. Evaluation of diffuse myocardial fibrosis in heart failure with cardiac magnetic resonance contrast-enhanced T1 mapping. J Am Coll Cardiol 2008;52:1574–80.

104. Chen Z, Sohal M, Voigt T, et al. Myocardial tissue characterization by cardiac magnetic resonance imaging using T1 mapping predicts ventricular arrhythmia in ischemic and non-ischemic cardiomyopathy patients with implantable cardioverter-defibrillators. Heart Rhythm 2015;12:792–801.

105. Puntmann VO, Carr-White G, Jabbour A, et al. T1-mapping and outcome in nonischemic cardiomyopathy: all-cause mortality and heart failure. JACC Cardiovasc Imaging 2016;9:40–50.

106. Leonardi S, Raineri C, De Ferrari GM, et al. Usefulness of cardiac magnetic resonance in assessing the risk of ventricular arrhythmias and sudden death in patients with hypertrophic cardiomyopathy. Eur Heart J 2009;30:2003–10.

107. Grun S, Schumm J, Greulich S, et al. Long-term follow-up of biopsy-proven viral myocarditis: predictors of mortality and incomplete recovery. J Am Coll Cardiol 2012;59:1604–15.

108. Shen MJ, Zipes DP. Role of the autonomic nervous system in modulating cardiac arrhythmias. Circ Res 2014;114:1004–21.

109. Lown B, Verrier RL. Neural activity and ventricular fibrillation. N Engl J Med 1976;294:1165–70.

110. Merlet P, Valette H, Dubois-Rande JL, et al. Prognostic value of cardiac metaiodobenzylguanidine imaging in patients with heart failure. J Nucl Med 1992;33:471–7.

111. Wakabayashi T, Nakata T, Hashimoto A, et al. Assessment of underlying etiology and cardiac sympathetic innervation to identify patients at high risk of cardiac death. J Nucl Med 2001;42: 1757–67.

112. Fallavollita JA, Heavey BM, Luisi AJ Jr, et al. Regional myocardial sympathetic denervation predicts the risk of sudden cardiac arrest in ischemic cardiomyopathy. J Am Coll Cardiol 2014;63:141–9.

113. Al Badarin FJ, Wimmer AP, Kennedy KF, et al. The utility of ADMIRE-HF risk score in predicting serious arrhythmic events in heart failure patients: incremental prognostic benefit of cardiac 123I-mIBG scintigraphy. J Nucl Cardiol 2014;21:756–62.

Biomarkers to Predict Cardiovascular Death

Devinder S. Dhindsa, MD, Jay Khambhati, MD, Pratik B. Sandesara, MD,
Danny J. Eapen, MD, Arshed A. Quyyumi, MD*

KEYWORDS

- Biomarkers • Cardiovascular death • Risk score • Risk stratification

KEY POINTS

- Risk prediction models in identifying the "vulnerable" patient at risk for cardiovascular death are presently limited.
- Pathway-specific biomarkers of inflammation, thrombosis, immune function, and cell stress improve risk prediction for cardiovascular death in patients with coronary artery disease and heart failure.
- Similarly, markers of inflammation, myocardial stretch, and others improve risk prediction in patients with heart failure.

Cardiovascular disease (CVD) is the leading cause of mortality worldwide.[1] Several population-based CVD risk models have been incorporated into guidelines to target primary prevention with the goal of appropriate risk stratification for at-risk individuals. Despite these models, a sizable gap in the current ability to risk stratify remains, as evidenced by most cases of sudden cardiac death (SCD) occurring in previously asymptomatic individuals in whom death can be the first manifestation of CVD.[2] Improving risk stratification is an important step in enhancing the ability to identify individuals who would benefit from prophylactic and preventative measures. One area of current investigation is the use of biomarkers to assist prediction of cardiovascular death. A useful biomarker (1) separates individuals with or without risk (discrimination), (2) stratifies individuals appropriately and thus potentially change clinical course (classification), and (3) denotes how well the predicted risk matches actual risk in the community (calibration).[3] Clinical tools such as the Framingham risk score predict long-term risk of coronary heart disease outcomes in the healthy population,[4,5] but fail to reliably predict risk of adverse outcomes in patients with established coronary artery disease (CAD).[6] Biomarkers that are surrogates for pathophysiologic processes associated with acute CAD progression to plaque instability, erosion, and rupture and possibly for arrhythmogenesis may be better predictors of future risk of cardiovascular death. This article considers biomarkers that have been shown to identify subjects at increased risk for cardiovascular death within the (1) general population, (2) in those with established CAD, and (3) in those with heart failure (HF) (**Fig. 1**).

BIOMARKERS OF CARDIOVASCULAR DEATH IN THE GENERAL POPULATION

Metabolic

Abnormal lipid profiles are central to many current risk prediction calculators, and do serve to identify subjects with increased likelihood of underlying CAD.[7] Although the Physicians Health Study did not find an association between plasma lipids and SCD,[8] possibly because of the low power of the

Disclosure Statement: None known.
Division of Cardiology, Department of Medicine, Emory University School of Medicine, 1462 Clifton Road Northeast, Suite 507, Atlanta, GA 30322, USA
* Corresponding author.
E-mail address: aquyyum@emory.edu

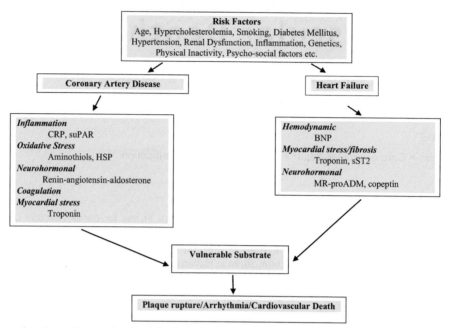

Fig. 1. Biomarkers in cardiovascular death in the heart failure and coronary artery disease population. BNP, brain natriuretic peptide; CRP, C-reactive protein; HSP, heat-shock proteins; MR-proADM, mid-regional proadrenomedullin; suPAR, soluble urokinase plasminogen activator receptor.

study, in a prospective evaluation of nearly 8000 British men, a 3.5-fold increased risk of SCD was observed between extreme quintiles in plasma lipids in subjects without any self-reported history of CAD.[9] Of note, SCD was defined as death within 1 hour of symptoms in these studies.

High-density lipoprotein cholesterol (HDL-C) is one such component of the lipid profile that is featured in several risk prediction models. In post hoc analyses of the Treating to New Targets (TNT) study and the Justification for the Use of Statins in Primary Prevention: An Intervention Trial Evaluating Rosuvastatin (JUPITER) trial, there was little to no association between HDL-C levels and adverse cardiovascular events in patients on statin therapy.[10] Although the robust prospective observational data links lower HDL-C levels and CVD, causality remains unestablished. Additionally, raising HDL, with such therapy as niacin and CETP inhibition, does not seem to affect outcomes.[11]

Other potential biomarkers for cardiovascular death are the nonesterified free fatty acids. Nonesterified free fatty acids are believed to be proarrhythmogenic because they modulate potassium and calcium channels and possibly have direct toxic effects.[12] In a nonischemic population of 5000 middle-aged men followed for 22 years in the Paris Prospective Study I, nonesterified free fatty acids were found to be independent risk factors for SCD (risk ratio [RR], 1.70; 95% confidence interval [CI], 1.21–2.13).[13]

Inflammatory and Prothrombotic Markers

High-sensitivity C-reactive protein (hsCRP) is an inflammatory marker that has been studied extensively in a variety of clinical contexts, including CAD.[3,14] HsCRP has been proposed as a useful biomarker for evaluation and for decision-making regarding treatment in asymptomatic subjects. In the JUPITER trial, asymptomatic individuals with elevated hsCRP and low-density lipoprotein cholesterol who were randomized to statin therapy had a 47% reduction in the risk of nonfatal myocardial infarction (MI), stroke, and cardiovascular death compared with those randomized to placebo.[15] Largely based on these data, the 2013 American College of Cardiology/American Heart Association Cholesterol Management guidelines advise consideration of hs-CRP use when treatment decision is uncertain in intermediate-risk groups.[16] However, when evaluated for its role in predicting SCD, the results have been mixed. In the Physician's Health Study, CRP was an independent predictor of SCD with an RR of 2.65 when comparing the highest with the lowest quartile.[8] However, in two other studies, the Nurses Health Study and the Prospective Epidemiological Study of Myocardial Infarction (PRIME) study, there were no observed associations between CRP levels and SCD.[17,18]

Lipoprotein phospholipase A₂, a novel lipid-related biomarker that plays a role in the depletion of oxidized phospholipids from lipoproteins, is also considered to reflect inflammation.[14] Lipoprotein phospholipase A$_2$ predicts presence of CAD in the general population after adjusting for traditional risk factors and CRP[14,19,20] and predicts 5-year cardiovascular mortality with a hazard ratio (HR) of 2.0 after adjustment for B-type natriuretic peptide (BNP) and hsCRP.[21]

Another marker of inflammation, interleukin (IL)-6, promotes release of CRP from the liver. In the PRIME study of nearly 10,000 European men followed for 10 years, elevated IL-6 was predictive of SCD (HR for highest and lowest tertiles, 3.06).[22] Other biomarkers that have been implicated in development of CAD and vulnerable plaque include myeloperoxidase, metalloproteinases, and IL-18.[3] The clinical utility of these biomarkers requires further investigation.

Renal Dysfunction

Renal dysfunction is another risk factor for the development of CAD. Cystatin C, a validated measure of renal insufficiency,[14] was independently associated with an elevated risk of SCD when comparing the highest with the lowest tertiles (HR, 2.67) in the Cardiovascular Health Study.[23] Microalbuminuria in individuals with or without diabetes mellitus is associated with an increase in cardiovascular death risk.[24–26] Secondary hyperparathyroidism and dysregulated vitamin D levels are also sequelae of renal dysfunction. In the German Diabetes and Dialysis study, 4-year follow-up of more than 1100 dialysis patients revealed an association between SCD and severe vitamin D deficiency.[27] Older patients with lower vitamin D and higher parathormone levels were also more likely to suffer from SCD in the absence of underlying CVD in the Cardiovascular Health Study.[28]

Electrolytes

Magnesium is known for its' membrane stabilizing effects. In the Atherosclerosis Risk in Communities cohort, serum magnesium concentrations were noted to have an inverse relationship to SCD (HR between extreme quartiles, 0.62; 95% CI, 0.42–0.03), a finding confirmed in the Nurses' Health Study Cohort.[29]

Myocardial Markers

The most widely used markers of myocardial stretch are the natriuretic peptides, namely BNP or N-terminal pro-BNP (NT-proBNP).[14,30] Natriuretic peptides are released from cardiac myocytes and their elevated levels were strongly linked with SCD in the Nurse's Health Study; for each standard deviation increment, the RR was 1.49,[18] a finding that was confirmed in men and women enrolled in the Cardiovascular Health Study. In a nested case-controlled analysis comprised of more than 5400 subjects followed for 16 years with an older white and African American cohort, the HR for SCD for NT-proBNP was 2.5.[31]

Troponin is a frequently used biomarker for the diagnosis of MI. Availability of the new generation of high-sensitivity assays enables detection of very low concentrations of circulating cardiac troponins. In contrast to the conventional troponin assays, the high-sensitivity troponin (hsTn) assays detect circulating troponin in the absence of myocardial necrosis. High levels of circulating hsTn have been associated with prevalent CAD and with adverse incident cardiovascular events in patients with stable CAD or the general and elderly population.[32–36] In a community-based cohort of men free of CVD, higher levels of hsTn were associated with increased risk of death (HR, 1.26 for those above a cutoff of troponin I >0.021 µg/mL) after adjustment of traditional risk factors.[37] De Lemos and colleagues[38] demonstrated that elevated levels of hsTn were linked with higher adjusted all-cause mortality ranging from 1.9% in those within the lowest quintile to 28.4% in those within the highest quintile. Importantly, higher levels of hsTn levels were also associated with structural abnormalities including left ventricular hypertrophy and left ventricular systolic dysfunction.

Multimarker Strategy

Because biomarkers representing a variety of different pathophysiologic processes all seem to predict incident cardiovascular death, strategies of combining these biomarkers into an aggregate multimarker score have been investigated. In a cohort of 1982 men without CVD followed for 13 years in the Quebec cardiovascular study, the combination of IL-6 and fibrinogen levels predicted risk of development of CVD.[39] In the Framingham Heart Study where 10 biomarkers were measured (CRP, BNP, N-terminal proatrial natriuretic peptide, aldosterone, renin, fibrinogen, D dimer, plasminogen-activator inhibitor type 1, homocysteine, urinary albumin/creatinine ratio), individuals with a multimarker score in the highest quintile compared with the two lowest quintiles had a four-fold greater risk of death.[40] In 27,347 postmenopausal women enrolled in the Women's Health Initiative, a multimarker score comprised of IL-6, D dimer, coagulation factor VIII, von Willebrand factor, and homocysteine predicted and improved risk classification.[41]

BIOMARKERS OF CARDIOVASCULAR DEATH IN CORONARY ARTERY DISEASE

CAD is linked to 80% or more of the episodes of reported SCD in developed countries and can be the first manifestation of cardiac disease in 20% to 25% of patients.[2] Not surprisingly, SCD and CAD share several traditional risk factors, including diabetes mellitus, hypertension, smoking, hyperlipidemia, and increased age.[42] The associated risk of SCD in individuals with CAD was 1.9- to 5.3-fold higher than those without CAD in the Framingham Heart Study.[43] Additionally, the rate of SCD is noted to be higher in the first 30 days post-MI.[44] However, the exact mechanism of SCD in CAD is likely to be multifactorial in origin. Although acute coronary occlusion caused by plaque rupture with resultant MI and fatal arrhythmia is a well-recognized cause of SCD, occlusive coronary thrombus was found in less than half of patients presenting with cardiac arrest by angiography or at autopsy,[2,45,46] and less than half of patients exhibit enzymatic evidence of MI following an arrest.[45] Nonetheless, microinfarctions caused by thrombi from ruptured or eroded plaques have been noted in greater than 50% of individuals presenting with SCD and likely provide the necessary substrate for sustained arrhythmia.[2,47] Unfortunately, identifying individuals at highest risk of SCD has proven to be a challenge, because implantable cardioverter-defibrillator placement even in the highly vulnerable period post-MI has not shown benefit.[48,49]

Inflammation

CRP is a well-studied marker of systemic inflammation with mixed evidence regarding the utility of this biomarker by itself in risk stratification for SCD. The Bypass Angioplasty Revascularization Investigation 2 Diabetes (BARI-2D) trial demonstrated a relationship between elevated CRP levels and cardiovascular events,[50] although this result was not replicated in the Veterans Affairs Diabetes Trial (VADT).[51] Nevertheless, hs-CRP has utility when combined with other biomarkers to risk stratify patients with CAD.[52–54]

The soluble urokinase plasminogen activator receptor (suPAR) is an emerging marker predicting risk of coronary and renal events. The urokinase plasminogen activator is a serine protease produced by smooth muscle cells, vascular endothelial cells, macrophages, monocytes, and fibroblasts, and when bound to its receptor, leads to the generation of plasmin.[55,56] Urokinase plasminogen activator receptor is involved in several functions including migration, adhesion, fibrinolysis, and cell proliferation.[57–59] Plasma suPAR reflects cellular shedding of urokinase plasminogen activator receptor, which is induced during inflammation; shedding seems to be free of circadian changes and is relatively stable during periods of acute stress.[60,61] SuPAR seems to predict incident CVD independent of the Framingham risk score in healthy populations.[62,63] In a population with suspected or known CAD, elevated levels of plasma suPAR were independently associated with the presence and severity of angiographic CAD and with an increased risk of cardiovascular death (HR, 4.2 in the highest quartile as compared with lowest quartile).[64] Moreover, in individuals presenting with ST-elevation MI or in the post–cardiac arrest population, elevated suPAR level was an independent predictor of all-cause mortality and recurrent MI.[65,66]

Oxidative Stress

Oxidative stress is an important initiating event in the pathogenesis of multiple conditions including CVD.[67] Plasma aminothiol antioxidants, cysteine and glutathione and their oxidized counterparts, cystine and glutathione disulfide, and their redox potentials can be quantified in plasma to assess systemic oxidative stress in vivo.[68] High plasma cystine and low glutathione levels were associated with increased mortality in subjects with CAD, a finding that was independent of, and additive to, other clinical risk measures and hsCRP levels.[52]

Cellular Stress

Heat shock proteins (HSPs), such as HSP70, are intracellular proteins that increase in response to cellular stress.[69] In cross-sectional studies, HSP70 levels were demonstrated to be significantly higher in patients without CAD patients than those with CAD, and inversely proportional to degree of atherosclerotic disease (measured by number of diseased vessels).[70] However, in a study of 3415 patients with suspected or known CAD undergoing cardiac catheterization, elevated HSP70 levels correlated with increased risk of cardiac death even after adjustment for clinical variables and hsCRP.[54]

Neurohormonal

Neurohormonal dysregulation including upregulation of the renin-angiotensin-aldosterone system accompanies atherosclerosis and HF. In the LURIC (LUdwigshafen RIsk and Cardiovascular Health) study of predominantly older white men referred for coronary angiography, elevated renin and aldosterone levels were associated with adverse cardiovascular events including HF and

SCD.[71,72] Additionally, increased aldosterone levels were associated with a higher risk of cardiac arrest in the post–ST-segment elevation MI population (comparing extreme quartiles: HR, 3.74).[73]

Hypercoagulability

The coagulation pathway biomarkers have been evaluated for their potential relationship to cardiac death. Elevated plasma levels of fibrin degradation products (FDPs), higher than the 75th percentile, were found to be independently associated with the risk of all-cause and cardiovascular death.[74] D dimer and von Willebrand factor levels were elevated in patients with acute MI and cardiovascular death, although this relationship was attenuated after adjustment for CRP.[75] In the BARI-2D study, elevated D dimer levels were associated with increased mortality, with every 10% increase in D dimer levels being associated with a 4% increased mortality rate, a relationship that was closely linked with CRP.[50]

Myocardial Markers

HsTn also identifies high-risk patients within the CAD population. Omland and colleagues[76] demonstrated a strong and graded increase in the cumulative incidence of cardiovascular death in those with higher hsTnT levels in the Prevention of Events with Angiotensin-Converting Enzyme Inhibitor (PEACE) trial (adjusted HR, 2.09 per unit increase in natural log of hsTnT level), findings that have been confirmed in several additional studies.[77–79] Low values of hsTn may have a strong negative predictive value, an area that requires further study.

Repair and Regeneration: Role of Progenitor Cells

Although risk factor–mediated injury to the vascular endothelium is well understood, the mechanisms underlying regeneration and the pivotal role of progenitor cells (PCs) in vascular repair and hence cardiovascular health has only recently been appreciated.[80–82] Endothelial PCs are mononuclear cells that originate primarily (but not exclusively) from the bone marrow and differentiate into endothelial cells in vitro and in vivo.[83,84] PCs reside primarily in bone marrow, circulate, and contribute to blood vessel formation during tissue repair.[83,85–96] Endogenous PCs contribute to re-endothelialization of tissues after endothelial injury, attenuating progression to frank atherosclerosis.[97–103] Circulating PCs are multilineage, but the most common circulating PCs are of hematopoietic and endothelial PCs that are capable of vascular repair, largely by their paracrine

activities.[104,105] Our recent studies have shown reduction in the number and migratory activity of PCs in patients with CAD compared with healthy subjects.[106–112] Endothelial dysfunction correlates with PC number and function.[106,110] Importantly, a low PC count seems to be an independent predictor of poor outcome in patients with CAD,[113,114] stroke, or acute lung injury.[112–116]

Multimarker Risk Score

Because multiple pathway-specific biomarkers have been associated with increased mortality risk in patients with CAD, recent studies have begun to investigate whether a combination of these biomarkers, which reflect activation of diverse pathophysiologic pathways, will provide better discrimination of risk of mortality in patients with CAD. Several pathways are involved and act synergistically in the development of atherosclerotic plaque and its progression to the stage of plaque instability and rupture. HsCRP was used to represent the inflammatory pathway, FDP levels to represent activation of the coagulation pathway, HSP70 was used as a marker of cellular stress, and suPAR represented immune activation and inflammation.[53] Using a biomarker risk score (BRS), Eapen and colleagues[74] showed that a combination of plasma levels of three of the previously mentioned markers, hs-CRP, HSP70, and FDPs was predictive for CVD events including death, independent of all clinical variables, such that subjects with elevated levels (beyond specific cutoff values) of all three biomarkers had a 5.2-fold increased risk of cardiovascular death compared with those without any elevations of biomarkers. In an extension of these findings, Ghasemzedah and colleagues[53] showed that elevation in circulating levels of all four of these biomarkers was associated with a 6.8-fold increase in risk for cardiovascular death and an 11.9-fold increased risk of all-cause death, as compared with those with no elevation in the levels of any biomarker. Thus, the 28% of subjects without elevation in any of the biomarkers had a 1.1% annual mortality rate compared with a mortality rate of 21% in the 2.6% of the total population with elevation of all four biomarkers (**Figs. 2 and 3**).

These results were reproduced in 2032 subjects with CAD and diabetes enrolled in the BARI-2D study and followed for 5 years for cardiovascular events. Biomarkers were measured at baseline and retested in 1304 subjects at 1-year. BRS was determined as the biomarker number greater than previously defined cutoff values (CRP >3 mg/L; HSP70 >0.313 ng/mL; and

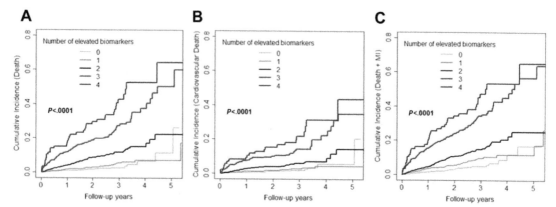

Fig. 2. Cumulative incidence plots for all-cause death (*A*), cardiovascular death (*B*), and all-cause death/MI (*C*), per category of the biomarker risk score.

FDP >1 µg/mL). Patients with a BRS of 3 had a four-fold increased risk of all-cause death and a 6.8-fold increased risk of cardiac death compared with those with a BRS of 0 (**Fig. 4**).[117]

After intensive medical therapy for a year, the average individual biomarker levels decreased with approximately 80% of patients decreasing their BRS. Importantly, the BRS recalibrated at 1 year also predicted risk. Those with 1-year BRS of 2 to 3 had a 4-year mortality rate of 21.1% versus 7.4% for those with BRS of 0 to 1 (*P*<.0001). Thus, not only was this BRS validated in terms of its ability to identify patients with CAD at very high near-term risk of MI/death, but the study showed that the BRS is modifiable by

intensification of medical therapy, can reclassify risk, and thus can be used to guide therapy to reduce mortality in CAD (**Fig. 5**).[117]

BIOMARKERS OF SUDDEN CARDIAC DEATH IN HEART FAILURE

One of the best available predictors of SCD is the presence of reduced left ventricular systolic function. In the Framingham Heart Study, individuals with HF have a 2.6- to 6.2-fold increased risk of SCD.[43] The only population (with the exception of those with rare genetic structural conditions and channelopathies) that has been identified as having a mortality benefit from primary

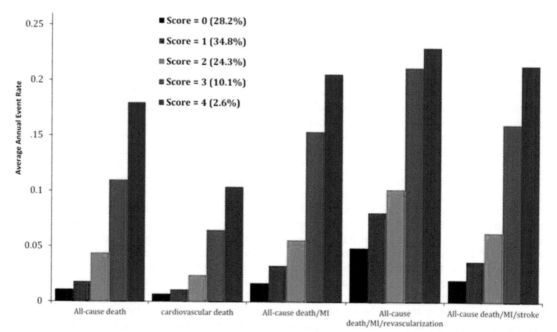

Fig. 3. Annual event rates of major adverse cardiovascular events in each category of the biomarker risk score.

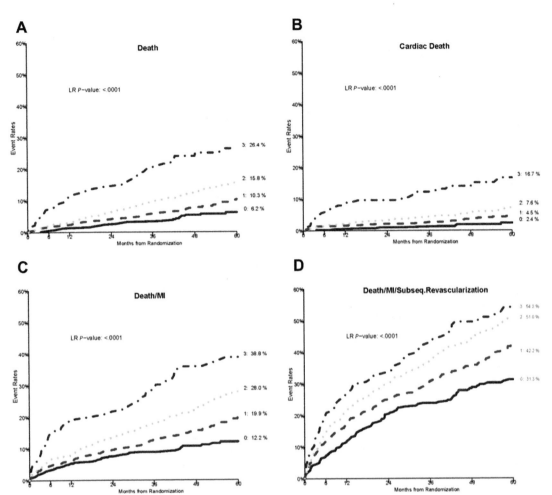

Fig. 4. Five-year cumulative incidence of event rates by number of positive biomarkers at baseline (Bari-2D study). This association is demonstrated with all-cause death (*A*), cardiac death (*B*), composite death/MI (*C*), and death/MI/revascularization (*D*).

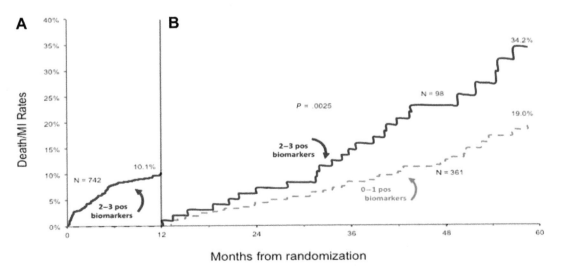

Fig. 5. Cumulative incidence of death/MI in those with the biomarker risk score of 2 to 3 at baseline (BARI-2D study). (*A*) Death/MI event curve during the first year of follow-up. (*B*) Event rates from year 2 to 5 in subjects in whom the BRS decreased to 0 or 1 compared with those in whom the BRS remained high at 2 or 3.

prophylactic implantable cardioverter-defibrillator placement are those with an ejection fraction less than 35% as evidenced in the Multicenter Automatic Defibrillator Implantation Trial (MADIT II) and Sudden Cardiac Death in Heart Failure Trial (SCD-HeFT).[118,119] In survivors of cardiac arrest with a left ventricular ejection fraction less than 30%, the risk of SCD exceeds 30% over 5 years.[119,120] Unfortunately, these easily identifiable high-risk individuals comprise a minority of individuals presenting with SCD, and therefore ejection fraction has poor sensitivity in identifying most individuals at risk for SCD.[121–123]

Hemodynamic Stress

BNP was independently associated with an elevated risk for SCD in patients with chronic HF in the Vienna Heart Failure Cohort[124] and in survivors of acute MI in the Multiple Risk Factor Analysis Trial.[125] In the Val-HeFT study, elevated NT-proBNP levels were correlated with an increased mortality risk (HR, 1.99).[126] In the Organized Program to Initiate Lifesaving Treatment in Hospitalized Patients with Heart Failure (OPTIMIZE-HF) trial, discharge BNP was a strong predictor of outcomes, including 1-year mortality (HR, 1.34; 95% CI, 1.28–1.40).[127]

Myocardial Stress

Cardiac troponin levels, measured by conventional and high-sensitivity assays, are predictors of mortality in HF. In the Acute Decompensated Heart Failure National Registry (ADHERE), a positive troponin by the conventional assay compared with those with normal levels on hospital admission was associated with increased in-hospital mortality (8.0% vs 2.7%).[128] In a stable HF population, elevated hsTn levels were associated with an increased mortality risk (HR, 2.1).[129] Changes in hsTn over time seems to be a robust predictor of future cardiovascular events.[130]

In response to cellular stress, soluble ST2 acts to promote myocardial hypertrophy, inflammation, and fibrosis through the ST2 receptor, an IL-1 receptor family member.[14] Soluble ST2 seems to be associated with HF and biomechanical overload rather than adverse events from CAD, and has been of particular interest for potential prognostication in HF.[131] In the MUSIC registry (MUerta Subita en Insuficiencia Cardiaca) of ambulatory patients with HF followed for 3 years, elevated soluble ST2 levels were independently associated with SCD.[42,132] Importantly, when combined with NT-proBNP levels, sST2 was found to provide additional incremental prognostic value for SCD risk stratification in HF.[133]

Neurohormonal

The sympathetic nervous system is dysregulated in individuals with HF. Mid-regional proadrenomedullin, a precursor to a vasodilator with inotropic properties, adrenomedullin, is a predictor of mortality in HF in addition to BNP.[134] Elevated copeptin levels, a propeptide fragment of arginine vasopressin, was associated with increased 90-day mortality, with an HR of 3.9 in those within the highest compared with lowest quartile, especially in those with concurrent hyponatremia (HR, 7.36).[135]

FUTURE DIRECTIONS

Although genome-wide association studies have identified numerous single-nucleotide polymorphisms that associate with CAD,[136–139] the discovered variants only explain a small fraction of risk and generally have not predicted risk of SCD.[140] Recent advances in gene expression analysis have also discovered transcriptomic signatures in peripheral blood that associate with presence and severity of CAD and risk of adverse events, possibly in a sex-specific manner.[141,142] In a recent study of 338 white patients with CAD, peripheral blood gene expression was measured on Illumina HT-12 (Illumina Inc., San Diego, CA) microarrays. A principal component score capturing covariance of 238 genes significantly predicted risk of cardiovascular death (HR, 8.5) after adjustment for traditional covariates.[143] Metabolomic, proteomic, and microRNA-based analyses are currently being explored to discover novel predictors of SCD.

SUMMARY

Use of biomarkers for risk stratification for SCD continues to evolve. It seems that a multimarker strategy for risk stratification using simple measures of circulating proteins and usual clinical risk factors, particularly in patients with known CAD, can be currently used to identify patients at near-term risk of death. Whether similar strategies in the general population will prove to be cost-effective needs to be investigated.

REFERENCES

1. Lozano R, Naghavi M, Foreman K, et al. Global and regional mortality from 235 causes of death for 20 age groups in 1990 and 2010: a systematic

analysis for the Global Burden of Disease Study. Lancet 2010;380:2095–128.

2. Zipes DP, Wellens HJJ. Sudden cardiac death. Circulation 1998;98:2334–51.

3. Havmoller R, Chugh SS. Plasma biomarkers for prediction of sudden cardiac death: another piece of the risk stratification puzzle? Circ Arrhythm Electrophysiol 2012;5:237–43.

4. Wilson PW, D'Agostino RB, Levy D, et al. Prediction of coronary heart disease using risk factor categories. Circulation 1998;97:1837–47.

5. Pencina MJ, D'Agostino RB Sr, Larson MG, et al. Predicting the 30-year risk of cardiovascular disease: the Framingham Heart Study. Circulation 2009;119:3078–84.

6. Shlipak MG, Ix JH, Bibbins-Domingo K, et al. Biomarkers to predict recurrent cardiovascular disease: the heart and soul study. Am J Med 2008; 121:50–7.

7. Castelli WP. Cholesterol and lipids in the risk of coronary artery disease: the Framingham Heart Study. Can J Cardiol 1988;4(Suppl A):5a–10a.

8. Albert CM, Ma J, Rifai N, et al. Prospective study of C-reactive protein, homocysteine, and plasma lipid levels as predictors of sudden cardiac death. Circulation 2002;105:2595–9.

9. Wannamethee G, Shaper AG, Macfarlane PW, et al. Risk factors for sudden cardiac death in middle-aged British men. Circulation 1995;91: 1749–56.

10. Boekholdt SM, Hovingh GK, Mora S, et al. Very low levels of atherogenic lipoproteins and the risk for cardiovascular events: a meta-analysis of statin trials. J Am Coll Cardiol 2014;64:485–94.

11. Boden WE, Probstfield JL, Anderson T, et al. Niacin in patients with low HDL cholesterol levels receiving intensive statin therapy. N Engl J Med 2011;365:2255–67.

12. Oliver MF, Opie LH. Effects of glucose and fatty acids on myocardial ischaemia and arrhythmias. Lancet 1994;343:155–8.

13. Jouven X, Charles MA, Desnos M, et al. Circulating nonesterified fatty acid level as a predictive risk factor for sudden death in the population. Circulation 2001;104:756–61.

14. Thomas MR, Lip GY. Novel risk markers and risk assessments for cardiovascular disease. Circ Res 2017;120:133–49.

15. Ridker PM, Danielson E, Fonseca FAH, et al. Rosuvastatin to prevent vascular events in men and women with elevated C-reactive protein. N Engl J Med 2008;359:2195–207.

16. Goff DC, Lloyd-Jones DM, Bennett G, et al. 2013 ACC/AHA guideline on the assessment of cardiovascular risk. A report of the American College of Cardiology/American Heart Association Task Force on practice guidelines. Circulation 2014;129:S49–73.

17. Korngold EC, Januzzi JL Jr, Gantzer ML, et al. Amino-terminal pro-B-type natriuretic peptide and high-sensitivity C-reactive protein as predictors of sudden cardiac death among women. Circulation 2009;119:2868–76.

18. Whang W, Kubzansky LD, Kawachi I, et al. Depression and risk of sudden cardiac death and coronary heart disease in women: results from the Nurses' Health Study. J Am Coll Cardiol 2009;53: 950–8.

19. Daniels LB, Laughlin GA, Sarno MJ, et al. Lipoprotein-associated phospholipase A2 is an independent predictor of incident coronary heart disease in an apparently healthy older population: the Rancho Bernardo Study. J Am Coll Cardiol 2008; 51:913–9.

20. Koenig W, Khuseyinova N, Löwel H, et al. Lipoprotein-associated phospholipase A2 adds to risk prediction of incident coronary events by C-reactive protein in apparently healthy middle-aged men from the general population. results from the 14-year follow-up of a large cohort from Southern Germany. Circulation 2004;110:1903–8.

21. Winkler K, Hoffmann MM, Winkelmann BR, et al. Lipoprotein-associated phospholipase A2 predicts 5-year cardiac mortality independently of established risk factors and adds prognostic information in patients with low and medium high-sensitivity C-reactive protein (the Ludwigshafen risk and cardiovascular health study). Clin Chem 2007;53: 1440–7.

22. Empana JP, Jouven X, Canoui-Poitrine F, et al. C-reactive protein, interleukin 6, fibrinogen and risk of sudden death in European middle-aged men: the PRIME study. Arterioscler Thromb Vasc Biol 2010;30:2047–52.

23. Deo R, Sotoodehnia N, Katz R, et al. Cystatin C and sudden cardiac death risk in the elderly. Circ Cardiovasc Qual Outcomes 2010;3:159–64.

24. Jager A, Kostense PJ, Ruhe HG, et al. Microalbuminuria and peripheral arterial disease are independent predictors of cardiovascular and all-cause mortality, especially among hypertensive subjects: five-year follow-up of the Hoorn Study. Arterioscler Thromb Vasc Biol 1999;19: 617–24.

25. Gerstein HC, Mann JF, Yi Q, et al. Albuminuria and risk of cardiovascular events, death, and heart failure in diabetic and nondiabetic individuals. JAMA 2001;286:421–6.

26. Brouwers FP, Asselbergs FW, Hillege HL, et al. Long-term effects of fosinopril and pravastatin on cardiovascular events in subjects with microalbuminuria: ten years of follow-up of Prevention of Renal and Vascular End-stage Disease Intervention Trial (PREVEND IT). Am Heart J 2011;161: 1171–8.

27. Drechsler C, Pilz S, Obermayer-Pietsch B, et al. Vitamin D deficiency is associated with sudden cardiac death, combined cardiovascular events, and mortality in haemodialysis patients. Eur Heart J 2010;31:2253–61.

28. Deo R, Katz R, Shlipak MG, et al. Vitamin D, parathyroid hormone, and sudden cardiac death: results from the cardiovascular health study. Hypertension 2011;58:1021–8.

29. Chiuve SE, Korngold EC, Januzzi JL Jr, et al. Plasma and dietary magnesium and risk of sudden cardiac death in women. Am J Clin Nutr 2011;93:253–60.

30. Hall C. Essential biochemistry and physiology of (NT-pro)BNP. Eur J Heart Fail 2004;6:257–60.

31. Patton KK, Sotoodehnia N, DeFilippi C, et al. N-terminal pro-B-type natriuretic peptide is associated with sudden cardiac death risk: the cardiovascular health study. Heart Rhythm 2011;8:228–33.

32. Everett BM, Brooks MM, Vlachos HEA, et al. Troponin and cardiac events in stable ischemic heart disease and diabetes. N Engl J Med 2015;373:610–20.

33. Neumann JT, Havulinna AS, Zeller T, et al. Comparison of three troponins as predictors of future cardiovascular events: prospective results from the FINRISK and BiomaCaRE studies. PLoS One 2014;9:e90063.

34. Sinning C, Keller T, Zeller T, et al, Gutenberg Health Study. Association of high-sensitivity assayed troponin I with cardiovascular phenotypes in the general population: the population-based Gutenberg health study. Clin Res Cardiol 2014;103:211–22.

35. White HD, Tonkin A, Simes J, et al, LIPID Study Investigators. Association of contemporary sensitive troponin I levels at baseline and change at 1 year with long-term coronary events following myocardial infarction or unstable angina: results from the LIPID Study (Long-term intervention with pravastatin in ischaemic disease). J Am Coll Cardiol 2014;63:345–54.

36. Ndrepepa G, Braun S, Schulz S, et al. High-sensitivity troponin T level and angiographic severity of coronary artery disease. Am J Cardiol 2011;108:639–43.

37. Zethelius B, Johnston N, Venge P. Troponin I as a predictor of coronary heart disease and mortality in 70-year-old men: a community-based cohort study. Circulation 2006;113:1071–8.

38. de Lemos JA, Drazner MH, Omland T, et al. Association of troponin t detected with a highly sensitive assay and cardiac structure and mortality risk in the general population. JAMA 2010;304:2503–12.

39. St-Pierre AC, Cantin B, Bergeron J, et al. Inflammatory markers and long-term risk of ischemic heart disease in men: a 13-year follow-up of the Quebec Cardiovascular Study. Atherosclerosis 2005;182:315–21.

40. Wang TJ, Gona P, Larson MG, et al. Multiple biomarkers for the prediction of first major cardiovascular events and death. N Engl J Med 2006;355:2631–9.

41. Kim HC, Greenland P, Rossouw JE, et al. Multimarker prediction of coronary heart disease risk: the women's health initiative. J Am Coll Cardiol 2010;55:2080–91.

42. Deo R, Albert CM. Epidemiology and genetics of sudden cardiac death. Circulation 2012;125:620–37.

43. Cupples LA, Gagnon DR, Kannel WB. Long- and short-term risk of sudden coronary death. Circulation 1992;85:I11–8.

44. Adabag AS, Therneau TM, Gersh BJ, et al. Sudden death after myocardial infarction. JAMA 2008;300:2022–9.

45. Greene HL. Sudden arrhythmic cardiac death: mechanisms, resuscitation and classification. The Seattle perspective. Am J Cardiol 1990;65:4b–12b.

46. Warnes CA, Roberts WC. Sudden coronary death: comparison of patients with to those without coronary thrombus at necropsy. Am J Cardiol 1984;54:1206–11.

47. Santini M, Lavalle C, Ricci RP. Primary and secondary prevention of sudden cardiac death: who should get an ICD? Heart 2007;93:1478–83.

48. Hohnloser SH, Kuck KH, Dorian P, et al. Prophylactic use of an implantable cardioverter–defibrillator after acute myocardial infarction. N Engl J Med 2004;351:2481–8.

49. Steinbeck G, Andresen D, Seidl K, et al. Defibrillator implantation early after myocardial infarction. N Engl J Med 2009;361:1427–36.

50. Sobel BE, Hardison RM, Genuth S, et al. Profibrinolytic, antithrombotic, and antiinflammatory effects of an insulin-sensitizing strategy in patients in the bypass angioplasty revascularization investigation 2 diabetes (BARI 2D) trial. Circulation 2011;124:695–703.

51. Koska J, Saremi A, Bahn G, et al. The effect of intensive glucose lowering on lipoprotein particle profiles and inflammatory markers in the Veterans Affairs Diabetes Trial (VADT). Diabetes Care 2013;36:2408–14.

52. Patel RS, Ghasemzadeh N, Eapen DJ, et al. Novel biomarker of oxidative stress is associated with risk of death in patients with coronary artery disease. Circulation 2016;133:361–9.

53. Ghasemzedah N, Hayek SS, Ko YA, et al. Pathway-specific aggregate biomarker risk score is associated with burden of coronary artery disease and predicts near-term risk of myocardial infarction and death. Circ Cardiovasc Qual Outcomes 2017;10(3) [pii:e001493].

54. Eapen DJ, Ghasemzadeh N, MacNamara JP, et al. The evaluation of novel biomarkers and the multiple biomarker approach in the prediction of cardiovascular disease. Curr Cardiovasc Risk Rep 2014;8:408.

55. Fuhrman B. The urokinase system in the pathogenesis of atherosclerosis. Atherosclerosis 2012; 222:8–14.

56. Waltz DA, Fujita RM, Yang X, et al. Nonproteolytic role for the urokinase receptor in cellular migration in vivo. Am J Respir Cell Mol Biol 2000;22: 316–22.

57. Madsen CD, Sidenius N. The interaction between urokinase receptor and vitronectin in cell adhesion and signalling. Eur J Cell Biol 2008;87:617–29.

58. Blasi F, Carmeliet P. uPAR: a versatile signalling orchestrator. Nat Rev Mol Cell Biol 2002;3: 932–43.

59. Madsen CD, Ferraris GM, Andolfo A, et al. uPAR-induced cell adhesion and migration: vitronectin provides the key. J Cell Biol 2007;177:927–39.

60. Thuno M, Macho B, Eugen-Olsen J. suPAR: the molecular crystal ball. Dis Markers 2009;27: 157–72.

61. Lyngbaek S, Marott JL, Sehestedt T, et al. Cardiovascular risk prediction in the general population with use of suPAR, CRP, and Framingham Risk Score. Int J Cardiol 2013;167(6):2904–11.

62. Kjellman A, Akre O, Gustafsson O, et al. Soluble urokinase plasminogen activator receptor as a prognostic marker in men participating in prostate cancer screening. J Intern Med 2011;269: 299–305.

63. Persson M, Engstrom G, Bjorkbacka H, et al. Soluble urokinase plasminogen activator receptor in plasma is associated with incidence of CVD. Results from the Malmo Diet and Cancer Study. Atherosclerosis 2012;220:502–5.

64. Eapen DJ, Manocha P, Ghasemzadeh N, et al. Soluble urokinase plasminogen activator receptor level is an independent predictor of the presence and severity of coronary artery disease and of future adverse events. J Am Heart Assoc 2014;3: e001118.

65. Lyngbæk S, Marott JL, Møller DV, et al. Usefulness of soluble urokinase plasminogen activator receptor to predict repeat myocardial infarction and mortality in patients with ST-segment elevation myocardial infarction undergoing primary percutaneous intervention. Am J Cardiol 2012;110: 1756–63.

66. Rundgren M, Lyngbaek S, Fisker H, et al. The inflammatory marker suPAR after cardiac arrest. Ther hypothermia Temp Manag 2015;5:89–94.

67. Harrison D, Griendling KK, Landmesser U, et al. Role of oxidative stress in atherosclerosis. Am J Cardiol 2003;91:7a–11a.

68. Jones DP, Liang Y. Measuring the poise of thiol/disulfide couples in vivo. Free Radic Biol Med 2009; 47:1329–38.

69. Delogu G, Signore M, Mechelli A, et al. Heat shock proteins and their role in heart injury. Curr Opin Crit Care 2002;8:411–6.

70. Zhu J, Quyyumi AA, Wu H, et al. Increased serum levels of heat shock protein 70 are associated with low risk of coronary artery disease. Arterioscler Thromb Vasc Biol 2003;23:1055–9.

71. Tomaschitz A, Pilz S, Ritz E, et al. Associations of plasma renin with 10-year cardiovascular mortality, sudden cardiac death, and death due to heart failure. Eur Heart J 2011;32: 2642–9.

72. Tomaschitz A, Pilz S, Ritz E, et al. Plasma aldosterone levels are associated with increased cardiovascular mortality: the Ludwigshafen risk and cardiovascular health (LURIC) study. Eur Heart J 2010;31:1237–47.

73. Beygui F, Collet J-P, Benoliel J-J, et al. High plasma aldosterone levels on admission are associated with death in patients presenting with acute ST-elevation myocardial infarction. Circulation 2006;114:2604–10.

74. Eapen DJ, Manocha P, Patel RS, et al. Aggregate risk score based on markers of inflammation, cell stress, and coagulation is an independent predictor of adverse cardiovascular outcomes. J Am Coll Cardiol 2013;62:329–37.

75. Wannamethee SG, Whincup PH, Shaper AG, et al. Circulating inflammatory and hemostatic biomarkers are associated with risk of myocardial infarction and coronary death, but not angina pectoris, in older men. J Thromb Haemost 2009;7: 1605–11.

76. Omland T, de Lemos JA, Sabatine MS, et al. Sensitive cardiac troponin t assay in stable coronary artery disease. N Engl J Med 2009;361: 2538–47.

77. Kavsak PA, Xu L, Yusuf S, et al. High-sensitivity cardiac troponin I measurement for risk stratification in a stable high-risk population. Clin Chem 2011;57: 1146–53.

78. McQueen MJ, Kavsak PA, Xu L, et al. Predicting myocardial infarction and other serious cardiac outcomes using high-sensitivity cardiac troponin T in a high-risk stable population. Clin Biochem 2013;46:5–9.

79. Koenig W, Breitling LP, Hahmann H, et al. Cardiac troponin T measured by a high-sensitivity assay predicts recurrent cardiovascular events in stable coronary heart disease patients with 8-year follow-up. Clin Chem 2012;58:1215–24.

80. Asahara T, Murohara T, Sullivan A, et al. Isolation of putative progenitor endothelial cells for angiogenesis. Science 1997;275:964–7.

81. Lin Y, Weisdorf DJ, Solovey A, et al. Origins of circulating endothelial cells and endothelial outgrowth from blood. J Clin Invest 2000;105:71–7.

82. Quyyumi AA. Endothelial function in health and disease: new insights into the genesis of cardiovascular disease. Am J Med 1998;105:32s–9s.

83. Urbich C, Dimmeler S. Endothelial progenitor cells: characterization and role in vascular biology. Circ Res 2004;95:343–53.

84. Urbich C, Dimmeler S. Endothelial progenitor cells functional characterization. Trends Cardiovasc Med 2004;14:318–22.

85. Springer ML, Chen AS, Kraft PE, et al. VEGF gene delivery to muscle: potential role for vasculogenesis in adults. Mol Cell 1998;2:549–58.

86. Asahara T, Kalka C, Isner JM. Stem cell therapy and gene transfer for regeneration. Gene Ther 2000;7:451–7.

87. Murohara T, Ikeda H, Duan J, et al. Transplanted cord blood-derived endothelial precursor cells augment postnatal neovascularization. J Clin Invest 2000;105:1527–36.

88. Urbich C, Heeschen C, Aicher A, et al. Relevance of monocytic features for neovascularization capacity of circulating endothelial progenitor cells. Circulation 2003;108:2511–6.

89. Takahashi T, Kalka C, Masuda H, et al. Ischemia- and cytokine-induced mobilization of bone marrow-derived endothelial progenitor cells for neovascularization. Nat Med 1999;5:434–8.

90. Risau W. Mechanisms of angiogenesis. Nature 1997;386:671–4.

91. Schaper W, Scholz D. Factors regulating arteriogenesis. Arterioscler Thromb Vasc Biol 2003;23:1143–51.

92. Subramaniyam V, Waller EK, Murrow JR, et al. Bone marrow mobilization with granulocyte macrophage colony-stimulating factor improves endothelial dysfunction and exercise capacity in patients with peripheral arterial disease. Am Heart J 2009;158(1):53–60.e1.

93. Crosby JR, Kaminski WE, Schatteman G, et al. Endothelial cells of hematopoietic origin make a significant contribution to adult blood vessel formation. Circ Res 2000;87:728–30.

94. Jackson KA, Majka SM, Wang H, et al. Regeneration of ischemic cardiac muscle and vascular endothelium by adult stem cells. J Clin Invest 2001;107:1395–402.

95. Kocher AA, Schuster MD, Szabolcs MJ, et al. Neovascularization of ischemic myocardium by human bone-marrow-derived angioblasts prevents cardiomyocyte apoptosis, reduces remodeling and improves cardiac function. Nat Med 2001;7:430–6.

96. Murayama T, Tepper O, Silver M, et al. Determination of bone marrow-derived endothelial progenitor cell significance in angiogenic growth factor-induced neovascularization in vivo. Exp Hematol 2002;30(8):967–72.

97. Shi Q, Rafii S, Wu MH, et al. Evidence for circulating bone marrow-derived endothelial cells. Blood 1998;92:362–7.

98. Peichev M, Naiyer AJ, Pereira D, et al. Expression of VEGFR-2 and AC133 by circulating human CD34+ cells identifies a population of functional endothelial precursors. Blood 2000;95:952–8.

99. Fujiyama S, Amano K, Uehira K, et al. Bone marrow monocyte lineage cells adhere on injured endothelium in a monocyte chemoattractant protein-1-dependent manner and accelerate re-endothelialization as endothelial progenitor cells. Circ Res 2003;93:980–9.

100. Griese DP, Ehsan A, Melo LG, et al. Isolation and transplantation of autologous circulating endothelial cells into denuded vessels and prosthetic grafts: implications for cell-based vascular therapy. Circulation 2003;108:2710–5.

101. Werner N, Priller J, Laufs U, et al. Bone marrow-derived progenitor cells modulate vascular reendothelialization and neointimal formation: effect of 3-hydroxy-3-methylglutaryl coenzyme a reductase inhibition. Arterioscler Thromb Vasc Biol 2002;22:1567–72.

102. Rauscher FM, Goldschmidt-Clermont PJ, Davis BH, et al. Aging, progenitor cell exhaustion, and atherosclerosis. Circulation 2003;108:457–63.

103. Gunsilius E, Duba H-C, Petzer AL, et al. Evidence from a leukaemia model for maintenance of vascular endothelium by bone-marrow-derived endothelial cells. Lancet 2000;355:1688–91.

104. Xu S, Zhu J, Yu L, et al. Endothelial progenitor cells: current development of their paracrine factors in cardiovascular therapy. J Cardiovasc Pharmacol 2012;59:387–96.

105. Shimada IS, Spees JL. Stem and progenitor cells for neurological repair: minor issues, major hurdles, and exciting opportunities for paracrine-based therapeutics. J Cell Biochem 2011;112:374–80.

106. Heiss C, Keymel S, Niesler U, et al. Impaired progenitor cell activity in age-related endothelial dysfunction. J Am Coll Cardiol 2005;45:1441–8.

107. Scheubel RJ, Zorn H, Silber R-E, et al. Age-dependent depression in circulating endothelial progenitor cells in patients undergoing coronary artery bypass grafting. J Am Coll Cardiol 2003;42:2073–80.

108. Vasa M, Fichtlscherer S, Adler K, et al. Increase in circulating endothelial progenitor cells by statin therapy in patients with stable coronary artery disease. Circulation 2001;103:2885–90.

109. Britten MB, Abolmaali ND, Assmus B, et al. Infarct remodeling after intracoronary progenitor cell treatment in patients with acute myocardial infarction (TOPCARE-AMI): mechanistic insights from serial

contrast-enhanced magnetic resonance imaging. Circulation 2003;108:2212–8.

110. Hill JM, Zalos G, Halcox JP, et al. Circulating endothelial progenitor cells, vascular function, and cardiovascular risk. N Engl J Med 2003;348:593–600.

111. Tepper OM, Galiano RD, Capla JM, et al. Human endothelial progenitor cells from type II diabetics exhibit impaired proliferation, adhesion, and incorporation into vascular structures. Circulation 2002; 106:2781–6.

112. Ghani U, Shuaib A, Salam A, et al. Endothelial progenitor cells during cerebrovascular disease. Stroke 2005;36:151–3.

113. Schmidt-Lucke C, Rossig L, Fichtlscherer S, et al. Reduced number of circulating endothelial progenitor cells predicts future cardiovascular events: proof of concept for the clinical importance of endogenous vascular repair. Circulation 2005; 111:2981–7.

114. Werner N, Kosiol S, Schiegl T, et al. Circulating endothelial progenitor cells and cardiovascular outcomes [see comment]. N Engl J Med 2005; 353:999–1007.

115. Fadini GP, de Kreutzenberg S, Agostini C, et al. Low CD34+ cell count and metabolic syndrome synergistically increase the risk of adverse outcomes. Atherosclerosis 2009;207:213–9.

116. Burnham EL, Taylor WR, Quyyumi AA, et al. Increased circulating endothelial progenitor cells are associated with survival in acute lung injury. Am J Respir Crit Care Med 2005;172(7): 854–60.

117. Ghasemzadeh N, Brooks M, Vlachos H, et al. An aggregate biomarker risk score predicts high risk of near-term myocardial infarction and death: findings from BARI 2D (Bypass angioplasty revascularization investigation 2 diabetes). J Am Heart Assoc 2017;6(7) [pii:e003587].

118. Moss AJ, Hall WJ, Cannom DS, et al. Improved survival with an implanted defibrillator in patients with coronary disease at high risk for ventricular arrhythmia. Multicenter Automatic Defibrillator Implantation Trial Investigators. N Engl J Med 1996; 335:1933–40.

119. Bardy GH, Lee KL, Mark DB, et al. Amiodarone or an implantable cardioverter–defibrillator for congestive heart failure. N Engl J Med 2005;352: 225–37.

120. Stevenson WG, Stevenson LW, Middlekauff HR, et al. Sudden death prevention in patients with advanced ventricular dysfunction. Circulation 1993;88:2953–61.

121. de Vreede-Swagemakers JJ, Gorgels AP, Dubois-Arbouw WI, et al. Out-of-hospital cardiac arrest in the 1990's: a population-based study in the Maastricht area on incidence, characteristics and survival. J Am Coll Cardiol 1997;30:1500–5.

122. Stecker EC, Vickers C, Waltz J, et al. Population-based analysis of sudden cardiac death with and without left ventricular systolic dysfunction: two-year findings from the Oregon Sudden Unexpected Death Study. J Am Coll Cardiol 2006;47: 1161–6.

123. Gorgels AP, Gijsbers C, de Vreede-Swagemakers J, et al. Out-of-hospital cardiac arrest–the relevance of heart failure. The Maastricht Circulatory Arrest Registry. Eur Heart J 2003;24:1204–9.

124. Berger R, Huelsman M, Strecker K, et al. B-Type Natriuretic peptide predicts sudden death in patients with chronic heart failure. Circulation 2002; 105:2392–7.

125. Tapanainen JM, Lindgren KS, Makikallio TH, et al. Natriuretic peptides as predictors of non-sudden and sudden cardiac death after acute myocardial infarction in the beta-blocking era. J Am Coll Cardiol 2004;43:757–63.

126. Cohn JN, Tognoni G. A Randomized trial of the angiotensin-receptor blocker valsartan in chronic heart failure. N Engl J Med 2001;345:1667–75.

127. Kociol RD, Horton JR, Fonarow GC, et al. Admission, discharge, or change in B-type natriuretic peptide and long-term outcomes: data from organized program to initiate lifesaving treatment in hospitalized patients with heart Failure (OPTIMIZE-HF) linked to Medicare claims. Circ Heart Fail 2011;4:628–36.

128. Peacock WF 4th, De Marco T, Fonarow GC, et al. Cardiac troponin and outcome in acute heart failure. N Engl J Med 2008;358:2117–26.

129. Latini R, Masson S, Anand IS, et al. Prognostic value of very low plasma concentrations of troponin T in patients with stable chronic heart failure. Circulation 2007;116:1242–9.

130. Masson S, Anand I, Favero C, et al. Serial measurement of cardiac troponin T using a highly sensitive assay in patients with chronic heart failure: data from 2 large randomized clinical trials. Circulation 2012;125:280–8.

131. Bhardwaj A, Januzzi JL Jr. ST2: a novel biomarker for heart failure. Expert Rev Mol Diagn 2010;10: 459–64.

132. Bayes-Genis A, de Antonio M, Vila J, et al. Head-to-head comparison of 2 myocardial fibrosis biomarkers for long-term heart failure risk stratification: ST2 versus galectin-3. J Am Coll Cardiol 2014;63: 158–66.

133. Pascual-Figal DA, Ordonez-Llanos J, Tornel PL, et al. Soluble ST2 for predicting sudden cardiac death in patients with chronic heart failure and left ventricular systolic dysfunction. J Am Coll Cardiol 2009;54:2174–9.

134. Maisel A, Mueller C, Nowak R, et al. Mid-region pro-hormone markers for diagnosis and prognosis in acute dyspnea: results from the

BACH (Biomarkers in Acute Heart Failure) trial. J Am Coll Cardiol 2010;55:2062–76.

135. Maisel A, Xue Y, Shah K, et al. Increased 90-day mortality in patients with acute heart failure with elevated copeptin: secondary results from the Biomarkers in Acute Heart Failure (BACH) study. Circ Heart Fail 2011;4:613–20.

136. Roberts R, Stewart AF. Genes and coronary artery disease: where are we? J Am Coll Cardiol 2012;60:1715–21.

137. Samani NJ, Erdmann J, Hall AS, et al. Genomewide association analysis of coronary artery disease. N Engl J Med 2007;357:443–53.

138. Schunkert H, Konig IR, Kathiresan S, et al. Large-scale association analysis identifies 13 new susceptibility loci for coronary artery disease. Nat Genet 2011;43:333–8.

139. Huertas-Vazquez A, Nelson CP, Guo X, et al. Novel loci associated with increased risk of sudden cardiac death in the context of coronary artery disease. PLoS One 2013;8:e59905.

140. Visscher PM, Brown MA, McCarthy MI, et al. Five years of GWAS discovery. Am J Hum Genet 2012;90:7–24.

141. Wingrove JA, Daniels SE, Sehnert AJ, et al. Correlation of peripheral-blood gene expression with the extent of coronary artery stenosis. Circ Cardiovasc Genet 2008;1:31–8.

142. Rosenberg S, Elashoff MR, Lieu HD, et al. Whole blood gene expression testing for coronary artery disease in nondiabetic patients: major adverse cardiovascular events and interventions in the PREDICT trial. J Cardiovasc Transl Res 2012;5:366–74.

143. Kim J, Ghasemzadeh N, Eapen DJ, et al. Gene expression profiles associated with acute myocardial infarction and risk of cardiovascular death. Genome Med 2014;6:40.

Cardiac Innervation and the Autonomic Nervous System in Sudden Cardiac Death

 CrossMark

William A. Huang, MD, Noel G. Boyle, MD, PhD,
Marmar Vaseghi, MD, PhD, FHRS*

KEYWORDS

- Autonomic • Innervation • Sympathetic • Parasympathetic • Sudden death
- Ventricular tachycardia • Ventricular fibrillation

KEY POINTS

- Cardiac neural control occurs at multiple levels, and each level has the capability to receive afferent neurotransmission and control efferent outflow to the heart.
- Sympathetic nervous system activation in myocardial infarction increases ventricular fibrillation/ventricular tachycardia (VT/VF) by providing both of the ingredients required for arrhythmogenesis: increased myocardial excitability and heterogeneous repolarization predisposing to reentry.
- Myocardial infarction remodels the sympathetic nervous system such that sympathetic activity is amplified, promoting VT/VF.
- Strategies for neuraxial modulation have aimed at decreasing sympathetic activity and augmenting parasympathetic tone, at various levels of cardiac neural control.
- Autonomic modulation has progressed from basic science to animal studies and human studies, although in clinical trials, some therapies have had mixed results.

INTRODUCTION

The autonomic nervous system controls every aspect of cardiac physiology. Autonomic imbalances, whether from central nervous system disorders such as in epilepsy[1] or from cardiac pathologic remodeling of the peripheral nervous system, can cause significant atrial and ventricular tachyarrhythmias and bradyarrhythmias. In this article, the role of the autonomic nervous system in sudden cardiac death (SCD) is reviewed with a particular focus on the levels at which neuromodulatory therapies may have proven benefit.

ANATOMY

The autonomic nervous system consists of sympathetic and parasympathetic branches. Neural processing occurs at several levels (**Fig. 1**). The intrinsic cardiac ganglia reside on the epicardium and receive postganglionic sympathetic and preganglionic parasympathetic connections. In the thorax, the extracardiac but intrathoracic ganglia, such as the stellate ganglia, the middle cervical ganglia, and the thoracic ganglia of T2-T4, also process neural information, controlling sympathetic outflow to the heart. Finally, sympathetic afferent information passes through the dorsal

Disclosure Statement: The authors have nothing to disclose.
UCLA Cardiac Arrhythmia Center, David Geffen School of Medicine at UCLA, 100 MP, Suite 660, Los Angeles, CA 90095, USA
* Corresponding author.
E-mail address: mvaseghi@mednet.ucla.edu

Card Electrophysiol Clin 9 (2017) 665–679
http://dx.doi.org/10.1016/j.ccep.2017.08.002
1877-9182/17/© 2017 Elsevier Inc. All rights reserved.

cardiacEP.theclinics.com

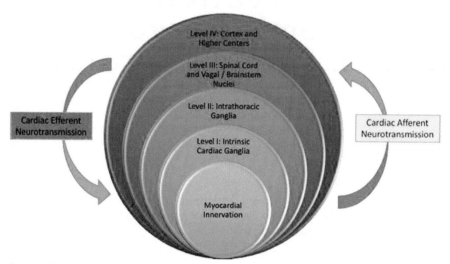

Fig. 1. Cardiac neural control occurs at multiple levels, and each level has the capability to receive afferent neurotransmission and control efferent outflow to the heart (directly or indirectly). Level I represents the intrinsic cardiac ganglia, located in the fat pads of the epicardium. Level II includes the stellate, middle cervical, and thoracic ganglia. Level III includes the spinal cord, vagal nerve, and brainstem nuclei. Level IV represents cortex and higher centers. Each level also demonstrates parallel processing of neural information.

root ganglia and reaches the spinal cord, where additional neural processing can take place. Some of this information is then sent to the brainstem and higher centers. At each level, afferent neurotransmission feeds back information to neurons that in turn affect efferent control of the heart, completing an independent neural circuit that modulates cardiac function. In addition, direct vagal afferent fibers originate from the myocardium and synapse via pseudounipolar neurons of the nodose ganglia in the nucleus tractus solitarius of the brainstem. Finally, although sympathetic efferent fibers originate in the thoracic ganglia and parasympathetic preganglionic fibers travel in the vagal trunk, it is important to note that there is significant intermixing of these fibers in the thorax so that most nerves reaching the heart in the mediastinum have mixed (sympathetic and parasympathetic) fibers.[2,3]

Sympathetic Efferent Neurotransmission

The journey of cardiac sympathetic preganglionic fibers originates in the central nervous system primarily in the brainstem, with modulation by higher centers such as the subthalamic and periaqueductal gray as well as rostral ventrolateral medulla.[4] These preganglionic fibers leave the spinal cord at the level of T1 to T4 and synapse in the right and left stellate ganglia, T2-T4 thoracic, and middle cervical ganglia. Postganglionic fibers then originate from these ganglia and travel along

epicardial vascular structures as dictated by embryologic growth cues of endothelin-1 and nerve growth factor (NGF) released by vascular smooth muscle cells, particularly along coronary veins and then arteries.[5,6] Therefore, sympathetic innervation is particularly dense around the sinus node and coronary sinus, with decreasing density from the base of the ventricle to the apex.[7] In addition, these fibers provide input to the numerous ganglionated subplexuses interspersed throughout bilateral atria and ventricles.[4,8] Most postganglionic sympathetic fibers, however, synapse directly onto the myocardium. The major neurotransmitter of the sympathetic nervous system is norepinephrine, which stimulates myocardial beta-receptors. Roles for additional neurotransmitters such as neuropeptide Y are currently under investigation.[9]

Parasympathetic Efferent Neurotransmission

Preganglionic cardiac parasympathetic efferent fibers begin in the nucleus ambiguus and dorsal motor nucleus of the brainstem and travel in the vagosympathetic trunk bilaterally.[10] These preganglionic fibers synapse within the intrinsic cardiac ganglia residing in fat pads on the heart.[11] Postganglionic neurons then provide direct innervation to the sinus node, atrioventricular node, and bilateral atria and ventricles.[12–15] Acetylcholine is the major neurotransmitter of the heart, stimulating muscarinic (predominantly

M2 and M3) receptors on the myocytes. However, important cotransmitters are released with vagal nerve stimulation (VNS), including nitric oxide and vasoactive intestinal peptide. Of note, although the vagal trunk consists of primarily efferent parasympathetic nerve fibers, evidence for dopaminergic fibers within the trunk also exists.[16,17] The role of these dopaminergic fibers remains to be elucidated. Importantly, most of the fibers of the vagal trunk are afferent (>80%).[18] The vagal nerve has the added complexity of providing dual autonomic and bidirectional flow of information via multiple neurotransmitter messengers.

Neural Afferent Neurotransmission

Afferent nerve fibers provide critical feedback from the myocardium and can be mechanosensory, chemosensory, or both.[4] Chemosensory neurons respond to a variety of stimuli, including hydrogen ions, potassium, bradykinin, oxygen radicals, adenosine, adenosine triphosphate, and arachidonic acid metabolites. These nerve fibers send information to the intrinsic cardiac ganglia, the intrathoracic ganglia, the dorsal root ganglia of the spinal cord, and via the nodose ganglia (the inferior ganglia of the vagosympathetic trunk) to the brainstem. Afferents arising from renal parenchyma and renal pelvis travel via the dorsal root ganglia of the spinal cord and can also modulate sympathetic outflow.[19] Of note, aortic and carotid body mechanosensory and chemosensory afferents appear to travel via the vagal trunk to the brain.[20,21]

Neural Circuits

Local circuit neurons in the intrathoracic and intracardiac ganglia serve as processors of afferent information. They provide local reflex arcs back to the heart through efferent nerves, fine tuning cardiac function on a beat-by-beat basis.[4,22,23] Orthotopic heart transplantation serves as a prime example of independent regulation with intact but isolated intracardiac ganglia.[24] Transection of the spinal cord at T1-T4 in a porcine model demonstrates the ability of the remaining neuronal networks to regulate cardiac function, independently of the central nervous system.[25] In addition to local information processing that occurs at the intrinsic cardiac ganglia, the local circuit neurons within these ganglia serve as important peripheral stations for processing neural information, receiving input from both the central nervous system (sympathetic and parasympathetic) and the myocardium.[26]

AUTONOMIC NERVOUS SYSTEM AND CARDIAC PATHOPHYSIOLOGY
Response to Sympathetic Activation

Norepinephrine stimulation of beta-adrenergic receptors causes downstream modulation of ion channels and calcium release, which culminates in increases in inotropy, chronotropy, lusitropy, and dromotropy in normal hearts. However, in the setting of structural heart disease, the electrophysiological effects of sympathetic activation predispose to sudden death.[27] The calcium-loading effects on the sarcoplasmic reticulum can create delayed afterdepolarizations that can initiate ventricular arrhythmias.[28] Action potential duration (APD) is shortened in areas of dense sympathetic innervation, and because of the heterogeneity of sympathetic innervation, APD dispersion increases. In ischemic cardiomyopathy, direct and indirect sympathetic activation with isoproterenol and nitroprusside in humans[29] and electrical stimulation of the stellate ganglia in porcine hearts has been shown to significantly increase dispersion of repolarization.[30] T-peak to T-end interval, a marker of SCD, correlates with dispersion of repolarization and is significantly increased with stellate ganglion stimulation in these studies. Of note, T-peak to T-end interval is not increased with uniform norepinephrine infusion in normal hearts, highlighting the nonuniform distribution of direct nerve activation.[31] The dispersion of repolarization sets the stage for functional blocks and promotes a substrate for reentrant arrhythmias. In addition, sympathetic stimulation in animal models has been shown to increase electrical restitution and electrical alternans and decrease ventricular effective refractory period (ERP) and ventricular fibrillation threshold (VFT).[32] Furthermore, the cotransmitters released with sympathetic stimulation, namely neuropeptide Y, have been shown to reduce vagal release of acetylcholine and increase ventricular fibrillation (VF) inducibility by acting directly on the myocardial Y1 receptor.[9] Other indirect effects of sympathetic activation include a neurally induced proinflammatory state, which confers negative remodeling of the myocardium.[33] The sympathetic activation that occurs with cardiac disease, along with structural changes such as connexin-43 downregulation and lateralization,[34,35] acts in concert to cause malignant ventricular arrhythmias that result in sudden death (**Fig. 2**).

Parasympathetic Activation

The primary method of increasing parasympathetic tone has been via stimulation of the vagal

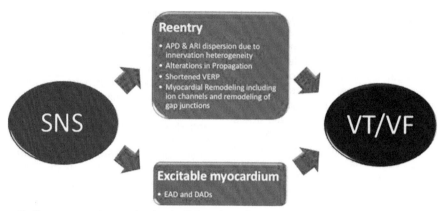

Fig. 2. Sympathetic nervous system activation in the setting of MI increases the risk of VT/VF by modulating the 2 primary criteria needed for initiation of arrhythmias, including conduction velocity and repolarization. Therefore, sympathetic activation creates both more excitable myocardium by initiating EADs and DADs and a substrate that is more likely to promote reentry. DAD, delayed after depolarization; EAD, early after depolarization; SNS, sympathetic nervous system; VERP, ventricular effective refractory period.

trunk. VNS has been shown to reduce slope of APD restitution, lengthen ventricular ERP, and raise VFT in various animal models, including rats, rabbits, pigs, cats, and dogs.[36–38] Furthermore, direct right and left VNS or indirect stimulation via phenylephrine infusion increases epicardial and endocardial ventricular APD, and ERP.[39] Unlike right and left thoracic ganglia stimulation, lateral differences are not evident when stimulating the vagal nerves.[37] The neurotransmitter conferring these beneficial effects include acetylcholine, which interacts with beneficial receptor subtypes, including muscarinic receptor subtype 3 and nicotinic receptor α7nAChR.[40] Nitric oxide release because of VNS also protects against ventricular arrhythmias.[41] Connexin-43, a gap junction protein that is decreased in myocardial infarction (MI), is preserved in the setting of VNS.[42] Other beneficial effects of parasympathetic activation include improvement of heart failure in animal models,[43] coronary vasodilation,[44–46] decrease in reactive oxygen radicals,[47] and reduction of inflammation.[48] Therefore, through several mechanisms, increasing parasympathetic tone protects against ventricular arrhythmias.

NEURAL REMODELING IN THE SETTING OF MYOCARDIAL INFARCTION
Denervation

MI can cause local denervation of sympathetic fibers and create electrical heterogeneity of the myocardium.[49] Local denervation of infarcted regions exhibits a blunted ability to shorten activation recovery interval (ARI) with stellate stimulation, contributing to ARI dispersion.[30] Denervation of myocardium increases beta-adrenergic sensitivity, calcium mishandling, and APD dispersion.[50,51]

Sympathetic denervation can be imaged with radioactive analogues of norepinephrine, namely 131I-meta-iodo-benzyguanidine, using single-photon emission computerized tomography or 11C-hydroxyephedrine using PET. Greater degree of denervation on these imaging modalities predicts SCD risk better than infarct size or ejection fraction (EF).[52,53] Furthermore, the denervation patterns seen on PET imaging correspond well with late gadolinium enhancement scar regions seen on MRI,[54] and the heterogeneity of innervation at the border zones correlate with increased ventricular arrhythmia inducibility.[55]

The reinnervation process is shaped by chemoattractants and chemorepellants with NGF playing a key role as a chemoattractant. In a heart failure rat model, myocardial NGF levels decrease in response to norepinephrine stimulation.[56] The reduced NGF levels decrease sympathetic innervation density in the myocardium, thus attenuating the synaptic input and equilibrating the myocardial exposure to higher sympathetic tone. Afferent innervation is also controlled by NGF. In a streptozocin-induced diabetic mice model, diabetes decreased NGF production and afferent signaling in the dorsal root ganglia. This cardiac sensory neuropathy predisposes to sudden death by means of clinically silent ischemia.[57] Other neurotrophic factors, such as Sema3a, act as a chemorepellant and thereby prevent innervation. Clinically, polymorphisms in the SEMA3A gene have been linked to unexplained cardiac arrest.[58] Sema3a overexpression in left stellate ganglion of ischemic rats has been shown to reduce nerve sprouting, attenuate the dephosphorylation of connexin 43, and reduce ventricular arrhythmia inducibility.[59] Similarly, Sema3a overexpression in the infarct border zones of rats reduces sympathetic innervation and ventricular tachycardia (VT) inducibility.[60] The mechanism behind the persistent postinfarction sympathetic denervation has been attributed to the chemorepellant effect of chondroitin sulfate proteoglycans (present in scar) binding with neuronal protein tyrosine phosphatase receptor σ, which is a key regulator of axonal growth depending on its ligand.[61] When this paired binding is prevented with intracellular sigma peptide, sympathetic innervation is restored and arrhythmia susceptibility is reduced.[51] In summary, pathologic patterns of denervation predispose to sudden death by creating proarrhythmic substrate. Understanding this pathophysiology has led to a few promising therapeutic molecular targets that focus on modulating reinnervation at the level of myocardium.

Hyperinnervation

Axonal damage and denervation is followed by attempts at reinnervation by the cardiac peripheral nerves. However, this process appears to be very heterogeneous. Reinnervation is observed in localized regions along border zones of infarcts and appears to proceed in a heterogeneous fashion likely determined by the underlying molecular milieu driving the innervation process. This heterogeneous hyperinnervation increases the dispersion of repolarization and provides the substrate for ventricular arrhythmias.[62] In explanted human hearts with history of VT, evidence of myocardial hyperinnervation at border zones of scar regions has been observed.[63] In addition, following MI, infusing NGF into the stellate ganglia to promote sympathetic nerve sprouting increases the incidence of ventricular arrhythmias and SCD in canine hearts.[64] Restoring appropriate reinnervation of the scar has been shown to decrease arrhythmias in a mouse model of MI.[51] Therefore, agents that promote homogeneous reinnervation may serve as an important cornerstone in autonomic clinical therapeutics.

Neural Remodeling of the Cardiac and Extracardiac Ganglia

In addition to neural remodeling at the level of the myocardium, ischemic and nonischemic cardiomyopathies are associated with remodeling of the extracardiac (stellate) ganglia. Human stellate ganglia from patients with structural heart disease have been shown to contain enlarged neurons,[65] and in a porcine infarct model, stellate ganglia contain less nonsympathetic neural populations, and more proarrhythmic neuropeptide Y activity.[66] In a canine infarct model, an increase in synaptic density of stellate ganglion neurons has been observed by measuring growth-associated protein 43 and synaptophysin.[67] Similar increases in sympathetic remodeling of stellate ganglia have been seen in patients with heart failure.[65] In a porcine infarct model, the degree of neural remodeling including increased neuronal size and neuronal nitric oxide synthase (nNOS) activity has been shown in the dorsal root, stellate, right atrial, and ventral interventricular ganglionated plexi.[68] Furthermore, the ability of neurons within the intrinsic cardiac ganglia to respond to various stimuli, such as preload reduction, is altered in the setting of MI.[26] Extracardiac ganglia remodeling plays an important role in modulating ventricular arrhythmias. **Fig. 3** provides a flow chart that represents the different effects of infarcted myocardium on remodeling the afferent and efferent limbs of the sympathetic nervous system.

NEURAXIAL MODULATION TO REDUCE RISK OF SUDDEN CARDIAC DEATH
Modulation of the Sympathetic Nervous System

Except for a few disorders such as LQT3 or Brugada, reducing the sympathetic activity is expected to reduce ventricular arrhythmias and SCD in the setting of structural heart disease.

Chemical blockade

The pharmacologic cornerstones of cardioprotective heart failure therapy in the past 2 decades block sympathetic activation with the use of beta-blockers,[69] angiotensin-converting enzyme inhibitors (ACEI),[70] angiotensin receptor blockers (ARB),[71] and aldosterone antagonists.[72] Beta-adrenergic receptor blockade has long-term improvement in heart failure and mortality.[73] ACEI and ARB effectively block the effect of angiotensin II, which is known to increase central nervous system sympathetic outflow and impair the baroreceptor pathways that restrain sympathetic outflow at the nucleus tractus solitarius.[74] Aldosterone antagonists have been shown to decrease myocardial norepinephrine content and increase VFT.[75] Statins, in addition to their cornerstone role in ischemic heart disease,[76] have been also implicated in reducing sympathetic outflow.[77] In the critical care

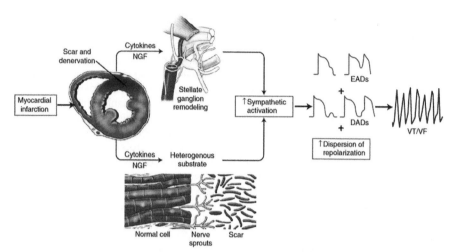

Fig. 3. Effects of MI on the cardiac sympathetic system. Infarcted myocardium stimulates release of signaling molecules including NGF that promote remodeling of the afferent and efferent nervous system such that sympathetic nervous activity is amplified. Remodeling of the nervous system occurs at all levels, including the intrinsic cardiac ganglia, the thoracic ganglia, and the higher centers. This along with denervation and nerve sprouting at the myocardial level further amplifies the substrate heterogeneity and ultimately increases risk of VT and VF. (*Adapted from* Vaseghi M, Ajijola O, Mahajan A. Sympathetic innervation denervation, and cardiac arrhythmias. In: Zipes D, Jalife J, eds. Cardiac electrophysiology: from cell to bedside. 6th ed. Philadelphia, PA: Elsevier Saunders; 2014:409–18; with permission).

setting of electrical storm, sedation and general anesthesia can reduce sympathetic activity and control ventricular arrhythmias.[78]

Cardiac resynchronization therapy

Cardiac resynchronization therapy (CRT) with biventricular pacing has been another cornerstone of heart failure therapy that modulates the autonomic nervous system. Using PET imaging, homogeneous sympathetic innervation has been shown to be increased in the myocardium of CRT responders.[79] In addition, although heart failure increases muscarinic receptor subtype 2 and its $G\alpha i$ counterpart, CRT upregulates known protective muscarinic receptor subtype 3.[80]

Thoracic epidural anesthesia

Reduction of sympathetic outflow from the spinal cord can be accomplished by injecting anesthetic agents into the thoracic epidural space. Reducing VF with thoracic epidural anesthesia (TEA) has been demonstrated in an ischemic rat model.[81] The initial human case report showed a dramatic reduction of a patient's electrical storm corresponding with the initiation of bupivacaine in the T1-T2 epidural space.[82] A subsequent case series of 8 patients who underwent TEA showed no adverse procedural outcomes, and 6 patients showed a significant decrease (>80%) in VT burden.[83] For patients in whom the procedure is not contraindicated because of anticoagulation,

TEA offers the advantages of emergency bedside initiation with minimal effects on hemodynamic parameters,[84] while bridging toward a more definitive therapy. In addition, there has been reported success with intrathecal clonidine in reducing ischemia-induced ventricular arrhythmias in a postinfarct canine model.[85]

Spinal cord stimulation

Spinal cord stimulation (SCS) has been approved in the United States for chronic pain and intractable angina.[86] Similar to TEA, SCS acts in the epidural space of T1-T4, but the nerves are modulated by electrical impulses rather than chemical deactivation. SCS modulates the autonomic innervation of the heart by reducing stellate ganglia activity,[87] increasing vagal tone,[88] altering intrinsic cardiac neuron activity,[89] and modifying sympathetic nerve sprouting in the myocardium.[90] In a postinfarct canine heart model with superimposed pacing-induced heart failure, SCS reduced ischemia driven VF from 59% to 23%.[91] Furthermore, intermittent chronic SCS in a similar model lowered VF because of ischemia and improved the EF compared with carvedilol, demonstrating benefit beyond conventional heart failure medical therapy.[92] Similar reductions in ventricular ectopy were observed in an ischemic porcine model, where SCS decreased dispersion of repolarization.[93] An initial case series of SCS in patients with heart failure showed benefit. SCS reduced VT/VF burden by at least 75% over a period of 4 months with a 2-month midpoint crossover design.[94] However, SCS has shown mixed results in human clinical trials of heart failure. The Thoracic Spinal Cord Stimulation for Heart Failure as a Restorative Treatment study showed safety and efficacy in New York Heart Association (NYHA) class III patients with EF 25% to 30%.[95] Determining the Feasibility of Spinal Cord Neuromodulation for the Treatment of Chronic Systolic Heart Failure study evaluated NYHA class III patients with EF ≤35% and showed no improvement in EF.[96] It is possible that the discrepant SCS clinical results of VT/VF versus HF can be explained by differences of how SCS was applied, including duration and frequency of stimulation.

Cardiac sympathetic denervation/ decentralization

Cardiac sympathetic denervation (CSD) can be achieved with surgical removal of stellate and T1-T4 ganglia via video-assisted thoracoscopic surgery.[78] Although this surgery does not interrupt all the thoracic sympathetic pathways to the heart, as the upper half of the stellate and the middle cervical ganglia remain intact, it has shown benefit in a variety of clinical settings. In a case series of 22 patients with long QT, catecholaminergic polymorphic VT, and idiopathic VT, 73% had a marked reduction in VT burden with 55% having complete cessation at median follow-up of 28 months with left CSD.[97] In the setting for VT storm and structural heart disease in 9 patients, 3 had complete cessation of VT and 2 had partial response.[83] The beneficial effects of bilateral CSD were reported in a case series of 41 patients, 17 of whom underwent unilateral and 27 of whom underwent bilateral.[98] Although both left and bilateral CSD significantly reduced the burden of ICD shocks in the year after the procedure compared with the 6 months prior, patients with bilateral CSD had a significantly greater ICD shock-free survival at 1 year. Therefore, for control of ventricular arrhythmias refractory to standard medical therapy, bilateral CSD serves as a promising therapeutic strategy. Risks of the procedure are less than 5% and include mild ptosis, pneumothorax, or hemothorax, and occasionally, vasopressor support after the procedure. Long-term side effects include a change in sweating pattern and sensation in approximately 10% to 15% of patients as well as neuropathic pain, which generally resolves within 6 months after the procedure.[98]

Emerging frontiers in animal models include molecular modification of the stellate ganglia. Delivering nNOS to hypertensive rats can improve impaired vagal tone[99] and attenuate hyperactive sympathetic tone.[100] Another therapeutic avenue includes reducing stellate activity with low-level VNS. By upregulating a hyperpolarizing small conductance calcium-activated potassium channel SK2 in dogs, neuronal firing of the sympathetic branch is effectively reduced with VNS.[101] The ability to translate nonsurgical methods to modify stellate activity can potentially provide the benefits without the complications of surgical CSD.

Renal sympathetic denervation

Renal afferent nerve fibers that modulate the sympathetic outflow can be reduced by catheter ablation of these fibers in the renal arteries, a procedure known as renal artery denervation (RDN). The first successful report of RDN for arrhythmias showed dramatic reductions of VT/VF burden for 2 patients with VT storm.[102] Similar benefit was seen in a refractory VT patient during the post-revascularization recovery after an ST elevation MI[103] and another who failed endocardial and epicardial ablation.[104] A case series of 4 patients with cardiomyopathy undergoing RDN showed safety and efficacy with reduction of VT burden from 11 VT episodes in the month preceding procedure to 0.3 per month following the procedure.[105] A subsequent case series of 10 patients with cardiomyopathies showed a dramatic reduction with 28.5 device shocks in the preceding 6 months and 0 shocks after renal denervation.[106] However, although RDN has shown antiarrhythmic benefit in case series of patients with refractory ventricular arrhythmias and structural heart disease, the inability to reach a prespecified clinical outcome in the SIMPLICITY-HTN3 trial[107] has highlighted the challenges of identifying precise targets and endpoints of ablation within the renal arteries.[78,108] There is much anticipation of the results from the current ongoing trials evaluating the efficacy of RDN to reduce ventricular arrhythmias, including RESCUE[109] and RESET-VT.[110]

Modulation of the Parasympathetic Nervous System

Vagal nerve stimulation

Augmenting the protective effects of the parasympathetic nervous system for controlling ventricular arrhythmias has been accomplished with VNS in animal models. Vagal nerve stimulators are implanted surgically akin to an implantable pacemaker with stimulation leads attached to the cervical the vagal trunk, adapted from US Food and Drug Administration–approved therapy for epilepsy and depression.[111,112] Side effects from the procedure include infection, dysphagia, hoarseness, cough, and pain.[86] A reduction in SCD from ventricular arrhythmias has been demonstrated with vagal stimulation in a healed infarct canine model subjected to repeat ischemia.[113] The first human cardiac application was described in 8 patients for the indication of heart failure using CardioFit stimulators (BioControl Medical Ltd., Yehud, Israel).[114] Subsequent human trials for heart failure have shown mixed results. ANTHEM-HF, a nonblinded trial for NYHA II-III patients with EF less than 40%, showed improvements in NYHA class and EF.[115] NECTAR-HF was a randomized blinded study, which showed no improvements with VNS with respect to objective parameters, such as EF, but improved clinical parameters such as NYHA class.[116] INOVATE-HF was a randomized study that further showed no benefit of mortality or worsening HF in NYHA III patients with EF ≤40%.[117] In many ways, VNS trials for heart failure share parallel lessons to the negative trials of SCS. As mentioned above, the vagosympathetic trunk contains both parasympathetic and sympathetic and afferent and efferent nerves. Different stimulation parameters can differentially engage these fibers,[118] and the effects of VNS is significantly increased when the vagosympathetic trunk is transected in animal studies,[119,120] demonstrating the powerful effects of afferent fiber activation on efferent effects. In addition, a case of a patient experiencing an increase in ventricular arrhythmias after VNS has been reported.[38] Therefore, the stimulation parameters used can significantly affect the outcomes of VNS and may account for the mixed human clinical trial results. With better characterization of the optimal dose of stimulation, VNS remains a promising option to apply to reduce VT/VF.

Tragus nerve stimulation

A less invasive method of stimulating the parasympathetic nervous system has been performed using tragus nerve stimulation.[86] A flat electrical clip is applied to the tragus, the anterior protuberance of the outer ear, and electrical stimulation is applied to the auricular branch of the vagal nerve. Much of the data on tragus nerve stimulation has focused on its beneficial effects for atrial fibrillation and atrial arrhythmias.[121] In addition, chronic tragus nerve stimulation in a canine model of healed MI demonstrated improved left ventricular remodeling.[122] A randomized trial of 40 patients demonstrated that tragus nerve stimulation suppressed pacing-induced atrial fibrillation, increased cycle length of atrial fibrillation, and decreased inflammatory cytokines.[123] The TREAT-AF trial will study the effects in a larger population.[124] It is possible that the anti-inflammatory and cardiac remodeling effect of tragus nerve stimulation could prove useful in treatment of heart failure and ventricular arrhythmias.

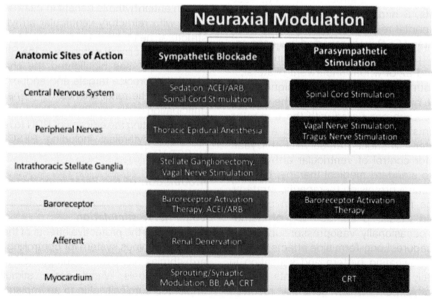

Fig. 4. Neuraxial modulation can be targeted at multiple levels of the cardiac autonomic nervous system, from the central nervous system to the neuromyocardial junction. Therapeutic goals generally include decreasing sympathetic activity and augmenting parasympathetic activity. AA, aldosterone antagonist; BB, beta-blocker.

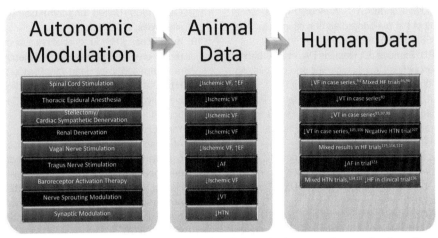

Fig. 5. Autonomic modulation therapies have translated from basic research to animal studies and human studies, although in clinical trials, some therapies have had mixed results. AF, atrial fibrillation; EF, ejection fraction; HF, heart failure; HTN, hypertension.

Baroreceptor activation therapy

Baroreflex sensitivity is significantly reduced in the setting of the heart failure, and patients with decreased baroreflex sensitivity have an increased risk of SCD.[125,126] Baroreceptor activation therapy (BAT) via electrical stimulation of the carotid bodies augments vagal tone[127] and decreases sympathetic outflow.[128] At the intrathoracic level, BAT-attenuated left stellate ganglia electrical activity (amplitude and frequency) in the setting of canine ischemia.[129] At the level of the intrinsic cardiac ganglia, BAT reduced anterior right ganglionated plexus electrical amplitude and frequency, decreased ability of the superior left ganglionated plexus to reduce sinus slowing, and reduced AF in dogs.[130] In canine models of ischemic cardiomyopathy, BAT has decreased ventricular arrhythmias, decreased slope of APD restitution, and lengthened ventricular ERP.[129,131,132] BAT has also been shown to decrease ischemia-driven inflammation, oxidative stress, and apoptosis and improve connexin-43 levels. Current human data have focused on the use of BAT for the treatment of hypertension and heart failure.[133] A phase III trial of the Rheos BAT system (CVRx, Inc., Minneapolis, MN, USA), which stimulates bilateral carotid bodies for resistant hypertension, has shown mixed results, failing to achieve prespecified endpoints but able to improve proportion of patients with SBP less than 140 mm Hg. The primary risk with this procedure was cranial nerve injury resulting in dysphonia, dysphagia, and localized numbness in 4.8% of patients.[134] Phase 2 trial results for resistant hypertension using Barostim (CVRx, Inc., Minneapolis, MN, USA), a smaller device with unilateral stimulation of the right carotid body, has shown similar reductions in blood pressure

without significant cranial nerve injury.[135] Barostim in heart failure patients with NYHA III and EF ≤35% showed improvements in NYHA class, 6-minute walk time, and quality-of-life scores.[136] Although BAT has not been used for treatment of ventricular arrhythmias, its potential promise for treatment of heart failure could lead to a reduction in ventricular arrhythmias. **Fig. 4** summarizes the neuraxial modulation targets and their relationship to the levels of cardiac innervation. The level of evidence of translating these various modalities from bench side to bedside is summarized in **Fig. 5**.

SUMMARY

Autonomic cardiac innervation plays a significant role in SCD, modulating the fabric of cardiac excitability and propagation. Significant neural remodeling in the setting of heart disease predisposes to malignant ventricular arrhythmias by causing alterations at the level of the myocardium, the intrinsic cardiac ganglia, extracardiac intrathoracic sympathetic ganglia, extrathoracic ganglia, spinal cord, and the brainstem, as well as the higher centers and the cortex. Therapeutic strategies at each of these levels have been used to restore the balance between the sympathetic and parasympathetic branches of the autonomic nervous system. Detailed characterization of this complex neural network will provide further important therapeutic insights into the treatment of SCD.

REFERENCES

1. van der Lende M, Surges R, Sander JW, et al. Cardiac arrhythmias during or after epileptic seizures. J Neurol Neurosurg Psychiatry 2016;87(1):69–74.

2. Phillips JG, Randall WC, Armour JA. Functional anatomy of the major cardiac nerves in cats. Anat Rec 1986;214(4):365–71.

3. Janes RD, Brandys JC, Hopkins DA, et al. Anatomy of human extrinsic cardiac nerves and ganglia. Am J Cardiol 1986;57(4):299–309.

4. Ardell JL, Andresen MC, Armour JA, et al. Translational neurocardiology: preclinical models and cardioneural integrative aspects. J Physiol 2016; 594(14):3877–909.

5. Manousiouthakis E, Mendez M, Garner MC, et al. Venous endothelin guides sympathetic innervation of the developing mouse heart. Nat Commun 2014;5:3918.

6. Nam J, Onitsuka I, Hatch J, et al. Coronary veins determine the pattern of sympathetic innervation in the developing heart. Development 2013; 140(7):1475–85.

7. Angelakos ET, King MP, Millard RW. Regional distribution of catecholamines in the hearts of various species. Ann N Y Acad Sci 1969;156(1): 219–40.

8. Armour JA, Murphy DA, Yuan BX, et al. Gross and microscopic anatomy of the human intrinsic cardiac nervous system. Anat Rec 1997;247(2): 289–98.

9. Herring N. Autonomic control of the heart: going beyond the classical neurotransmitters. Exp Physiol 2015;100(4):354–8.

10. Waxman SG. Clinical neuroanatomy. 27th edition. New York: McGraw-Hill Education/Medical; 2013.

11. Shen MJ, Zipes DP. Role of the autonomic nervous system in modulating cardiac arrhythmias. Circ Res 2014;114(6):1004–21.

12. Pauza DH, Skripka V, Pauziene N, et al. Morphology, distribution, and variability of the epicardiac neural ganglionated subplexuses in the human heart. Anat Rec 2000;259(4):353–82.

13. Coote JH. Myths and realities of the cardiac vagus. J Physiol 2013;591(17):4073–85.

14. Rysevaite K, Saburkina I, Pauziene N, et al. Immunohistochemical characterization of the intrinsic cardiac neural plexus in whole-mount mouse heart preparations. Heart Rhythm 2011; 8(5):731–8.

15. Ulphani JS, Cain JH, Inderyas F, et al. Quantitative analysis of parasympathetic innervation of the porcine heart. Heart Rhythm 2010;7(8):1113–9.

16. Randall WC, Priola DV, Pace JB. Responses of individucal cardiac chambers to stimulation of the cervical vagosympathetic trunk in atropinized dogs. Circ Res 1967;20(5):534–44.

17. Seki A, Green HR, Lee TD, et al. Sympathetic nerve fibers in human cervical and thoracic vagus nerves. Heart Rhythm 2014;11(8):1411–7.

18. Jänig W. The integrative action of the autonomic nervous system: neurobiology of homeostasis.

Cambridge (United Kingdom): Cambridge University Press; 2006.

19. Xu B, Zheng H, Liu X, et al. Activation of afferent renal nerves modulates RVLM-projecting PVN neurons. Am J Physiol Heart Circ Physiol 2015;308(9): H1103–11.

20. Llewellyn-Smith IJ, Verberne AJM. Central regulation of autonomic functions. 2nd edition. New York: Oxford University Press; 2011.

21. Andresen MC, Peters JH. Comparison of baroreceptive to other afferent synaptic transmission to the medial solitary tract nucleus. Am J Physiol Heart Circ Physiol 2008;295(5):H2032–42.

22. Armour JA. Potential clinical relevance of the 'little brain' on the mammalian heart. Exp Physiol 2008; 93(2):165–76.

23. Beaumont E, Salavatian S, Southerland EM, et al. Network interactions within the canine intrinsic cardiac nervous system: implications for reflex control of regional cardiac function. J Physiol 2013; 591(18):4515–33.

24. Vaseghi M, Lellouche N, Ritter H, et al. Mode and mechanisms of death after orthotopic heart transplantation. Heart Rhythm 2009;6(4):503–9.

25. Yamakawa K, Howard-Quijano K, Zhou W, et al. Central vs. peripheral neuraxial sympathetic control of porcine ventricular electrophysiology. Am J Physiol Regul Integr Comp Physiol 2016;310(5): R414–21.

26. Rajendran PS, Nakamura K, Ajijola OA, et al. Myocardial infarction induces structural and functional remodelling of the intrinsic cardiac nervous system. J Physiol 2016;594(2):321–41.

27. Habecker BA, Anderson ME, Birren SJ, et al. Molecular and cellular neurocardiology: development, cellular and molecular adaptations to heart disease. J Physiol 2016;594(14):3853–75.

28. Myles RC, Wang L, Kang C, et al. Local beta-adrenergic stimulation overcomes source-sink mismatch to generate focal arrhythmia. Circ Res 2012;110(11):1454–64.

29. Vaseghi M, Lux RL, Mahajan A, et al. Sympathetic stimulation increases dispersion of repolarization in humans with myocardial infarction. Am J Physiol Heart Circ Physiol 2012;302(9): H1838–46.

30. Ajijola OA, Yagishita D, Patel KJ, et al. Focal myocardial infarction induces global remodeling of cardiac sympathetic innervation: neural remodeling in a spatial context. Am J Physiol Heart Circ Physiol 2013;305(7):H1031–40.

31. Yagishita D, Chui RW, Yamakawa K, et al. Sympathetic nerve stimulation, not circulating norepinephrine, modulates T-peak to T-end interval by increasing global dispersion of repolarization. Circ Arrhythm Electrophysiol 2015;8(1): 174–85.

32. Ng GA, Brack KE, Patel VH, et al. Autonomic modulation of electrical restitution, alternans and ventricular fibrillation initiation in the isolated heart. Cardiovasc Res 2007;73(4):750–60.

33. Janig W. Sympathetic nervous system and inflammation: a conceptual view. Auton Neurosci 2014; 182:4–14.

34. Dhein S, Hagen A, Jozwiak J, et al. Improving cardiac gap junction communication as a new antiarrhythmic mechanism: the action of antiarrhythmic peptides. Naunyn Schmiedebergs Arch Pharmacol 2010;381(3):221–34.

35. Jiang H, Hu X, Lu Z, et al. Effects of sympathetic nerve stimulation on ischemia-induced ventricular arrhythmias by modulating connexin43 in rats. Arch Med Res 2008;39(7): 647–54.

36. Brack KE, Patel VH, Coote JH, et al. Nitric oxide mediates the vagal protective effect on ventricular fibrillation via effects on action potential duration restitution in the rabbit heart. J Physiol 2007; 583(Pt 2):695–704.

37. Martins JB, Zipes DP. Effects of sympathetic and vagal nerves on recovery properties of the endocardium and epicardium of the canine left ventricle. Circ Res 1980;46(1):100–10.

38. Huang WA, Shivkumar K, Vaseghi M. Device-based autonomic modulation in arrhythmia patients: the role of vagal nerve stimulation. Curr Treat Options Cardiovasc Med 2015;17(5):379.

39. Ellenbogen KA, Smith ML, Eckberg DL. Increased vagal cardiac nerve traffic prolongs ventricular refractoriness in patients undergoing electrophysiology testing. Am J Cardiol 1990; 65(20):1345–50.

40. Zhao M, He X, Bi XY, et al. Vagal stimulation triggers peripheral vascular protection through the cholinergic anti-inflammatory pathway in a rat model of myocardial ischemia/reperfusion. Basic Res Cardiol 2013;108(3):345.

41. Brack KE, Coote JH, Ng GA. Vagus nerve stimulation protects against ventricular fibrillation independent of muscarinic receptor activation. Cardiovasc Res 2011;91(3):437–46.

42. Wu W, Lu Z. Loss of anti-arrhythmic effect of vagal nerve stimulation on ischemia-induced ventricular tachyarrhythmia in aged rats. Tohoku J Exp Med 2011;223(1):27–33.

43. Hamann JJ, Ruble SB, Stolen C, et al. Vagus nerve stimulation improves left ventricular function in a canine model of chronic heart failure. Eur J Heart Fail 2013;15(12):1319–26.

44. Feigl EO. Parasympathetic control of coronary blood flow in dogs. Circ Res 1969;25(5):509–19.

45. Henning RJ, Sawmiller DR. Vasoactive intestinal peptide: cardiovascular effects. Cardiovasc Res 2001;49(1):27–37.

46. Zhao G, Shen W, Xu X, et al. Selective impairment of vagally mediated, nitric oxide-dependent coronary vasodilation in conscious dogs after pacing-induced heart failure. Circulation 1995;91(10): 2655–63.

47. Shinlapawittayatorn K, Chinda K, Palee S, et al. Low-amplitude, left vagus nerve stimulation significantly attenuates ventricular dysfunction and infarct size through prevention of mitochondrial dysfunction during acute ischemia-reperfusion injury. Heart Rhythm 2013;10(11): 1700–7.

48. Bonaz B, Sinniger V, Pellissier S. Anti-inflammatory properties of the vagus nerve: potential therapeutic implications of vagus nerve stimulation. J Physiol 2016;594(20):5781–90.

49. Nori SL, Gaudino M, Alessandrini F, et al. Immunohistochemical evidence for sympathetic denervation and reinnervation after necrotic injury in rat myocardium. Cell Mol Biol 1995; 41(6):799–807.

50. Inoue H, Zipes DP. Results of sympathetic denervation in the canine heart: supersensitivity that may be arrhythmogenic. Circulation 1987;75(4): 877–87.

51. Gardner RT, Wang L, Lang BT, et al. Targeting protein tyrosine phosphatase sigma after myocardial infarction restores cardiac sympathetic innervation and prevents arrhythmias. Nat Commun 2015;6: 6235.

52. Malhotra S, Fernandez SF, Fallavollita JA, et al. Prognostic significance of imaging myocardial sympathetic innervation. Curr Cardiol Rep 2015; 17(8):62.

53. Fallavollita JA, Heavey BM, Luisi AJ Jr, et al. Regional myocardial sympathetic denervation predicts the risk of sudden cardiac arrest in ischemic cardiomyopathy. J Am Coll Cardiol 2014;63(2): 141–9.

54. de Haan S, Rijnierse MT, Harms HJ, et al. Myocardial denervation coincides with scar heterogeneity in ischemic cardiomyopathy: a PET and CMR study. J Nucl Cardiol 2016;23(6):1480–8.

55. Zhou Y, Zhou W, Folks RD, et al. I-123 mIBG and Tc-99m myocardial SPECT imaging to predict inducibility of ventricular arrhythmia on electrophysiology testing: a retrospective analysis. J Nucl Cardiol 2014;21(5):913–20.

56. Kimura K, Kanazawa H, Ieda M, et al. Norepinephrine-induced nerve growth factor depletion causes cardiac sympathetic denervation in severe heart failure. Auton Neurosci 2010;156(1–2):27–35.

57. Ieda M, Kanazawa H, Ieda Y, et al. Nerve growth factor is critical for cardiac sensory innervation and rescues neuropathy in diabetic hearts. Circulation 2006;114(22):2351–63.

58. Nakano Y, Chayama K, Ochi H, et al. A nonsynonymous polymorphism in semaphorin 3A as a risk factor for human unexplained cardiac arrest with documented ventricular fibrillation. PLoS Genet 2013;9(4):e1003364.

59. Yang LC, Zhang PP, Chen XM, et al. Semaphorin 3a transfection into the left stellate ganglion reduces susceptibility to ventricular arrhythmias after myocardial infarction in rats. Europace 2016; 18(12):1886–96.

60. Chen RH, Li YG, Jiao KL, et al. Overexpression of Sema3a in myocardial infarction border zone decreases vulnerability of ventricular tachycardia post-myocardial infarction in rats. J Cell Mol Med 2013;17(5):608–16.

61. Chien PN, Ryu SE. Protein tyrosine phosphatase sigma in proteoglycan-mediated neural regeneration regulation. Mol Neurobiol 2013; 47(1):220–7.

62. Li CY, Li YG. Cardiac sympathetic nerve sprouting and susceptibility to ventricular arrhythmias after myocardial infarction. Cardiol Res Pract 2015; 2015:698368.

63. Cao JM, Fishbein MC, Han JB, et al. Relationship between regional cardiac hyperinnervation and ventricular arrhythmia. Circulation 2000;101(16): 1960–9.

64. Cao JM, Chen LS, KenKnight BH, et al. Nerve sprouting and sudden cardiac death. Circ Res 2000;86(7):816–21.

65. Ajijola OA, Wisco JJ, Lambert HW, et al. Extracardiac neural remodeling in humans with cardiomyopathy. Circ Arrhythm Electrophysiol 2012;5(5): 1010–116.

66. Ajijola OA, Yagishita D, Reddy NK, et al. Remodeling of stellate ganglion neurons after spatially targeted myocardial infarction: neuropeptide and morphologic changes. Heart Rhythm 2015;12(5): 1027–35.

67. Han S, Kobayashi K, Joung B, et al. Electroanatomic remodeling of the left stellate ganglion after myocardial infarction. J Am Coll Cardiol 2012; 59(10):954–61.

68. Nakamura K, Ajijola OA, Aliotta E, et al. Pathological effects of chronic myocardial infarction on peripheral neurons mediating cardiac neurotransmission. Auton Neurosci 2016;197:34–40.

69. Packer M, Fowler MB, Roecker EB, et al. Effect of carvedilol on the morbidity of patients with severe chronic heart failure: results of the carvedilol prospective randomized cumulative survival (COPERNICUS) study. Circulation 2002;106(17): 2194–9.

70. Effect of enalapril on survival in patients with reduced left ventricular ejection fractions and congestive heart failure. The SOLVD Investigators. N Engl J Med 1991;325(5):293–302.

71. Cohn JN, Tognoni G. Valsartan Heart Failure Trial I. A randomized trial of the angiotensin-receptor blocker valsartan in chronic heart failure. N Engl J Med 2001;345(23):1667–75.

72. Pitt B, Zannad F, Remme WJ, et al. The effect of spironolactone on morbidity and mortality in patients with severe heart failure. Randomized Aldactone Evaluation Study Investigators. N Engl J Med 1999;341(10):709–17.

73. Effect of metoprolol CR/XL in chronic heart failure: metoprolol CR/XL randomised intervention trial in congestive heart failure (MERIT-HF). Lancet 1999; 353(9169):2001–7.

74. Arnold AC, Gallagher PE, Diz DI. Brain reninangiotensin system in the nexus of hypertension and aging. Hypertens Res 2013;36(1):5–13.

75. Cittadini A, Monti MG, Isgaard J, et al. Aldosterone receptor blockade improves left ventricular remodeling and increases ventricular fibrillation threshold in experimental heart failure. Cardiovasc Res 2003; 58(3):555–64.

76. Cannon CP, Braunwald E, McCabe CH, et al. Intensive versus moderate lipid lowering with statins after acute coronary syndromes. N Engl J Med 2004; 350(15):1495–504.

77. Millar PJ, Floras JS. Statins and the autonomic nervous system. Clin Sci 2014;126(6):401–15.

78. Tung R, Shivkumar K. Neuraxial modulation for treatment of VT storm. J Biomed Res 2015;29(1): 56–60.

79. Martignani C, Diemberger I, Nanni C, et al. Cardiac resynchronization therapy and cardiac sympathetic function. Eur J Clin Invest 2015;45(8): 792–9.

80. DeMazumder D, Kass DA, O'Rourke B, et al. Cardiac resynchronization therapy restores sympathovagal balance in the failing heart by differential remodeling of cholinergic signaling. Circ Res 2015;116(10):1691–9.

81. Blomberg S, Ricksten SE. Thoracic epidural anaesthesia decreases the incidence of ventricular arrhythmias during acute myocardial ischaemia in the anaesthetized rat. Acta Anaesthesiol Scand 1988;32(3):173–8.

82. Mahajan A, Moore J, Cesario DA, et al. Use of thoracic epidural anesthesia for management of electrical storm: a case report. Heart Rhythm 2005;2(12):1359–62.

83. Bourke T, Vaseghi M, Michowitz Y, et al. Neuraxial modulation for refractory ventricular arrhythmias: value of thoracic epidural anesthesia and surgical left cardiac sympathetic denervation. Circulation 2010;121(21):2255–62.

84. Hasenbos M, Liem TH, Kerkkamp H, et al. The influence of high thoracic epidural analgesia on the cardiovascular system. Acta Anaesthesiol Belg 1988;39(1):49–54.

85. Issa ZF, Ujhelyi MR, Hildebrand KR, et al. Intra-thecal clonidine reduces the incidence of ischemia-provoked ventricular arrhythmias in a canine postinfarction heart failure model. Heart Rhythm 2005;2(10):1122–7.

86. Hou Y, Zhou Q, Po SS. Neuromodulation for cardiac arrhythmia. Heart Rhythm 2016;13(2): 584–92.

87. Wang S, Zhou X, Huang B, et al. Spinal cord stimulation protects against ventricular arrhythmias by suppressing left stellate ganglion neural activity in an acute myocardial infarction canine model. Heart Rhythm 2015;12(7):1628–35.

88. Olgin JE, Takahashi T, Wilson E, et al. Effects of thoracic spinal cord stimulation on cardiac autonomic regulation of the sinus and atrioventricular nodes. J Cardiovasc Electrophysiol 2002;13(5): 475–81.

89. Foreman RD, Linderoth B, Ardell JL, et al. Modulation of intrinsic cardiac neurons by spinal cord stimulation: implications for its therapeutic use in angina pectoris. Cardiovasc Res 2000;47(2): 367–75.

90. Liao SY, Liu Y, Zuo M, et al. Remodelling of cardiac sympathetic re-innervation with thoracic spinal cord stimulation improves left ventricular function in a porcine model of heart failure. Europace 2015;17(12):1875–83.

91. Issa ZF, Zhou X, Ujhelyi MR, et al. Thoracic spinal cord stimulation reduces the risk of ischemic ventricular arrhythmias in a postinfarction heart failure canine model. Circulation 2005;111(24): 3217–20.

92. Lopshire JC, Zhou X, Dusa C, et al. Spinal cord stimulation improves ventricular function and reduces ventricular arrhythmias in a canine postinfarction heart failure model. Circulation 2009; 120(4):286–94.

93. Odenstedt J, Linderoth B, Bergfeldt L, et al. Spinal cord stimulation effects on myocardial ischemia, infarct size, ventricular arrhythmia, and noninvasive electrophysiology in a porcine ischemia-reperfusion model. Heart Rhythm 2011; 8(6):892–8.

94. Grimaldi R, de Luca A, Kornet L, et al. Can spinal cord stimulation reduce ventricular arrhythmias? Heart Rhythm 2012;9(11):1884–7.

95. Tse HF, Turner S, Sanders P, et al. Thoracic spinal cord stimulation for heart failure as a restorative treatment (SCS HEART study): first-in-man experience. Heart Rhythm 2015;12(3): 588–95.

96. Zipes DP, Neuzil P, Theres H, et al. Determining the feasibility of spinal cord neuromodulation for the treatment of chronic systolic heart failure: the DEFEAT-HF Study. JACC Heart Fail 2016;4(2): 129–36.

97. Hofferberth SC, Cecchin F, Loberman D, et al. Left thoracoscopic sympathectomy for cardiac denervation in patients with life-threatening ventricular arrhythmias. J Thorac Cardiovasc Surg 2014;147(1): 404–9.

98. Vaseghi M, Gima J, Kanaan C, et al. Cardiac sympathetic denervation in patients with refractory ventricular arrhythmias or electrical storm: intermediate and long-term follow-up. Heart Rhythm 2014;11(3): 360–6.

99. Heaton DA, Li D, Almond SC, et al. Gene transfer of neuronal nitric oxide synthase into intracardiac ganglia reverses vagal impairment in hypertensive rats. Hypertension 2007;49(2):380–8.

100. Li D, Wang L, Lee CW, et al. Noradrenergic cell specific gene transfer with neuronal nitric oxide synthase reduces cardiac sympathetic neurotransmission in hypertensive rats. Hypertension 2007; 50(1):69–74.

101. Shen MJ, Hao-Che C, Park HW, et al. Low-level vagus nerve stimulation upregulates small conductance calcium-activated potassium channels in the stellate ganglion. Heart Rhythm 2013;10(6): 910–5.

102. Ukena C, Bauer A, Mahfoud F, et al. Renal sympathetic denervation for treatment of electrical storm: first-in-man experience. Clin Res Cardiol 2012; 101(1):63–7.

103. Hoffmann BA, Steven D, Willems S, et al. Renal sympathetic denervation as an adjunct to catheter ablation for the treatment of ventricular electrical storm in the setting of acute myocardial infarction. J Cardiovasc Electrophysiol 2013; 24(10):1175–8.

104. Scholz EP, Raake P, Thomas D, et al. Rescue renal sympathetic denervation in a patient with ventricular electrical storm refractory to endo- and epicardial catheter ablation. Clin Res Cardiol 2015; 104(1):79–84.

105. Remo BF, Preminger M, Bradfield J, et al. Safety and efficacy of renal denervation as a novel treatment of ventricular tachycardia storm in patients with cardiomyopathy. Heart Rhythm 2014;11(4): 541–6.

106. Armaganijan LV, Staico R, Moreira DA, et al. 6-Month outcomes in patients with implantable cardioverter-defibrillators undergoing renal sympathetic denervation for the treatment of refractory ventricular arrhythmias. JACC Cardiovasc Interv 2015;8(7):984–90.

107. Bakris GL, Townsend RR, Liu M, et al. Impact of renal denervation on 24-hour ambulatory blood pressure: results from SYMPLICITY HTN-3. J Am Coll Cardiol 2014;64(11):1071–8.

108. Kandzari DE, Bhatt DL, Brar S, et al. Predictors of blood pressure response in the SYMPLICITY HTN-3 trial. Eur Heart J 2015;36(4):219–27.

109. REnal SympathetiC Denervation to sUpprEss Tachyarrhythmias in ICD Recipients (RESCUE). Available at: https://clinicaltrials.gov/ct2/show/NCT01747837?term=NCT01747837&rank=1. Accessed June 24, 2016.

110. REnal Sympathetic dEnervaTion as an Adjunct to Catheter-based VT Ablation (RESET-VT). Available at: https://clinicaltrials.gov/ct2/show/NCT01858194?term=NCT01858194&rank=1. Accessed June 24, 2016.

111. Klooster DC, de Louw AJ, Aldenkamp AP, et al. Technical aspects of neurostimulation: focus on equipment, electric field modeling, and stimulation protocols. Neurosci Biobehav Rev 2016;65: 113–41.

112. Chatterjee NA, Singh JP. Novel interventional therapies to modulate the autonomic tone in heart failure. JACC Heart Fail 2015;3(10):786–802.

113. Vanoli E, De Ferrari GM, Stramba-Badiale M, et al. Vagal stimulation and prevention of sudden death in conscious dogs with a healed myocardial infarction. Circ Res 1991;68(5):1471–81.

114. Schwartz PJ, De Ferrari GM, Sanzo A, et al. Long term vagal stimulation in patients with advanced heart failure: first experience in man. Eur J Heart Fail 2008;10(9):884–91.

115. Premchand RK, Sharma K, Mittal S, et al. Extended follow-up of patients with heart failure receiving autonomic regulation therapy in the ANTHEM-HF study. J Card Fail 2016;22(8):639–42.

116. Zannad F, De Ferrari GM, Tuinenburg AE, et al. Chronic vagal stimulation for the treatment of low ejection fraction heart failure: results of the NEural Cardiac TherApy foR Heart Failure (NECTAR-HF) randomized controlled trial. Eur Heart J 2015; 36(7):425–33.

117. Gold MR, Van Veldhuisen DJ, Hauptman PJ, et al. Vagus nerve stimulation for the treatment of heart failure: the INOVATE-HF trial. J Am Coll Cardiol 2016;68(2):149–58.

118. Yoo PB, Lubock NB, Hincapie JG, et al. High-resolution measurement of electrically-evoked vagus nerve activity in the anesthetized dog. J Neural Eng 2013;10(2):026003.

119. Yamakawa K, Rajendran PS, Takamiya T, et al. Vagal nerve stimulation activates vagal afferent fibers that reduce cardiac efferent parasympathetic effects. Am J Physiol Heart Circ Physiol 2015; 309(9):H1579–90.

120. Ardell JL, Rajendran PS, Nier HA, et al. Central-peripheral neural network interactions evoked by vagus nerve stimulation: functional consequences on control of cardiac function. Am J Physiol Heart Circ Physiol 2015;309(10):H1740–52.

121. Yu L, Scherlag BJ, Li S, et al. Low-level transcutaneous electrical stimulation of the auricular branch of the vagus nerve: a noninvasive approach to treat the initial phase of atrial fibrillation. Heart Rhythm 2013;10(3):428–35.

122. Wang Z, Yu L, Wang S, et al. Chronic intermittent low-level transcutaneous electrical stimulation of auricular branch of vagus nerve improves left ventricular remodeling in conscious dogs with healed myocardial infarction. Circ Heart Fail 2014;7(6): 1014–21.

123. Stavrakis S, Humphrey MB, Scherlag BJ, et al. Low-level transcutaneous electrical vagus nerve stimulation suppresses atrial fibrillation. J Am Coll Cardiol 2015;65(9):867–75.

124. Transcutaneous Electrical Vagus Nerve Stimulation to Suppress Atrial Fibrillation (TREAT-AF). Available at: https://clinicaltrials.gov/ct2/show/NCT02548754. Accessed July 27, 2016.

125. Exner DV, Kavanagh KM, Slawnych MP, et al. Noninvasive risk assessment early after a myocardial infarction the REFINE study. J Am Coll Cardiol 2007;50(24):2275–84.

126. De Ferrari GM, Sanzo A, Bertoletti A, et al. Baroreflex sensitivity predicts long-term cardiovascular mortality after myocardial infarction even in patients with preserved left ventricular function. J Am Coll Cardiol 2007;50(24):2285–90.

127. Eckberg DL, Fletcher GF, Braunwald E. Mechanism of prolongation of the R-R interval with electrical stimulation of the carotid sinus nerves in man. Circ Res 1972;30(1):131–8.

128. Heusser K, Tank J, Engeli S, et al. Carotid baroreceptor stimulation, sympathetic activity, baroreflex function, and blood pressure in hypertensive patients. Hypertension 2010;55(3):619–26.

129. Liao K, Yu L, Yang K, et al. Low-level carotid baroreceptor stimulation suppresses ventricular arrhythmias during acute ischemia. PLoS One 2014;9(10):e109313.

130. Liao K, Yu L, Zhou X, et al. Low-level baroreceptor stimulation suppresses atrial fibrillation by inhibiting ganglionated plexus activity. Can J Cardiol 2015;31(6):767–74.

131. Sheng X, Chen M, Huang B, et al. Cardioprotective effects of low-level carotid baroreceptor stimulation against myocardial ischemia-reperfusion injury in canine model. J Interv Card Electrophysiol 2016; 45(2):131–40.

132. Liao K, Yu L, He B, et al. Carotid baroreceptor stimulation prevents arrhythmias induced by acute myocardial infarction through autonomic modulation. J Cardiovasc Pharmacol 2014; 64(5):431–7.

133. Victor RG. Carotid baroreflex activation therapy for resistant hypertension. Nat Rev Cardiol 2015;12(8): 451–63.

134. Bisognano JD, Bakris G, Nadim MK, et al. Baroreflex activation therapy lowers blood pressure in patients with resistant hypertension: results from the double-

blind, randomized, placebo-controlled rheos pivotal trial. J Am Coll Cardiol 2011;58(7):765–73.

135. Hoppe UC, Brandt MC, Wachter R, et al. Minimally invasive system for baroreflex activation therapy chronically lowers blood pressure with pacemaker-like safety profile: results from the Barostim neo trial. J Am Soc Hypertens 2012; 6(4):270–6.

136. Abraham WT, Zile MR, Weaver FA, et al. Baroreflex activation therapy for the treatment of heart failure with a reduced ejection fraction. JACC Heart Fail 2015;3(6):487–96.

Sudden Cardiac Death in Ischemic Heart Disease
Pathophysiology and Risk Stratification

Nabil El-Sherif, MD[a,b,*], Mohamed Boutjdir, PhD[b], Gioia Turitto, MD[c]

KEYWORDS

- Electrophysiologic surrogates of sudden cardiac death • Biomarkers of sudden cardiac death
- Genomics of sudden cardiac death • Noninvasive variables of sudden cardiac death

KEY POINTS

- Electrophysiological surrogates for sudden cardiac death in ischemic heart disease include measures of conduction disorders, dispersion of repolarization, and of autonomic system.
- Arrhythmic risk for sudden cardiac death in ischemic heart disease could be modified by specific biomarkers, genomics, and noninvasive variables.
- The ultimate goal of management of sudden cardiac death should go beyond optimal use of the ICD to primarily identify novel methods for risk stratification, risk modification, and prevention of sudden cardiac death that could be applied to the general public at large.

INTRODUCTION

Sudden cardiac death (SCD) is a major public health problem in the United States and worldwide. It is estimated that each year in the United States 360,000 persons die of unexpected SCD in emergency departments or before reaching a hospital.[1] The current management of SCD is directed at a relatively small percentage of the total population at risk and primarily at those patients already known to be at increased risk by conventional criteria. Pharmaceutical strategies to prevent SCD have been largely ineffective. Because device therapy (implantable cardioverter-defibrillator [ICD]) is designed to rescue patients once an event has already occurred, primary SCD prevention has become one of today's most critical public health challenges. Current conventional risk stratifiers for SCD have shown low positive predictive power

either alone or in different combinations. As of 2005, the main criterion for primary ICD prophylaxis for SCD has been the presence of organic heart disease and depressed left ventricular ejection fraction (LVEF). Unfortunately, a depressed LVEF may be a good marker for total cardiac mortality, but is not specific for SCD, resulting in a significant redundancy of this strategy. The cost to the health care system of sustaining this approach would be substantial. For the immediate future, attempts to optimize the selection process for primary ICD prophylaxis that goes beyond depressed LVEF must continue.

The present article reviews the most recent pathophysiology and risk stratification of SCD in ischemic heart disease, and its management beyond the current single criterion of depressed LVEF.

Supported in part by REAP and MERIT grants from the VA Central Office Research Program, Washington, DC.
[a] State University of New York, Downstate Medical Center, Brooklyn, NY, USA; [b] New York Harbor VA Healthcare System, 800 Poly Place, Brooklyn, NY 11209, USA; [c] New York Presbyterian – Brooklyn Methodist Hospital, Brooklyn, NY, USA
* Corresponding author. New York Harbor VA Healthcare System, 800 Poly Place, Brooklyn, NY 11209.
E-mail address: nelsherif@aol.com

PATHOPHYSIOLOGY OF SUDDEN CARDIAC DEATH IN ISCHEMIC HEART DISEASE

SCD is a worldwide leading cause of all deaths (15%-20%). The majority of SCD occurs in patients with atherosclerotic coronary artery disease (CAD; 65%–85%).[2] However, there is considerable evidence that traditional markers of CAD, such as hypertension, obesity, smoking, diabetes, and lipid abnormalities, are not specific enough to identify patients at high risk for SCD.[3] Patients with similar risk factors for CAD may suffer from SCD or nonfatal ischemic events. The reason for this difference is not clear.

Arrhythmic SCD can be due to ventricular fibrillation (VF)/ventricular tachycardia (VT) or asystole/pulseless electrical activity events. The largest experience on the incidence of VT/VF during an acute ST-segment elevation myocardial infarction (STEMI) in the thrombolytic era comes from the GUSTO-1 trial (Global Utilization of Streptokinase and Tissue Plasminogen Activator for Occluded Coronary Arteries) of 40,895 patients who were treated with thrombolytic therapy.[4] The overall incidence of sustained VT/VF was 10.2%: 3.5% developed VT, 4.1% developed VF, and 2.7% developed both VT and VF. Approximately 80% to 85% of these arrhythmias occurred in the first 48 hours. However, in the era of primary PCI, the incidence of ventricular arrhythmias seems to be lower.[5]

Sustained VT/VF are less common in patients with an acute non-ST elevation myocardial infarction (MI) or unstable angina as illustrated in a pooled analysis of 4 major trials of more than 25,000 such patients.[6] VT/VF occurring within 24 to 48 hours of acute MI are thought to be epiphenomena of the MI and are not associated with worse prognosis after hospital discharge.

However, not all SCDs are due to arrhythmia. Nonarrhythmic causes are found by autopsy in 50% of SCD cases in patients with recent MI, and there is autopsy evidence of acute coronary events in 54% of SCD cases with CAD and even in 5% of SCD cases in patients without CAD.[7] In 97% of cases, acute MI was no diagnosed clinically antemortem. Postmortem MRI results in a higher diagnosis of preacute infarction as a possible cause of SCD.[8,9]

It is important to understand the cascade that relates the distal events of atherosclerosis to the proximal event of SCD (**Fig. 1**). Risk markers for SCD in CAD are likely to cluster under factors that may directly facilitate the development of acute coronary syndromes, specifically those factors that may facilitate transient triggering events, including plaque rupture, enhanced thrombogenesis, and coronary artery spasm.[10,11] There are significant data showing correlation between SCD and:

1. Markers of plaque vulnerability, such as heritable alterations of specific matrix metalloproteinases[12];
2. Markers of enhanced thrombogenesis, such as increased D-dimer, increased apolipoprotein-B, and decreased apolipoprotein-A1,[13] as well as

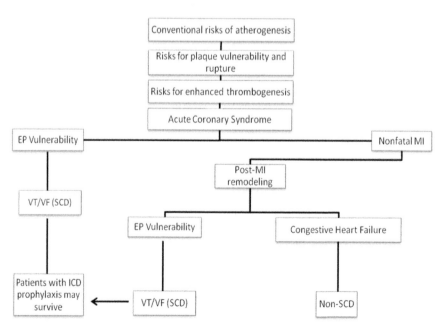

Fig. 1. CAD and SCD cascade. CAD, coronary artery disease; EP, electrophysiologic; ICD, implantable cardioverter-defibrillator; MI, myocardial infarction; SCD, sudden cardiac death; VT/VF, ventricular tachycardia/ventricular fibrillation.

polymorphism in platelet glycoprotein receptors[14];

3. Genetic variations that predispose to vasospasm, such as variations in the vascular endothelial nitric oxide synthetase system[15,16]; and

4. Markers of inflammatory response, such as C-reactive protein.[17]

Acute coronary syndrome can result either in early electrophysiologic vulnerability leading to fatal ventricular tachyarrhythmia and SCD (unless the patient has a prior ICD) or in nonfatal MI. In patient who survive a nonfatal MI, the heart undergoes a complex post-MI remodeling process that in the long run results in increased electrophysiologic vulnerability, fatal ventricular tachyarrhythmia, and SCD or in progressive deterioration of ventricular systolic function, ischemic cardiomyopathy, congestive heart failure, and non-SCD.

REMODELING AFTER MYOCARDIAL INFARCTION AND SUDDEN CARDIAC DEATH

Patients who suffer from a nonfatal MI as well as those who survive SCD in the setting of acute MI later undergo post-MI remodeling. Post-MI remodeling is a complex and time-dependent process

that involves structural, biochemical, neurohormonal, and electrophysiologic alterations. The acute loss of myocardium results in an abrupt increase in loading conditions that induces a unique pattern of remodeling involving the infarcted border zone and remote noninfarcted myocardium.[18] Post-MI remodeling is associated with time-dependent dilatation, distortion of ventricular shape, and hypertrophy of the noninfarcted myocardium. After a variable period of compensatory hypertrophy, deterioration of contractile function may develop, resulting in congestive heart failure. The role of continuous loss of cardiomyocytes to apoptosis in the noninfarcted myocardium, the negative consequences of remodeling of the interstitial matrix, the downregulation of the beta-adrenergic receptor G protein–adenylyl cyclase pathway and the L-type calcium current, and the alterations in calcium regulated excitation–contraction coupling are some of the major mechanisms involved in the transition to decompensated congestive heart failure of the post-MI heart.

In recent years, the understanding of the signal transduction pathways for cardiac remodeling in the post-MI heart[19,20] has provided opportunities for novel therapeutic interventions. **Fig. 2**

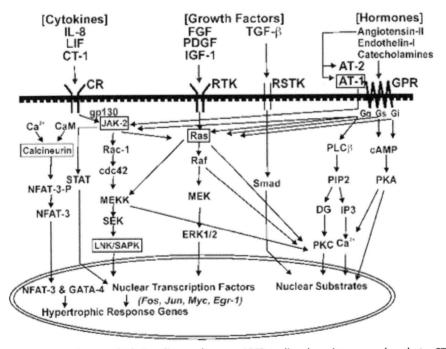

Fig. 2. Post-myocardial infarction (MI) signaling pathways. cAMP, cyclic adenosine monophosphate; CT1, cardiotropin1; FGF, fibroblast growth factor; GPR, G protein-coupled kinase receptors; IGF, insulinlike growth factor; IL, interleukin; JAK, Janus kinase; MEKK, MAP/Erk kinase kinase; LIF, leukemia inhibitory factor; NFAT, nuclear factor of activated T cell; PDGF, platelet-derived growth factor; PKA, protein kinase A; RSTK, receptor serine/threonine kinase; RTK, receptor tyrosine kinase; SEK, somatic embryogenesis receptor-like kinase; TGF, transforming growth factor. (*Modified from* Hefti MA, Harder BA, Eppenberger HM, et al. Signaling pathways in cardiac myocyte hypertrophy. J Mol Cell Cardiol 1997;29:2873–92; with permission of Elsevier.)

illustrates a proposed scheme for post-MI signaling pathways.[21,22] Many of these pathways were shown to be activated either in response to ischemia–reperfusion stimuli or to a stretch stimulus using different experimental models and sometimes noncardiac cell systems. However, cell membrane receptors and intracellular signaling proteins are highly conserved between mammalian species and the triggering events for cellular hypertrophy in humans are likely to resemble closely those in the various animal models used. The diagram shows that a cascade of successive transduction steps allows signal enhancement and diversification at branching points and thus permits combinatorial interactions between multiple pathways. Although multiple signaling pathways may act in synergistic, antagonistic, or permissive ways, some key pathways may play a dominant role.

There is a plethora of experimental and clinical evidence showing that the renin–angiotensin system and the B-adrenergic system play major roles in post-MI remodeling.[22] This explains the beneficial role of angiotensin-converting enzyme inhibitors, angiotensin II type-1 receptor antagonists,

and beta-blockers in the post-MI period. More recently, other signaling pathways, for example, the calcineurin pathway,[23] and the Janus kinase–signal transducer and activator of transcription[24] signaling pathway were also found to play a significant role in post-MI remodeling. Pharmaceutical agents that can block these pathways may provide new therapeutic modalities in the post-MI period.

CURRENT RISK STRATIFICATION OF SUDDEN CARDIAC DEATH IN ISCHEMIC HEART DISEASE

Current risk stratification of SCD in ischemic heart disease could be grouped into the following 3 categories (**Fig. 3**):

1. Electrophysiologic surrogates;
2. Functional/contractile surrogates; and
3. Modifiers of arrhythmic death that includes biomarkers, genomics, and several noninvasive clinical variables.

The electrophysiologic surrogates include measures of conduction disorders, measures of dispersion of repolarization, and measures of

Electrophysiological Surrogates

A) Measures of Conduction Disorders
(ECG-derived):
  - QRS duration, QRS fractionation, Signal Average ECG
  - Myocardial scan assessment (MRI, SPECT, PET)

B) Measures of dispersion of repolarization
(ECG-derived):
  - QT dispersion/variability
  - QRS-T angle
  - T peak-end interval, T peak-end/QT ratio
  - Early repolarization
  - T-wave alternans

C) Measures of autonomic system
(ECG-derived):
  - Heart Rate Variability
  - Heart Rate Turbulence
(Imaging):
  - SPECT (MIBG)
  - PET
    (^{11}C-*meta*-hydroxyephedrine)

D) Others
  - Ambulatory ECG monitoring
  - Electrophysiological study

Functional/Contractile Surrogate

  - NYH class
  - LVEF

Modifiers of Arrhythmic Risk

A) Biomarkers
  - C-reactive protein
  - Interleukin-6
  - Tumor necrosis factor - α receptor II
  - Pro-BNP
  - Cardiac troponin T

B) Genomics
  - Heritability of SCD, familial aggregation
  - Genetic risk variants of CAD
  - Genetic susceptibility to ischemic VF:
    • Common variants with modest effect
    • Rare variants with strong effect

C) Noninvasive Clinical Variables
  - Age >70 y
  - Renal Insufficiency
  - Diabetes
  - Obesity
  - AF
  - LVEF ≤20%
  - NYHA Class III

Fig. 3. Risk stratification of sudden cardiac death. AF, atrial fibrillation; BNP, brain natriuretic peptide; CAD, coronary artery disease; ECG, electrocardiograph; LVEF, left ventricular ejection fraction; MIBG, 123-iodine metaiodobenzylguanidine; NYHA, New York Heart Association; SCD, sudden cardiac death.

autonomic imbalance. These 3 categories represent the current understanding of the electrophysiologic mechanisms that underlie the initiation of VT/VF.

There are at least 2 shortcomings in the application of risk stratification of SCD.[25] One is that most of the risk stratifiers are applied in a dichotomous fashion, whereas the risk of a complex electrophysiologic entity like VT/VF is continuous. Second, many of the risk stratifiers are not fixed and can change over time. For example, in both the REFINE (Risk Estimation Following Infarction Noninvasive Evaluation) and CHARISMA (Clopidogrel for High Atherothrombotic Risk and Ischemic Stabilization, Management, and Avoidance) studies, measures of impaired autonomic function assessed within the first month after MI were poorly predictive of SCD. These measures became predictive when measured at 2 to 4 months.[26,27]

SURROGATE MEASURES OF CONDUCTION DISORDERS

Reduced left ventricular (LV) systolic function assessed as LVEF, as well as wall motion abnormalities, are crude markers of myocardial scar. Nevertheless, reduced LVEF remains the main criterion for prophylactic ICD, with the current understanding that it is a better assessor of total cardiac mortality than arrhythmic death. In contrast, there are several electrocardiography (ECG)-derived criteria that can better assess myocardial scarring. Prolonged QRS duration can reflect the presence of area of slow conduction and has been associated with the risk of SCD in the general population.[28,29] Fractionation of the QRS complex of the ECG is another marker of myocardial scar and may be useful for risk stratification for SCD VT/VF.[30] In a cohort of 361 ICD recipients with LV dysfunction, a fragmented QRS was a strong predictor of ventricular arrhythmias, whereas QRS duration was a better predictor of overall mortality.[31]

The signal-averaged (SA) ECG is more sensitive in detecting late ventricular activation from areas of heterogeneous scar.[32] In an early study, serial recording of the SA ECG was obtained from 156 patients with acute MI up to 5 days (phase 1), 6 to 31 days (phase 2), and 31 to 60 days (phase 3) after the infarction. The study showed that a positive SA ECG in phase 2 has the most significant relation to arrhythmic events in the first year after an MI.[33] However, the positive predictive value of an abnormal SA ECG has generally been insufficient for risk prediction in patients with ischemic heart disease.[34]

IMAGING AND QUANTIFICATION OF MYOCARDIAL SCAR

Both the scar extent and infarct core have been associated predominantly with monomorphic VT, whereas the periinfarction zone has been associated with polymorphic VT. Single photon emission computed tomography (SPECT) and PET imaging can identify myocardial scars by visualizing areas with reversible perfusion defects. In contrast, cardiac MRI is able to identify myocardial scars by delayed enhancement imaging after gadolinium administration. It has a much greater spatial resolution than SPECT or PET imaging.[35] Cardiac MRI is capable of differentiating heterogeneous scar, which appears as intermediate density delayed enhancement from dense scar.[36] Several studies have shown that the burden of heterogeneous scar is an independent predictor of VT/VF, ICD therapy, and overall mortality.[37,38]

SURROGATE MEASURES OF DISPERSION OF REPOLARIZATION

Almost all surrogate measures of dispersion of repolarization are derived from the 12-lead ECG. Dynamic changes in the QT interval including QT variability have been associated with SCD and overall mortality.[39]

$T_{peak-end}$ (T_{p-end}) and T_{p-end}/QT ratio are proposed to represent transmural dispersion of repolarization, and may predict the risk of malignant tachyarrhythmias. A T_{p-end} of greater than 0.1 and a T_{p-end}/QT ratio of greater than 0.3 was found to predict ventricular tachyarrhythmias within 24 hours of STEMI in a prospective case-control study.[40]

Early repolarization (ER) is defined as at least 1 mm (0.1 mV) of the QRS–ST junction above the baseline level in at least 2 inferior or lateral ECG leads.[41] Previously, ER was thought to be a benign feature of 12-lead ECG, but was linked to idiopathic VF by Haissaguerre and colleagues in 2008.[42] The clinical relevance of ER in the general population is low, given the high prevalence and low absolute risk. However, in acute STEMI, ER was found to be associated with a significant increase in risk of ventricular tachyarrhythmias in the acute post-MI phase (<72 hours), irrespective of LVEF and level of cardiac enzymes.[43,44]

Finally, an important measure of dispersion of ventricular repolarization is μV T-wave alternans (TWA), especially discordant alternans. Studies evaluating the usefulness of TWA in risk stratification for arrhythmic death have produced mixed results.[45,46] However, a more recent position paper that reviewed the different techniques of measuring TWA has supported its overall predictive usefulness for arrhythmic events.[47]

SURROGATE MEASURES OF AUTONOMIC FUNCTION

Autonomic neural influences, especially increased adrenergic and decreased cholinergic activity, can modulate the susceptibility to SCD after an MI. Resting heart rate has been shown to be an independent risk factor for SCD in middle-aged men.[48] There are data showing the heritability of heart rate variation.[49] Adrenergic agonists are known to trigger ventricular arrhythmias, and their circulating levels have similar diurnal patterns as SCD events.[50] Genetic polymorphism of β-adrenergic receptors have been associated with increased susceptibility to SCD in ischemic heart disease.[51] The association between plasma nonesterified fatty acids and SCD may be related to increased adrenergic tone or the effect on ion channel and transporters.[52] Further, mental stress was found to be associated with lateralization of midbrain activity, resulting in imbalanced activity in right and left cardiac sympathetic nerves and increased dispersion of repolarization, predisposing to arrhythmia.[53] Recently, a third type of β-adrenergic receptors, β-3 adrenergic receptors, was found in the human heart.[54] In both failing and post-MI myocardium, β-3 adrenergic receptors stimulation may have protective effects against β-1 and β-2 catecholaminergic stimulation.[55] This makes β-3 adrenergic receptors an attractive target for pharmacologic therapy of cardiac arrhythmias related to cardiac sympathetic nerve stimulation.

Heart rate variability (HRV) has been the most extensively investigated measure of autonomic tone. Loss of vagal tone leads to a decrease in the spontaneous variation in heart rate. Assessing the usefulness of HRV for the prediction of SCD and VT/VF is clouded by the numerous potential techniques used to quantify HRV (time domain indices, frequency domain indices, and nonlinear analyses).[56] Diminished HRV has been associated with both SCD and nonsudden death in MI and in chronic LV dysfunction, independent of LVEF.[57] The poor specificity of HRV to predict SCD and VT/VF may limit its use in risk stratification.[25]

Heart rate turbulence (HRT) has been evaluated as another noninvasive and reproducible measure of autonomic function. HRT quantifies the short-term variation in heart rate after a spontaneous ventricular premature beat. HRT has been shown to predict overall mortality, independent of LVEF, after MI.[58] In the REFINE study of patients after MI, HRT was also independently predictive of fatal

or nonfatal cardiac arrest.[26] Therefore, HRT may be more specific for SCD and VT/VF than HRV.

IMAGING OF CARDIAC SYMPATHETIC INNERVATION

An estimate of cardiac sympathetic innervation could be obtained using 123-iodine metaiodobenzylguanidine SPECT planar images. Myocardial uptake relative to mediastinum can be quantified, providing an estimate of the cardiac sympathetic innervation. A heart-to-mediastinum ratio of greater than 1.6 identified a group of heart failure patients at increased risk of VT/VF.[59] Furthermore, on SPECT images, the presence of regional abnormalities in 123-iodine metaiodobenzylguanidine uptake has been associated with high cumulative rate of ventricular arrhythmia in ICD patients.[60] Advances in SPECT and PET imaging can allow for visualization of cardiac sympathetic function of the LV. Using norepinephrine analogs, both PET and SPECT can identify areas of relative sympathetic denervation. In the prospective PARAPET study (Prediction of Arrhythmic Events with Positron Emission Tomography) of patients with ischemic cardiomyopathy receiving an ICD, the amount of viable but denervated myocardium was independently predictive of the development of VT or arrhythmic death.[61]

AMBULATORY MONITORING

Ambulatory ECG monitoring is attractive as a risk stratification tool because of its ubiquitous availability and ease of interpretation. Numerous trials have evaluated interventions, including drug and ICD therapy, to reduce mortality in patients with frequent PVCs or nonsustained VT after an MI or in the presence of LV dysfunction. The majority have shown a reduction in SCD and VT/VF, but no impact on overall mortality.[62,63] Thus, the role of ambulatory monitoring in risk stratification of arrhythmic death remains ill-defined.[25]

ELECTROPHYSIOLOGIC STUDY

Although programmed ventricular stimulation may predict future occurrence of monomorphic VT, it has limited ability to predict polymorphic VT or VF.

In the MUSTT study (Multicenter Unsustained Tachycardia Trial), the positive predictive value of electrophysiologic testing was high, but the negative predictive value was modest. Even in noninducible patients, the rate of cardiac arrest or SCD was relatively high (12% at 2 years).[64] In contrast, in the ABCD trial (Alternans Before Cardioverter Defibrillator) the combination of a negative TWA and negative electrophysiologic study identified a low-risk group with an event rate of 2.3% at 2 years in a population similar to the MUSTT population.[46] However, because of the invasive nature of electrophysiologic testing, and its modest negative predictive value, its role in the overall stratification of SCD in ischemic heart disease is limited.

BIOMARKERS

Biomarkers may be useful in refining the risk of SCD and VT/VF in the general population, particularly in individuals at an intermediate or high risk of CAD. However, large-scale, comprehensive studies of biomarkers are lacking. Biomarkers for inflammation, neurohumoral activation, and cardiac injury have been studied in patients with primary prevention ICD to predict appropriate shocks, a surrogate marker for SCD, and all-cause mortality. The PROSE-ICD trial (Prospective Observational Study of Implantable Cardioverter Defibrillators) investigated 5 potential biomarkers: C-reactive protein, interleukin-6, tumor necrosis factor-a receptor II, pro-brain natriuretic peptide, and cardiac troponin T. All markers were associated with a significant increase in all-cause mortality, but only interleukin-6 had an association with predicting appropriate shock therapy.[65]

GENOMICS

Several studies have demonstrated a familial aggregation of SCD, suggesting a possible influence of genetic factors. The first of these studies was published in 1998 and showed that a family history of MI or primary cardiac arrest was associated independently with an increased risk of primary cardiac arrest.[66] The observational Paris Prospective Study I confirmed that parental SCD is an independent risk factor for SCD in middle-aged men. A family history of SCD on either the paternal or maternal side of family was associated with a nearly 2-fold increased risk of SCD, and if both parents had a history of SCD, there was a 9-fold increased risk of dying suddenly.[67] These 2 studies did not distinguish between different phenotypes of SCD, that is, arrhythmic versus nonarrhythmic SCD. In contrast, the AGNES study (Arrhythmia Genetics in the NEtherlandS study) was the first to suggest an association between family history of SCD and VF caused by first STEMI.[68] However, little is known about the exact genetic component that increases the vulnerability of VF caused by MI in the general population. The genetic components are likely to involve both common variants with modest effect and rare variants with stronger effects.[69] Several studies have examined the association between common and rare genetic variables and SCD (see the review by Glinge

and colleagues[70]). However, only a few of the variants identified in these studies have been replicated, and many do not have yet a clear functional implication. The genetic component of VF and SCD following MI has been investigated using either candidate gene or genome-wide association studies. Some of the reasons for the lack of replication among genetic studies of SCD and VF may have to do with the fact that the effect of the risk of an allele may differ between populations, because of gene–gene interaction or gene–environment interaction.[71] Future research may also need to incorporate epigenetics for better understanding of the complex phenotype of VF and SCD. Last, but not least, a recent study showed that a score formed by the most significant genetic risk variant for CAD is associated significantly with the occurrence of CAD-related out-of-hospital cardiac arrest.[72]

NONINVASIVE CLINICAL RISK VARIABLES

A striking finding in the multivariable risk stratification is the degree of consistency among predictor variables.[73] The relative risk variables in the prospective randomized clinical trials include atrial fibrillation, age greater than 70 years, New York Heart Association functional class III, creatinine greater than 1.3 or blood urea nitrogen greater than 26 mg/dL, a QRS duration of greater than 120 ms, and an LVEF of less than 20%. Ideally, a multicenter randomized clinical trial could be conducted to test a multivariable risk stratification model. However, at least in the United States, such a randomized clinical trial is unlikely to succeed because ICD implantation is currently a class I guideline for patients with an LVEF of less than 35%.[73] An alternate method is to conduct a prospective observational comparative study. In such a study, patients receiving ICDs for primary prevention of SCD under current guidelines would be characterized by a number of noninvasive risk markers and followed prospectively; their survival would be compared with a group of patients matched for demographic characteristics who do not receive ICDs.[73] Because ICD implantation rate among eligible population can be as low as 7% in 1 study,[74] it may not be difficult to recruit a matching group. The low implantation rate probably reflects a perceived low benefit-to-cost ratio for the device.

A subanalysis of the MADIT-II study (Multicenter Automatic Defibrillator Implantation Trial) helps to explain the value of such a prospective observational study. In MADIT-II, patients with severe renal dysfunction (defined as blood urea nitrogen >50 mg/dL or creatinine >2.5 mg/dL) had very high mortality and did not derive benefit from ICD implantation. When these patients were excluded from subsequent analysis, patients with no risk factors (defined as age >70 years, atrial fibrillation, creatinine >1.3 mg/dL or blood urea nitrogen >26 mg/dL, New York Heart Association functional class III, and QRS duration >120 ms) had a very low risk of total mortality and did not derive a survival benefit from the ICD. Patient with more than 3 risk factors had very high mortality, owing primarily to nonarrhythmic death, and also did not derive benefit from the ICD. Only patients with 1 or 2 risk factors had the ICD improve their mortality.[75]

SUMMARY

The immediate future goals for risk stratification and management of SCD post-MI could be summarized as follows. (1) Identification of novel clinical, electrophysiologic, biochemical, and genetic markers for SCD including assessment of the functional consequences of sequence variants identified in human genetic studies as well as relevant environmental-genetic interactions. (2) Identification of a battery of a relatively limited number of incrementally cumulative low to intermediate risk variants and development of a "signature" combination of risk markers of SCD. However, we should not be surprised if the positive predictive value of some of the new risk markers, similar to conventional risk markers, will be relatively low, especially if these are applied to large populations who are at low risk. (3) One way of reducing the redundancy in the use of ICD implantation that is currently based solely on reduced LVEF is to identify those ICD-eligible patients with either very low or very high noninvasive clinical risk variables who may not benefit from ICD implantation. (4) Identification of novel pharmacologic, nonpharmacologic, and behavioral approaches for risk modification and prevention of SCD. (5) A wider collaboration among different academic and industrial institutions by sharing research results as well as resources such as clinical data, and blood and other tissues from biorepository centers. The ultimate goal is not only to change the current direction of management strategy of SCD away from increased ICD use, but primarily to identify novel methods for risk stratification, risk modification, and prevention of SCD that could be applied to the general public at large.

REFERENCES

1. Mozaffarian D, Anker SD, Anand I, et al. Prediction of mode of death in heart failure: the Seattle heart failure model. Circulation 2007;116:392–8.

2. American Heart Association. Heart and stroke statistical update. Dallas (TX): American Heart Association; 2001.

3. Braunwald E. Shattuck Lecture. Cardiovascular medicine at the turn of the millennium: triumphs, concerns and opportunities. N Engl J Med 1997; 377:1360–9.

4. Newby KH, Thompson T, Stebbins A, et al. Sustained ventricular arrhythmias in patients receiving thrombolytic therapy: incidence and outcome. The GUSTO Investigators. Circulation 1998;98:2567–73.

5. Jabbari R, Risgaard B, Fosbol EL, et al. Factors associated with and outcomes after ventricular fibrillation before and during primary angioplasty in patients with ST-segment elevation myocardial infarction. Am J Cardiol 2015;116:678–85.

6. Al-Khatib SM, Granger CB, Huang Y, et al. Sustained ventricular arrhythmias among patients with acute coronary syndrome with no-ST segment elevation: incidence, predictors, and outcomes. Circulation 2002;106:309–12.

7. Pouleur AC, Barkoudah E, Uno H, et al. Pathogenesis of sudden unexpected death in a clinical trial of patients with myocardial infarction and left ventricular dysfunction, heart failure, or both. Circulation 2010;122:597–602.

8. Jackowski C, Schwendener N, Grabherr S, et al. Post-mortem cardiac 3-T magnetic resonance imaging visualization of sudden cardiac death? J Am Coll Cardiol 2013;62:617–29.

9. Wellens HJ, Schwartz PJ, Lindemans FW, et al. Risk stratification of sudden cardiac death: current status and challenges for the future. Eur Heart J 2014;35: 1642–51.

10. Spooner PM, Albert C, Benjamin EL, et al. Sudden cardiac death, genes, and arrhythmogenesis: consideration of new population and mechanistic approaches from a National Heart Lung, and Blood Institute Workshop, part I. Circulation 2001;103: 2361–4.

11. Spooner PM, Albert C, Benjamin EL, et al. Sudden cardiac death, genes, and arrhythmogenesis: consideration of new population and mechanistic approaches from a National Heart, Lung, and Blood Institute Workshop, part II. Circulation 2001;103: 2447–52.

12. Gnasso A, Motti C, Irace C. Genetic variation in human stromelysin gene promoter and common carotid geometry in healthy male subjects. Arterioscler Thromb Vasc Biol 2000;20:1600–5.

13. Moss AJ, Goldstein RE, Marder VJ, et al. Thrombogenic factors and recurrent coronary events. Circulation 1999;99:2517–22.

14. Weiss EJ, Bray PF, Tayback M, et al. A polymorphism of a platelet glycoprotein receptor as an inherited risk factor for coronary thrombosis. N Engl J Med 1996;334:1090–4.

15. Nakayama M, Yasue H, Yoshimura M, et al. T786→C mutation in the 5'-flanking region of the endothelial nitric oxide synthase gene is associated with coronary spasm. Circulation 1999;99:2864–70.

16. Wang XL, Sim AS, Wang MX, et al. Genotype dependent and cigarette specific effects on endothelial nitric oxide synthase gene expression and enzyme activity. FEBS Lett 2000;471:45–50.

17. Albert CM, Ma J, Rifai N, et al. Prospective study of C-reactive protein, homocysteine, and plasma lipid levels as predictors of sudden cardiac death. Circulation 2002;105:2595–9.

18. St John Sutton MG, Sharpe N. Left ventricular remodeling after myocardial infarction. Pathophysiology and Therapy. Circulation 2000;101:2981–8.

19. Qin D, Zang ZH, Caref EB, et al. Cellular and ionic basis of arrhythmias in post infarction remodeled ventricular myocardium. Circ Res 1996;79:461–73.

20. Gidh-Jain M, Huang B, Jain P, et al. Differential expression of voltage-gated K+ channel genes in left ventricular remodeled myocardium after experimental myocardial infarction. Circ Res 1996;79:669–75.

21. El-Sherif N, Turitto G. Risk stratification and management of sudden cardiac death: a new paradigm. J Cardiovasc Eletrophysiol 2003;14:1–7.

22. Hefti MA, Harder BA, Eppenberger HM, et al. Signaling pathways in cardiac myocyte hypertrophy. J Mol Cell Cardiol 1997;29:2873–92.

23. Deng L, Huang B, Qin D, et al. Calcineurin inhibition ameliorates structural, contractile, and electrophysiological consequences of post-infarction remodeling. J Cardiovasc Electrophysiol 2001;12:1055–61.

24. El-Adawi H, Deng L, Tramontano A, et al. The functional role of the JAK-STAT pathway in post infarction remodeling. Cardiovasc Res 2003;58:126–35.

25. Deyell MW, Krahn AD, Goldberger JJ, et al. Sudden cardiac death risk stratification. Circ Res 2015;116:1907–18.

26. Exner DV, Kavanagh KM, Slawnych MP, et al, for the REFINE Investigators. Noninvasive risk assessment early after a myocardial infarction: the REFINE study. J Am Coll Cardiol 2007;50:2275–84.

27. Huikuri HV, Raatikainen MJ, Moerch-Joergensen R, et al, Cardiac Arrhythmias and Risk Stratification After Acute Myocardial Infarction Study Group. Prediction of fatal or near-fatal cardiac arrhythmia events in patients with depressed left ventricular function after an acute myocardial infarction. Eur Heart J 2009;30:689–98.

28. Aro AL, Anttonen O, Tikkanen JT, et al. Intraventricular conduction delay in a standard 12-lead electrocardiogram as a predictor of mortality in the general population. Circulation 2011;124:704–10.

29. Kurl S, Makikallio TH, Rautaharju P, et al. Duration of QRS complex in resting electrocardiogram is a predictor of sudden cardiac death in men. Circulation 2012;125:2588–94.

30. Chatterjee S, Changawala N. Fragmented QRS complex: a novel marker of cardiovascular disease. Clin Cardiol 2010;38:68–71.

31. Das MK, Maskoun W, Shen C, et al. Fragmented QRS on twelve-lead electrocardiogram predicts arrhythmic events in patients with ischemic and nonischemic cardiomyopathy. Heart Rhythm 2010;7:74–80.

32. Steinberg JS, Berbari EJ. The signal-averaged electrocardiogram: update on clinical application. J Cardiovasc Electrophysiol 1996;7:972–88.

33. El-Sherif N, Ursell SN, Bekheit S, et al. Prognostic significance of the signal-averaged ECG depends on the time of recording in the postinfarction period. Am Heart J 1989;118:256–64.

34. Goldberger JJ, Cain ME, Hohnloser SH, et al, American Heart Association, American College of Cardiology Foundation, Heart Rhythm Society. American Heart Association/American College of Cardiology Foundation/Heart Rhythm Society Scientific Statement on Noninvasive Risk Stratification Techniques for Identifying Patients at Risk for Sudden Cardiac Death. A scientific statement from the American Heart Association Council on Clinical Cardiology Committee on Electrocardiography and Arrhythmias and Council on Epidemiology and Prevention. J Am Coll Cardiol 2008;52:1179–99.

35. van der Bijl P, Delgado V, Bax JJ, et al. Noninvasive imaging markers associated with sudden cardiac death. Trends Cardiovasc Med 2016;26:348–60.

36. Perez-David E, Arenal A, Rubio-Guivernau JL, et al. Noninvasive identification of ventricular tachycardia-related conducting channels using contrast-enhanced magnetic resonance imaging in patients with chronic myocardial infarction: comparison of signal intensity scar mapping and endocardial voltage mapping. J Am Coll Cardiol 2011;57:184–94.

37. Roes SD, Borleffs CJ, van der Geest RJ, et al. Infarct tissue heterogeneity assessed with contrast-enhanced MRI predicts spontaneous ventricular arrhythmia in patients with ischemic cardiomyopathy and implantable cardioverter-defibrillator. Circ Cardiovasc Imaging 2009;2:183–90.

38. Schmidt A, Azevedo CF, Cheng A, et al. Infarct tissue heterogeneity by magnetic resonance imaging identifies enhanced cardiac arrhythmia susceptibility in patients with left ventricular dysfunction. Circulation 2007;115:2006–14.

39. Piccirillo G, Magri D, Matera S, et al. QT variability strongly predicts sudden cardiac death in asymptomatic subjects with mild or moderate left ventricular systolic dysfunction: a prospective study. Eur Heart J 2007;28:1344–50.

40. Shenthar J, Deora S, Rai M, et al. Prolonged Tpeak-end and Tpeak-end/QT ratio as predictors of malignant ventricular arrhythmias in the acute phase of ST-segment elevation myocardial infarction: a prospective case-control study. Heart Rhythm 2015; 12:484–9.

41. Behr E, Ensam B. New approaches to predicting the risk of sudden death. Clin Med 2016;16:283–9.

42. Haissaguerre M, Derval N, Sacher F, et al. Sudden cardiac arrest associated with early repolarization. N Engl J Med 2008;358:2016–23.

43. Patel RB, Ilkhanoff I, Ng J, et al. Clinical characteristics and prevalence of early repolarization associated with ventricular arrhythmias following acute ST-elevation myocardial infarction. Am J Cardiol 2012;110:615–20.

44. Rudic B, Veltmann C, Kuntz E, et al. Early repolarization pattern is associated with ventricular fibrillation in patients with acute myocardial infarction. Heart Rhythm 2012;9:1295–330.

45. Gold MR, Ip JH, Costantini O, et al. Role of microvolt T-wave alternans in assessment of arrhythmia vulnerability among patients with heart failure and systolic dysfunction: primary results from the T-wave alternans sudden cardiac death in heart failure trial substudy. Circulation 2008; 118:2022–8.

46. Costantini O, Hohnloser SH, Kirk MM, et al, ABCD Trial Investigators. The ABCD (Alternans Before Cardioverter Defibrillator) Trial: strategies using T-wave alternans to improve efficiency of sudden cardiac death prevention. J Am Coll Cardiol 2009; 53:471–9.

47. Verrier RL, Klingenheben T, Malik M, et al. Microvolt T-wave alternans: physiological basis, methods of assessment, and clinical utility-consensus guideline by International Society of Holter and Noninvasive Electrocardiology. J Am Coll Cardiol 2011;58: 1309–24.

48. Jouven X, Zureik M, Desnos M, et al. Resting heart rate as a predictive risk factor for sudden death in middle aged men. Cardiovasc Res 2001;50: 373–8.

49. Singh JP, Larson MG, O'Donnell CJ, et al. Heritability of heart rate variability: the Framingham heart study. Circulation 1999;99:2251–4.

50. Muller JE. Circadian variation and triggering of acute coronary events. Am Heart J 1999;137(Pt 2):51–8.

51. Jaillon P, Simon T. Genetic polymorphism of beta-adrenergic receptors and mortality in ischemic heart disease. Therapie 2007;62:1–7.

52. Jouven X, Charles MA, Desnos M, et al. Circulating nonesterified fatty acid level as a predictive risk factor for sudden cardiac death in the population. Circulation 2001;104:756–61.

53. Critchley HD, Taggart P, Sutton PM, et al. Mental stress and sudden cardiac death: asymmetric

midbrain activity as a linking mechanism. Brain 2005;128:75–85.

54. Gauthier C, Tavernier G, Charpentier F, et al. Functional beta3-adrenergic receptors in the human heart. J Clin Invest 1996;98:556–62.

55. Vadim VF, Ilya TL. Is beta3-adrenergic receptors a new target for treatment of post-infarct ventricular tachyarrhythmias and prevention of sudden cardiac death. Heart Rhythm 2008;5:298–9.

56. Heart rate variability: standards of measurement, physiological interpretation and clinical use. Task Force of the European Society of Cardiology and the North American Society of Pacing and Electrophysiology. Circulation 1996;93: 1043–65.

57. La Rovere MT, Pinna GD, Maestri R, et al. Short-term heart rate variability strongly predicts sudden cardiac death in chronic heart failure patients. Circulation 2003;107:565–70.

58. Schmidt G, Malik M, Barthel P, et al. Heart-rate turbulence after ventricular pre- mature beats as a predictor of mortality after acute myocardial infarction. Lancet 1999;353:1390–6.

59. Jacobson AF, Senior R, Cerqueira MD, et al. Myocardial iodine-123 meta-iodobenzylguanidine imaging and cardiac events in heart failure. Results of the prospective ADMIRE-HF (AdreView Myocardial Imaging for Risk Evaluation in Heart Failure) study. J Am Coll Cardiol 2010;55:2212–21.

60. Boogers MJ, Borleffs CJ, Henneman MM, et al. Cardiac sympathetic denervation assessed with 123-iodine metaiodobenzylguanidine imaging predicts ventricular arrhythmias in implantable cardioverter-defibrillator patients. J Am Coll Cardiol 2010;55: 2769–77.

61. Fallavollita JA, Heavey BM, Luisi AJ, et al. Regional myocardial sympathetic denervation predicts the risk of sudden cardiac arrest in ischemic cardiomyopathy. J Am Coll Cardiol 2014;63:141–9.

62. Cairns JA, Connolly SJ, Roberts R, et al. Randomised trial of outcome after myocardial infarction in patients with frequent or repetitive ventricular premature depolarisations: CAMIAT. Canadian Amiodarone Myocardial Infarction Arrhythmia Trial Investigators. Lancet 1997;349:675–82.

63. Hohnloser SH, Kuck KH, Dorian P, et al, DINAMIT Investigators. Prophylactic use of an implantable cardioverter-defibrillator after acute myocardial infarction. N Engl J Med 2004;351:2481–8.

64. Buxton AE, Lee KL, Fisher JD, et al. A randomized study of the prevention of sudden death in patients with coronary artery disease. Multicenter Unsustained Tachycardia Trial Investigators. N Engl J Med 1999;341:1882–90.

65. Cheng A, Zhang Y, Blasco-Colmenares E, et al. Protein biomarkers identify patients unlikely to benefit

from primary prevention implantable cardioverter defibrillators: findings from the Prospective Observational Study of Implantable Cardioverter Defibrillators (PROSE-ICD). Circ Arrhythm Electrophysiol 2014;7:1084–91.

66. Friedlander Y, Siscovick DS, Weinmann S, et al. Family history as a risk factor for primary cardiac arrest. Circulation 1998;97:155–60.

67. Jouven X, Desnos M, Guerot C, et al. Predicting sudden death in the population: the Paris prospective study I. Circulation 1999;99:1978–83.

68. Dekker LR. Familial sudden death is an important risk factor for primary ventricular fibrillation: a case-control study in acute myocardial infarction patients. Circulation 2006;114:1140–5.

69. Bodmer W, Bonilla C. Common and rare variants in multifactorial susceptibility to common diseases. Nat Genet 2008;40:695–701.

70. Glinge C, Sattler S, Jabbari R, et al. Epidemiology and genetics of ventricular fibrillation during acute myocardial infarction. J Geriatr Cardiol 2016;13:789–97.

71. Manolio TA, Collins FS, Cox NJ, et al. Finding the missing heritability of complex diseases. Nature 2009;461:747–53.

72. Hernesneimi JA, Lyytikkainen L-P, Oksala N, et al. Predicting sudden cardiac death using common genetic risk variants for coronary artery disease. Eur Heart J 2015;36:1669–75.

73. Buxton AE, Waks JW, Shen C, et al. Risk stratification for sudden cardiac death in North America-current perspectives. J Electrocardiol 2016;49:817–23.

74. Borleffs CJ, Wilde AA, Cramer MJ, et al. Clinical implementation of guidelines for cardioverter-defibrillator implantation: lost in translation? Neth Heart J 2007;15:129–32.

75. Goldberger I, Vyas AK, Hall WJ, et al. Risk stratification for primary implantation of a cardioverter-defibrillator in patients with ischemic left ventricular dysfunction. J Am Coll Cardiol 2008;51:288–96.

Ventricular Arrhythmias and Sudden Cardiac Death

Pok Tin Tang, BM BCh, BA[a], Mohammad Shenasa, MD[b], Noel G. Boyle, MD, PhD[a],*

KEYWORDS

- Ventricular arrhythmia • Sudden cardiac death • Ventricular tachycardia • Ventricular fibrillation

KEY POINTS

- Ventricular arrhythmias remain a significant cause of sudden cardiac death (SCD), and knowledge of their cause and high-risk features is important. SCD occurs when the interaction between vulnerable substrates and acute triggers results in sustained ventricular tachycardia (VT) progressing to ventricular fibrillation (VF).
- Ischemic cardiomyopathy is the most common cause of ventricular arrhythmias associated with structural heart disease, followed by nonischemic dilated cardiomyopathy. In these, left ventricular ejection fraction (LVEF) is most commonly used to assess risk of SCD.
- Due to the use of angiotensin converting enzyme inhibitors and angiotensin II receptor blockers, which exert an antifibrotic effect on the heart, and improved revascularization, a paradigm shift is emerging. Today, more than 50% of SCD occurs in individuals with normal LVEF. This phenomenon is due to the lack of reliable markers for risk stratification in this patient population. New strategies, particularly in imaging, are being developed that may aid this in future.
- In the absence of structural heart disease, ventricular arrhythmias raise the suspicion of primary arrhythmic syndromes. These are a heterogeneous group of disorders, including long QT syndrome and Brugada syndrome, where risk stratification is difficult and is mostly performed based on the history and clinical features.
- Better understanding of the substrates underlying VT/VF, their interactions with triggers, the process underlying arrhythmogenesis, and the events leading up to sudden death will improve risk stratification and potentially identify novel therapeutic targets for prevention of SCD.

INTRODUCTION

Ventricular arrhythmias are a major contributor to sudden cardiac death (SCD) as the initial recorded rhythm, with estimates of their prevalence varying from 30% to 75% of out-of-hospital cardiac arrests despite recent increases in the incidence of pulseless electrical activity[1,2] (**Fig. 1**). Not all ventricular arrhythmias result in SCD, which is thought to result from the interaction between a vulnerable myocardial substrate caused by an underlying disease process, and an acute trigger. Here, the authors aim to review the role of ventricular arrhythmias in SCD, first by approaching the substrates that support ventricular arrhythmias, then by exploring features of these substrates and the acute triggers that may lead to SCD. The large majority of cases of SCD are associated with structural heart disease, whether known or discovered after resuscitated cardiac arrest or post-mortem.

[a] UCLA Cardiac Arrhythmia Center, UCLA Health System, David Geffen School of Medicine at UCLA, Los Angeles, CA 90095, USA; [b] Heart & Rhythm Medical Group, San Jose, CA 95128, USA
* Corresponding author. David Geffen School of Medicine at UCLA, 100 UCLA Medical Plaza, Suite 660, Los Angeles, CA 90095-1679.
E-mail address: NBoyle@mednet.ucla.edu

Card Electrophysiol Clin 9 (2017) 693–708
http://dx.doi.org/10.1016/j.ccep.2017.08.004
1877-9182/17/© 2017 Elsevier Inc. All rights reserved.

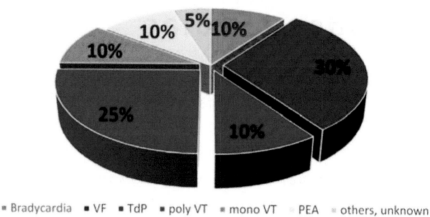

Fig. 1. Distribution of arrhythmias documented as the first rhythm in out-of-hospital SCD. Mono VT, monomorphic ventricular tachycardia; PEA, pulseless electrical activity; poly VT, polymorphic ventricular tachycardia; TdP, torsades de pointes. (*From* Israel CW. Mechanisms of sudden cardiac death. Ind Heart J 2014;66:S11; with permission.)

Of these, coronary artery disease is the greatest contributor, followed by the nonischemic cardiomyopathies (**Fig. 2**).

ISCHEMIC CARDIOMYOPATHY

In ischemic heart disease, the two main mechanisms of SCD are ventricular arrhythmias related to acute myocardial ischemia (covered elsewhere) and scar-related ventricular tachycardia (VT), associated with a previous myocardial infarction (MI).

In the post-MI period, myocyte death leads to fibrosis, while surviving populations of myocytes undergo electrical remodeling through gap junction changes. Electrical heterogeneity results in anisotropic conduction within cardiac tissue, forming localized regions of slow conduction that are the basis for macro-reentrant circuits and arrhythmogenesis.[3] In keeping with this, animal models of the infarct border zone, a highly heterogeneous region lying between normal myocardium and infarct, have been shown to possess these characteristics and are able to support reentrant arrhythmias[4]; in humans, scar heterogeneity on imaging has been shown to be the strongest predictor of spontaneous ventricular arrhythmias.[5,6]

In addition, the autonomic nervous system exerts significant influence on the electrical properties of the heart, and autonomic dysregulation has also been shown to play a prominent role in the genesis of ventricular arrhythmias leading to SCD.[7] A recent study showed that changes to the intrinsic cardiac nervous system occur after MI, the most apparent being the development of differential afferent innervation of the core infarct region (reduced) compared with border zone and healthy myocardium (preserved). In addition, the

authors of the study also observed morphologic and neurochemical remodeling of intracardiac ganglia, as well as altered neuronal responses to changes in cardiac loading.[8] These changes likely play an important role in governing electrical and structural remodeling of the post-MI myocardium that then predisposes to SCD.

The left ventricular ejection fraction (LVEF) is widely used for the assessment of risk of SCD in ischemic heart disease, and many studies have shown not only that reduced LVEF leads to an increased risk of SCD, but also that this can be lowered with implantable cardioverter-defibrillator (ICD) implantation.[9] An LVEF less than 30% to 35% is usually used as a cutoff for implantation. However, challenges in identifying those at high risk of SCD remain. First, few patients with reduced LVEF experience SCD, as evidenced by lower rates of ICD discharges for VT or ventricular fibrillation (VF) than in ICD implantation trials[10]; additionally, most cases of SCD in ischemic heart disease occur in patients with normal or moderately reduced LVEF (**Box 1**).[11]

As a result, there has been considerable interest in identifying other risk markers of SCD. The MUSTT trial showed that in patients with coronary artery disease and reduced LVEF, SCD risk was significantly lower in those where it was not possible to induce VT during electrophysiological study compared with those where VT was inducible.[12] Many other markers have been suggested, including ventricular ectopy, microvolt T-wave alternans, QRS duration, signal-averaged electrographic parameters, or indicators of autonomic tone, such as baroreflex sensitivity, heart rate turbulence, and heart rate variability.[13] However, these have not been unequivocally shown to be superior to LVEF as selection criteria for ICD

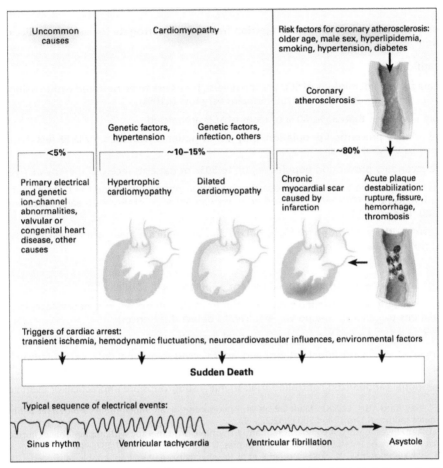

Fig. 2. The pathophysiology, cause, and epidemiology of SCD. (*From* Huikuri HV, Castellanos A, Myerburg RJ. Sudden death due to cardiac arrhythmias. N Engl J Med 2001;345:1475; with permission.)

implantation. QRS fragmentation, detectable on 12-lead electrocardiogram (ECG), may signify conduction delay, and some studies support its utility in risk prediction.[14–16] However, its sensitivity and specificity may be affected by interobserver variability, and the recognition that it can in some cases be a normal variant[17,18]; more in-depth characterization of the morphologies of fragmented QRS may yet improve its reliability for widespread use.[19]

Recently, advances in imaging technology have paved the way for studies to investigate their utility for risk stratification in structural heart disease. Late gadolinium enhancement cardiac magnetic resonance (LGE-CMR) has emerged as the gold-standard investigation in detecting myocardial fibrosis, because of its high sensitivity. Indeed, the extent of the peri-infarct zone as measured by LGE-CMR appears to be strongly linked to risk of SCD.[6,20,21] However, LGE-CMR is still limited by length of study, cost, and the need for administration of contrast.

Beyond LGE-CMR, other imaging techniques have also shown promise for the assessment of SCD risk. In keeping with the proposed role of the sympathetic nervous system in arrhythmogenesis, demonstrations of reduced sympathetic innervation of the heart by myocardial iodine-123 meta-iodobenzylguanidine imaging and 11C-meta-hydroxyephedrine PET have both been associated with an increased risk of SCD.[22,23] Reduced right ventricular ejection fraction (RVEF) has recently been suggested as an additional indicator. Specifically, it appeared to contribute incrementally to assessment by LVEF: the association between RVEF ≤45% and SCD was particularly strong in patients with LVEF greater than 35%, a group in whom SCD risk stratification has proved difficult.[24]

NONISCHEMIC CARDIOMYOPATHY

Nonischemic cardiomyopathy consists of a broad group of conditions, including idiopathic dilated

---

Box 1
Limitations of the use of left ventricular ejection fraction as a surrogate for sudden cardiac death risk stratification

1. Risk stratification

   - The cause and epidemiology of SCD are too diverse for its risk to be captured within a single parameter. Currently, absolute survival rate remains very low (<10%).
   - By using LVEF less than 35%, 80% of cases of SCD are missed.
   - In the primary prevention population, only 5% of patients with ICDs for LVEF less than 35% will experience VT/VF per year.[a]
   - In the secondary prevention population, up to 50% of patients received therapy at 1 year.[b]
   - SCD is highest in the early post–myocardial infarction period; however, the ICDs in acute myocardial infarction trial (DINAMIT) showed no improvement in mortality with early placement of ICDs (at 6–40 days after MI).[c]
   - The current risk stratification for VT/VF/SCD in clinical practice remains primitive: there is a need for novel risk markers.

2. Trials

   - Lack of homogeneity within enrolled patient populations in studies.
   - Only a small number of enrolled patients suffer from SCD (low event rate necessitates large patient populations to generate the power required to detect differences).
   - Lack of analysis of what happens to individual patients.
   - Incomplete data on individual patients and lack of access to original data, particularly in long-term trials.
   - Conventional randomized controlled trials in many subgroups are impractical or even impossible.

   [a]SCD-HeFT trial: Bardy GH, Lee KL, Mark DB, et al. Amiodarone or an implantable cardioverter-defibrillator for congestive heart failure. N Eng J Med 2005;352:225–37.
   [b]AVID trial: AVID Investigators, A comparison of antiarrhythmic-drug therapy with implantable defibrillators in patients resuscitated from near-fatal ventricular arrhythmias. N Engl J Med 1997;337:1576–84.
   [c]DINAMIT trial: Hohnloser SH, Kuck KH, Dorian P, et al. Prophylactic use of an implantable cardioverter-defibrillator after acute myocardial infarction. N Engl J Med 2004;351:2481–8.

---

cardiomyopathy (DCM), which is discussed here, but also cardiomyopathy associated with valvular heart disease, chronic ethanol and drug abuse, viral infections, Chagas disease, and others. Different causes of nonischemic cardiomyopathy can lead to the same or different types and morphologies of VT, which can occur in the same patient (**Fig. 3**).

As in ischemic cardiomyopathy, LVEF has been shown to be the most robust measure for stratifying risk of SCD in nonischemic cardiomyopathy and is widely used. Although multiple trials of ICD therapy based on LVEF in nonischemic cardiomyopathy failed to demonstrate statistically significant reductions in total mortality, a meta-analysis of 7 large-scale primary and secondary prevention trials showed that ICD implantation in nonischemic cardiomyopathy with reduced LVEF led to significant mortality reduction.[25] As a result, risk stratification in nonischemic cardiomyopathy remains primarily driven by LVEF.

However, the recently published DANISH trial may signal that a reappraisal of this approach is needed. The trial showed that prophylactic ICD implantation in symptomatic nonischemic cardiomyopathy led to half the incidence of SCD at 8 years compared with "usual clinical care". However, all-cause mortality was not significantly lowered,[26] again highlighting the need for more accurate risk prediction, to better balance the benefits of ICD implantation against its effects on morbidity and all-cause mortality.

In DCM, both focal scar tissue and diffuse, irregular fibrosis-containing myocytes with irregular hypertrophy have been observed. Left ventricular dilatation is also present, which leads to structural and electrical remodeling. Compared with ischemic cardiomyopathy, the knowledge of the mechanisms underlying arrhythmogenesis in DCM is less clear, but it appears that monomorphic sustained VT occurs through macro-reentrant circuits around scars.

A recent meta-analysis sought to quantify the role of 12 potential risk-stratifying markers in predicting SCD in DCM. These markers could be grossly categorized as autonomic parameters

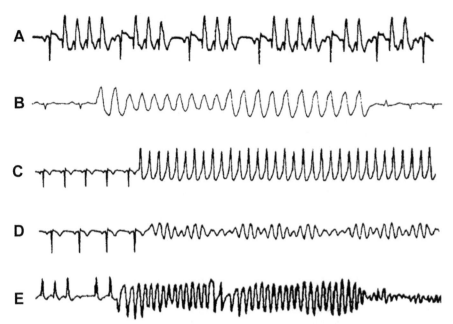

Fig. 3. The ventricular tachyarrhythmias. (*A*) Repetitive bursts of monomorphic VT, (*B*) nonsustained VT, (*C*) sustained monomorphic VT; (*D*) polymorphic VT, (*E*) degeneration of VT to VF. (*From* Shenasa M, Borggrefe M, Haverkamp W, et al. Ventricular tachycardia. Lancet 1993;341:1513; with permission.).

(baroreflex sensitivity, heart rate turbulence, heart rate variability), functional parameters (left-ventricular end-diastolic diameter, LVEF), arrhythmia-based parameters (electrophysiology study, nonsustained VT), depolarization parameters (QRS duration/left bundle branch block, QRS fragmentation, signal-averaged ECG), and repolarization parameters (T-wave alternans and QRS-T angle, although only one study was available in the latter).[27] Notably, in this study, none of the autonomic markers was significantly associated with risk. Although only addressed in 2 of the 45 studies in the meta-analysis, fragmented QRS complex appeared to be strongly correlated to SCD risk, consistent with earlier studies of QRS fragmentation in combined study populations of ischemic and nonischemic cardiomyopathy.[15]

Another meta-analysis of 29 studies investigated the use of LGE-CMR as a marker of risk. This suggested that in patients with DCM, LGE-CMR could be a significant predictor of SCD risk, as denoted by arrhythmic endpoints including SCD, VF, sustained VT, and appropriate ICD therapies.[28] However, these studies may have been subject to selection bias because they were all observational. There was also variation among study protocols, and a lack of explicit exclusion of patients with history of arrhythmia. A different study suggested that the distribution of LGE-CMR may also be significant: midwall fibrosis appears to be linked with increased risk.[29,30]

Reduced RVEF in DCM showed strong predictive capability for SCD in a post hoc subgroup analysis of a recent study covered earlier. However, this is a result that requires further investigation in a larger study population.[24]

One study suggested that a subset of DCM patients express an "arrhythmogenic phenotype," defined as presentation in early disease (study population was within 7 months of diagnosis) with syncope or Holter-detected ventricular arrhythmias ($\geq$5 beats nonsustained ventricular tachycardia [NSVT] at $\geq$150 bpm, $\geq$1000 premature ventricular contractions [PVCs] per 24 hours, or $\geq$50 couplets per 24 hours) in the absence of overt heart failure. The investigators found that 38% of their study population (cases of familial or suspected familial DCM) met these criteria, and that this subgroup was at greater risk of SCD, sustained VT, and VF.[31] The study also found that a positive family history of SCD or sustained VT/VF was a significant predictor for SCD. However, it is important to note that the study was largely limited to patients with familial forms of DCM and excluded patients who may have had milder disease.

HYPERTROPHIC CARDIOMYOPATHY

Although hypertrophic cardiomyopathy (HCM) is the cause in a significant number of cases of SCD, especially in younger populations, SCD is a relatively rare occurrence in HCM. The SCD risk in HCM is approximately 1.5% per year,[32] and most HCM patients have a normal life expectancy. Rapid monomorphic VT and VF are the arrhythmias associated with SCD in this population, based on electrograms recorded in ICD-aborted SCD events.[33] These are often triggered by PVCs,[34] but sinus tachycardia and atrial fibrillation have also been described as triggers.

Structural changes in the left ventricle again appear to underlie arrhythmogenesis in HCM. Ultimately, the picture is of cardiomyocyte disarray and fibrosis, which likely predisposes to ventricular arrhythmias and SCD by generating reentrant circuits in a similar manner to scars in ischemic and nonischemic cardiomyopathy. The exact cause of fibrosis is not known; however, some mechanisms have been described. Disorganized patterns of myocyte arrangement may play a role. It has also been noted that some degree of small vessel disease exists in HCM, which may contribute to remodeling and fibrosis by causing bursts of stress-induced ischemia.[35] Some serum biomarkers indicative of a profibrotic state are elevated in HCM, which can precede onset of clinically detectable left ventricular hypertrophy and may be an important predictor of death.[36]

Low LVEF is uncommon in HCM (except at a late stage, when heart failure develops), and as a result, different risk factors are used for stratification of SCD risk. In HCM patients, 50% of death is due to end-stage heart failure, whereas the other half is due to arrhythmias. The principal clinical features associated with increased risk of SCD include the following: (i) family history of HCM-related SCD in first-degree relatives, (ii) unexplained syncope, (iii) NSVT, (iv) abnormal blood pressure response to exercise, and (v) extreme LV hypertrophy, defined as septal thickness greater than 3.0 cm.[33] The risk conferred by these features is significant, as has been investigated in large international registries of ICDs implanted in patients with HCM at risk of SCD. Appropriate ICD shocks occurred at a rate of 5.5% per year: 11% per year in the secondary prevention cohort and 4% per year in the primary prevention cohort.[37]

Within the Maron classification of HCM based on distribution of hypertrophy, apical HCM has been noted to have a more benign prognosis.[38,39] Other structural features have also been investigated. LV apical aneurysm (not within the classification) is associated with increased risk of SCD, although its prevalence is relatively low and so studies have been based on small patient populations.[40] Left ventricular outflow tract obstruction is a disputed marker of risk: some consider it to be a risk factor,[41] whereas others describe the effect to be modest with a low positive predictive value,[42] or even not present at all.[43]

Recent advances in cardiac magnetic resonance (CMR) have been of interest to the HCM field, because fibrosis is recognized as a key factor in HCM-related SCD. However, studies of LGE-CMR in HCM have not been conclusive thus far[44–48]: for example, one study found late gadolinium enhancement (LGE) to be an independent risk factor for SCD on univariate analysis, but the effect was lost on multivariate analysis.[45] A current ongoing trial, "HCMR—Novel Markers of Prognosis in Hypertrophic Cardiomyopathy trial" (NCT01915615) is due for completion in 2018. This study aims to assess for CMR-based predictors of SCD in a multicenter population of 2750 subjects over a 5-year follow-up period. As the study should be adequately powered for the low event rate in HCM, it may provide definitive insights into the role of LGE and other markers as independent predictors of outcome in HCM.[49]

Fig. 4 shows an example of LGE detected by CMR in a patient with HCM and VT.

One potential limitation of LGE-CMR is its reliance on regional heterogeneity, which gives its high sensitivity in detecting local fibrosis. This is an advantage in ischemic cardiomyopathy, but in diseases such as HCM (and DCM), where diffuse fibrosis is also present, its sensitivity is reduced.[50] T1 mapping is another CMR technique that appears promising in future evaluation of HCM, because it assesses general expansion of the extracellular space, allowing it to better detect diffuse fibrosis.[51] However, there are still questions over its application that need to be answered before further investigation into its risk-stratifying capabilities can occur.[51]

ARRHYTHMOGENIC RIGHT VENTRICULAR CARDIOMYOPATHY

Arrhythmogenic right ventricular cardiomyopathy (ARVC) is a heritable disorder that is characterized by replacement of the right ventricular myocardium by fibrofatty tissue and is a significant cause of SCD in young populations and athletes. An early regional study in Italy over a period of 7 years showed that undiagnosed ARVC was found in 20% of cases of SCD in those under 35 years of age,[52] although a more recent study of autopsies for SCD in the under-35 age group in Denmark found that 5% were due to ARVC[53] (**Fig. 5**).

Most mutations identified in association with ARVC are related to cell-cell adhesion structures, localizing to the desmosome. Changes in cell-cell

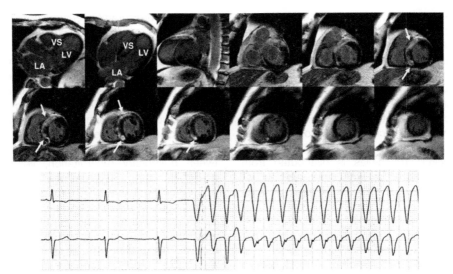

Fig. 4. Images from a patient with HCM. (*top*) CMR imaging showing areas of late gadolinium enhancement (*arrows*). (*bottom*) Holter electrocardiography recorded an episode of sustained VT during syncope that led to hospital admission. LA, left atrium; LV, left ventricle, VS, ventricular septum. (*From* Greulich S, Schumm J, Grün S, et al. Incremental value of late gadolinium enhancement for management of patients with hypertrophic cardiomyopathy. Am J Cardiol 2012;110:1208; with permission.)

adhesion lead to myocyte uncoupling, death, and development of the ARVC phenotype, characterized by fatty infiltration, fibrosis, and thinning of the right ventricular wall, usually occurring within a region defined by the posterior base, infundibulum, and apex, referred to as the "triangle of dysplasia."[54] These changes can also occur in the left ventricle, although uncommonly so. Arrhythmias most likely occur by slowed intraventricular conduction, and the formation of macroreentrant circuits related to the regions of dysplasia.[55] These range from ventricular

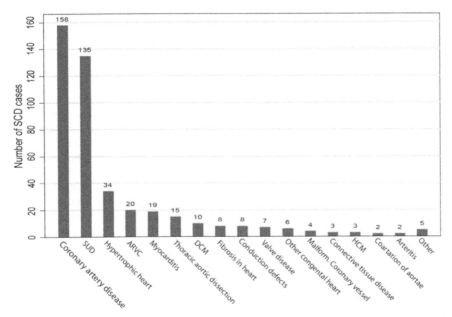

Fig. 5. Causes of SCD from 439 autopsies conducted in Denmark from 2007 to 2009, on patients with SCD from ages 1 to 49. SUD, sudden unexplained death. (*From* Risgard B, Winkel, BG, Jabbari R, et al. Burden of sudden cardiac death in persons aged 1 to 49 years: nationwide study in Denmark. Circ Arrhythm Electrophysiol 2014;7:209; with permission.)

premature beats to VT, characteristically with a left bundle branch block pattern, which can degenerate to VF. Some individuals are gene mutation carriers, and it has been shown that phenotypic expression of ARVC is required for the development of malignant arrhythmias and SCD.[56]

Estimations of mortality differ between studies, but are considered to lie between 0.1% and 3.6% per year.[57] A recent observational study of 301 ARVC patients suggested that risk of life-threatening arrhythmias is distributed from adolescence to later life, with a rate ranging between 1.5 and 4.0 per 100 person-years, peaking at the ages of 21 to 40 years.[58]

Risk markers in ARVC can be separated into multiple categories based on the level of risk conferred. A history of prior cardiac arrest or of sustained VT is the most significant predictor of SCD risk in ARVC.[59,60] Other major factors include a history of unexplained syncope or nonsustained VT, and severe ventricular dysfunction.[60–63] Men have a greater tendency for arrhythmias than women.[64] Some minor risk factors have been identified, although only in small-scale trials and occasionally with conflicting data. These risk factors include the amount and distribution of scarring,[55] frequent PVCs,[64] T-wave inversion beyond the right precordial leads,[64,65] and the presence of multiple desmosomal gene mutations.[66]

Interactions with the sympathetic nervous system are significant in ARVC. Ventricular arrhythmias and SCD are often triggered by adrenergic stimulation, and SCD can often occur during, or immediately after exercise.[67] In addition, exercise is also a significant long-term modifying factor of SCD in ARVC, by promoting development and progression of the disease phenotype. This likely occurs via acute loading of the right ventricle, leading to myocyte uncoupling and death, allowing progression of the pathologic changes described. In support of this, participation in sports increases long-term risk of SCD,[58,68] and a significant proportion of SCD in athletes is due to ARVC.[67,69]

REPAIRED CONGENITAL HEART DISEASE

Patients with repaired congenital heart disease are a population that are also at risk of ventricular arrhythmias and SCD (Elizabeth D. Sherwin and Charles I. Berul's article, "Sudden Cardiac Death in Children and Adolescents," in this issue). However, this is a group in whom risk stratification is difficult because of the heterogeneity of defects, small numbers of cases, and changing repair techniques, as evidenced in the field of ventricular arrhythmias in repaired Tetralogy of Fallot (TOF),

one of the more common repaired congenital heart diseases.[70] A recent study characterized the electrophysiological properties of anatomic isthmuses in repaired TOF, one substrate for ventricular arrhythmias in these patients, which are located in relation to ventricular patches and incision sites. The study found that slow conducting isthmuses as detected on electrophysiological testing was a risk factor for the development of VT.[71] Another study demonstrated a significant association between pulmonary regurgitation, ventricular arrhythmias, and SCD in the repaired TOF population, likely due to RV remodeling secondary to prolonged valve incompetence.[72] This has since been recognized as a major contributor to SCD in repaired TOF and not only has allowed those with repaired TOF and at high risk to be identified, but also indicates that pulmonary valve replacement or repair might improve long-term survival.

BRUGADA SYNDROME

Brugada syndrome is an inherited ion channel disorder resulting in an increased risk of SCD, despite an apparently structurally normal heart. The risk of SCD in symptomatic cases of Brugada syndrome is 10% in the first 4 years after presentation with symptoms.[73,74] Individuals with asymptomatic Brugada syndrome have a lower risk of arrhythmia, with an event incidence of 0.5% per year, than those presenting with syncope or sudden cardiac arrest.[75] In Brugada syndrome-related SCD, short-coupled ventricular premature beats evolve into polymorphic VT and finally degenerate to VF.

SCN5A, which codes for the sodium channel Nav1.5, is the most commonly affected gene. However, there is considerable genetic heterogeneity in Brugada syndrome; not all mutations in SCN5A result in Brugada syndrome, and many cases of Brugada syndrome are not associated with known sodium channel gene mutations. In more recent times, there has been interest in an anatomic substrate of the ECG patterns seen in Brugada syndrome, as a potential arrhythmogenic source. Consequent to this, the right ventricular outflow tract (RVOT) and upper RV anterior wall have been shown to be functionally important in the generation of VF and sudden death in Brugada syndrome,[76–78] and small-scale studies have detected region-specific structural abnormalities, such as epicardial fibrosis.[79]

Recent thinking in the field has sought to integrate these two known abnormalities to generate a unified narrative of arrhythmogenesis, proposing that ion channel mutations may be modifiers of core abnormalities in the RVOT region.[80] However, there is still no consensus on the pathogenesis of Brugada syndrome.

There is also no agreement on the mechanism underlying arrhythmogenesis, VF, and SCD in Brugada syndrome. Two prominent ideas are the slow conduction hypothesis, and the repolarization hypothesis.[81] The slow conduction hypothesis suggests that slowed conduction in the RVOT region leads to the generation of reentry circuits, and appears to be supported by the effectiveness of ablative therapy.[76–78] In the repolarization hypothesis, the generation of transmural gradients in the right ventricle leads to increased phase 2 reentry and the generation of ventricular arrhythmias.

Some predictors of risk of SCD in Brugada syndrome include (i) spontaneous type I ECG pattern, (ii) previous syncope, (iii) history of sinus node dysfunction, (iv) male gender, and (v) inducible ventricular arrhythmias during programmed electrical stimulation.[75,82,83] Other risk factors have also been identified, although not as consistently as those already listed, including family history of SCD,[74,84–86] and fever-induced type 1 Brugada syndrome.[87]

ECG features such as QRS fragmentation,[88] and presence of a wide/large S wave in lead I in spontaneous type I pattern patients (reflective of RVOT conduction delay),[89] appear to be associated with increased risk (**Fig. 6**). Of note, the latter appears to mark out the highest risk patients among those with a spontaneous type I pattern, already a high-risk group. Genetic analysis may also aid risk stratification in the future. Small studies have suggested that some genetic variants in Brugada syndrome carry greater arrhythmic risk than others.[90] A retrospective study found that nonsense mutations compared with functioning missense mutations led to more clinically severe phenotype; however, the rate of aborted SCD was similar.[91]

Many triggers of the Brugada pattern have been identified in Brugada syndrome, which may give indications as to the underlying pathogenic mechanisms. These triggers include fever,[87] sodium channel blockers,[92] vagotonic agents, and even large meals.[93] SCD tends to occur during sleep, or at rest.[94]

However, with greater awareness of Brugada syndrome, new diagnoses are being made of increasingly mild forms, for which these risk factors are less relevant. A retrospective study of a large registry in Brussels and Barcelona (447 patients) indicated that aborted SCD, spontaneous type I pattern, and inducible arrhythmias had become less common in new diagnoses made over the last 10 years,[95] which highlights the need to develop new risk-stratifying features for a new generation of Brugada syndrome patients.

LONG QT SYNDROME

Long QT syndrome (LQTS) results from mutations in potassium (LQT1 and 2) and sodium (mainly LQT3) channels that lead to prolongation of the QT_c interval. Regional prolongation of action potential duration can lead to spatiotemporal

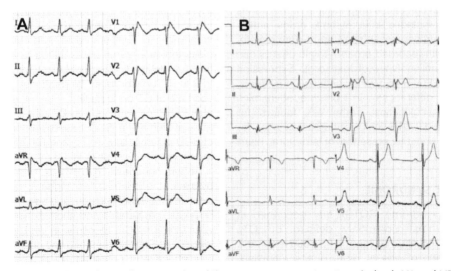

Fig. 6. ECGs in Brugada syndrome demonstrating: (*A*) spontaneous type I pattern in leads V1 and V2, (*B*) QRS fragmentation in leads II, III, aVF, V1, and V2. (*From* Sieira J, Brugada P. Brugada syndrome: defining the risk in asymptomatic patients. Arrhythm Electrophysiol Rev 2016;5:166; with permission.)

dispersion of repolarization, which, combined with the generation of early afterdepolarizations, cause sudden death through the development of torsades de pointes and VF.[96,97]

There are currently as many as 15 described subtypes of genetic LQTS, but LQT1 to LQTS3 are the most clinically significant and are described here. LQT1 is the most common subtype, accounting for 30% to 35% of cases of LQTS. SCD is often associated with sympathetic activity, such as emotional stress and physical activity, in particular simming.[98,99] LQT2, responsible for 25% to 30% of cases, is also driven by adrenergic stimuli: in this case, emotional stress and auditory stimuli are the characteristic triggers.[99,100] LQT3, found in 5% to 10% of cases, mainly causes SCD during bradycardias, but ventricular arrhythmias do occur in LQT3 and are associated with a particularly high risk of SCD, especially during sleep.[99]

The annual risk of SCD across the LQTS population is low, at around 0.15%.[101,102] However, this increases significantly in the presence of certain risk factors. The markers of highest SCD risk in LQTS are a prolonged QT_c interval greater than 500 ms, a history of recent syncope, and male gender.[101–103]

LQTS can also be induced by many drug classes, in a subtype termed "acquired LQTS," which likely represents interactions between drugs and the potassium channels involved in repolarization, such as the hERG channel, responsible for the rapid delayed rectifier potassium current. In some cases, patients with mutations for congenital LQTS but without prolonged QT interval at rest are "unmasked" by drug treatment. The range of drugs that can cause drug-induced LQTS varies greatly and includes antiarrhythmic drugs, antibiotics, and antidepressants; an up-to-date registry of drugs with recorded proarrhythmic effects can be found online (www.qtdrugs.org). Expression of acquired LQTS also varies between individuals, reflecting differences in pharmacodynamics and pharmacokinetics; some risk factors for drug-induced LQTS include increasing age, female sex, and the presence of structural heart disease.[104]

SHORT QT SYNDROME

Short QT syndrome (SQTS), first described in 2000, is most commonly defined by QT_c ≤330 ms, or alternatively, QT_c <360 ms, and the presence of one or more of the following: (i) history of cardiac arrest or syncope, (ii) family history of SCD at 40 or younger, or (iii) family history of SQTS.[105] The triggers of SCD are heterogeneous, with most occurring during rest, but a proportion of SCD occurs during exercise as well.[106] The mutations identified are gain-of-function mutations in potassium channels,[107–109] and arrhythmogenesis likely occurs due to the R-on-T phenomenon, triggered by PVCs.

Initial studies appeared to indicate a low risk of SCD in SQTS. However, these were retrospective and based on middle-aged patients,[110,111] and more recently, the risk is considered higher. In a study of a 73-patient registry, the largest SQTS cohort to date, SCD was the presenting symptom in 40% of index cases. The annual event rate was highest at 4% in the first year of life, and 1.3% thereafter up to age 40, by which time 41% had experienced an episode of SCD. A history of SCD on initial presentation appeared to lead to a much higher risk of further SCD at an observed annual rate of 10.6%, compared with 0.4% in those without history of SCD, and was also the only predictor of recurrence at follow-up.[106] The trend toward early SCD might explain why previous studies had reported low rates of mortality in SQTS. In keeping with this, another recent study has also reported a higher risk of SCD with shortened QT intervals.[112]

CATECHOLAMINERGIC POLYMORPHIC VENTRICULAR TACHYCARDIA

Catecholaminergic polymorphic ventricular tachycardia (CPVT) is a rare arrhythmogenic disease that most commonly manifests in the pediatric population. The principal mutations in CPVT are those affecting cardiac ryanodine receptor (RyR2), calquestrin (CASQ2), and ankyrin B, which appear to be linked through their role in calcium homeostasis. Calcium leak, particularly during diastole when under stress, leads to the generation of delayed afterdepolarizations. This can trigger a polymorphic bidirectional VT in the absence of QT prolongation, which then degenerates to VF. All patients with CPVT are considered to be at high risk of SCD, based both on high rates of SCD in family studies,[113] and on the number of appropriate SCD shocks in case series.[114]

Arrhythmogenesis in CPVT is markedly driven by sympathetic influences: triggers such as exercise, isoproterenol infusion, and adrenergic stimulation are predictable and characteristic, and it is very rare for SCD to occur at rest without any trigger.[114] Early studies showed that ß-blockade was effective in prevention of SCD,[113] although this has not been consistently replicated, with recent studies showing incomplete protection.[114,115]

EARLY REPOLARIZATION PATTERNS

Early repolarization (ER) patterns are often found in young men and have generally been considered benign. However, experimental studies have appeared to show that phase 2 reentry can be induced in the presence of ER pattern and may trigger polymorphic VT or VF,[116] supported by descriptions of SCD in the presence of ER patterns.[117]

Despite this, the risk of SCD does not appear to be great in this population. In one study, ER patterns were found in 1% of athletes undergoing screening for sports participation. In those with ER patterns and structurally normal hearts on initial evaluation, there was only 1 case of SCD (out of 81 athletes) over an average follow-up of 9 years. ER patterns may have been associated with structural heart disease in some instances, as evidenced by cases detected on initial evaluation, but also a small proportion of subjects who then went on to develop cardiomyopathies.[118] In these cases, the risk of SCD may be higher.

Some identified high-risk ER patterns include horizontal or descending ST segment $\geq$0.1 mV,[119] ST elevation $\geq$0.1 mV in inferior leads,[120] ST elevation $\geq$0.2 mV in inferior leads with horizontal/descending ST segment,[119] and slurring or notching of the ST segment.[121] However, the most significant features in assessing a patient with an ER pattern are most likely previous syncope or aborted SCD, and family history of SCD.

IDIOPATHIC VENTRICULAR TACHYCARDIA

In the structurally normal heart with VT, idiopathic VT is the most common cause of arrhythmia. This is primarily divided into two clinical entities, outflow tract VT (typically left bundle branch block and inferior axis) and fascicular VT (often right bundle branch block and left superior axis), both of which are usually associated with a good prognosis if treated. However, there are cases of apparent idiopathic VT who can go on to develop cardiac arrest and are therefore at increased risk of SCD. Features that appear to be linked to an increased risk include very rapid VT, short initial coupling interval, polymorphic VT, and Purkinje triggers.[122,123]

FUTURE DIRECTIONS

Ventricular arrhythmias are associated with a broad range of disease processes, leading to a varied group of substrates that are responsive to different acute triggers. Significant challenges remain in the understanding and management of these diseases, despite the progress that has already been made.

Further work is required to identify risk-stratifying markers in patients with known substrates. ICD implantation can be associated with morbidity effects such as lead infection, and inappropriate shocks. Improved risk stratification will allow the benefits of ICD implantation to be better quantified, aiding the risk-benefit analysis guiding decisions for implantation. The development and validation of disease-specific risk-prediction models may form useful guides for management options.

Expanding the knowledge of the mechanisms of SCD is also important. Many triggers for ventricular arrhythmias and SCD are known, such as electrolyte disturbances, ischemia, mechanical stretch and loading,[124] and changes in the autonomic nervous system,[7] but the interactions between triggers and vulnerable substrates are not always clear. Our understanding of the process of VT degeneration to VF is also unclear. Knowledge of how these events occur and cause SCD may allow identification of potential new methods of SCD prevention.

Advances in medical therapy, developments in pacemaker and ICD technology, and evolution of catheter ablation have achieved reductions in the risk of mortality from ventricular arrhythmias. Further elucidation of the interactions between acute triggers and vulnerable substrates, and how this leads to SCD, will lead to continued improvements in these management options, and the development of new therapies in combating SCD in ventricular arrhythmias. An example of this is the recent development of sympathetic modulation in the management of certain patients with ventricular arrhythmias.[125]

SUMMARY

Ventricular arrhythmias are associated with a broad range of conditions and remain an important cause of SCD. Current knowledge of risk markers helps identify a proportion of patients at risk, who benefit from available treatments such as beta-blockers and ICDs.

Despite recent progress, the current risk stratification models are imperfect. In the future, imaging and genetics, combined with current and new risk-stratification parameters, may help to better detect at-risk patients and to implement additional preventative therapies.

REFERENCES

1. Bayés de Luna A, Coumel P, Leclerq JF. Ambulatory sudden cardiac death: mechanisms of

production of fatal arrhythmia on the basis of data from 157 cases. Am Heart J 1989;117:151–9.

2. Girotra S, Nallamothu BK, Sepertus JA, et al. Trends in survival after in-hospital cardiac arrest. N Engl J Med 2012;367:1912–20.

3. Arenal A, Hernandez J, Perez-David E, et al. Do the spatial characteristics of myocardial scar tissue determine the risk of ventricular arrhythmias? Cardiovasc Res 2012;94(2):324–32.

4. Rutherford SL, Trew ML, Sands GB, et al. High-resolution 3-dimensional reconstruction of the infarct border zone: impact of structural remodeling on electrical activation. Circ Res 2012;111(3):301–11.

5. Roes SD, Borleffs CJ, van der Geest RJ, et al. Infarct tissue heterogeneity assessed with contrast-enhanced MRI predicts spontaneous ventricular arrhythmia in patients with ischemic cardiomyopathy and implantable cardioverter-defibrillator. Circ Cardiovasc Imaging 2009;2(3):183–90.

6. Watanabe E, Abbasi SA, Heydari B, et al. Infarct tissue heterogeneity by contrast-enhanced magnetic resonance imaging is a novel predictor of mortality in patients with chronic coronary artery disease and left ventricular dysfunction. Circ Cardiovasc Imaging 2014;7(6):887–94.

7. Fukuda K, Kanazawa H, Aizawa Y, et al. Cardiac innervation and sudden cardiac death. Circ Res 2015;116(12):2005–19.

8. Rajendran PS, Nakamura K, Ajijola OA, et al. Myocardial infarction induces structural and functional remodelling of the intrinsic cardiac nervous system. J Physiol 2016;594(2):321–41.

9. Moss AJ, Zareba W, Jackson Hall W, et al. Prophylactic implantation of a defibrillator in patients with myocardial infarction and reduced ejection fraction. N Engl J Med 2002;346:877–83.

10. Sabbag A, Suleiman M, Laish-Farkash A, et al. Contemporary rates of appropriate shock therapy in patients who receive implantable device therapy in a real-world setting: from the Israeli ICD registry. Heart Rhythm 2015;12(12):2426–33.

11. Huikuri H, Castellanos A, Myerburg RJ. Sudden death due to cardiac arrhythmias. N Engl J Med 2001;345:1473–82.

12. Buxton AE, Lee KL, DiCarlo L, et al. Electrophysiologic testing to identify patients with coronary artery disease who are at risk for sudden death. Multicenter Unsustained Tachycardia Trial Investigators. N Engl J Med 2000;342:1937–45.

13. Dagres N, Hindricks G. Risk stratification after myocardial infarction: is left ventricular ejection fraction enough to prevent sudden cardiac death? Eur Heart J 2013;34(26):1964–71.

14. Das MK, Saha C, El Masry H, et al. Fragmented QRS on a 12-lead ECG: a predictor of mortality and cardiac events in patients with coronary artery disease. Heart Rhythm 2007;4(11):1385–92.

15. Das MK, Maskoun W, Shen C, et al. Fragmented QRS on twelve-lead electrocardiogram predicts arrhythmic events in patients with ischemic and nonischemic cardiomyopathy. Heart Rhythm 2010;7(1):74–80.

16. Das MK, Khan B, Jacob S, et al. Significance of a fragmented QRS complex versus a Q wave in patients with coronary artery disease. Circulation 2006;113(21):2495–501.

17. Terho HK, Tikkanen JT, Junttila JM, et al. Prevalence and prognostic significance of fragmented QRS complex in middle-aged subjects with and without clinical or electrocardiographic evidence of cardiac disease. Am J Cardiol 2014;114(1):141–7.

18. Wang DD, Buerkel DM, Corbett JR, et al. Fragmented QRS complex has poor sensitivity in detecting myocardial scar. Ann Noninvasive Electrocardiol 2010;15:308–14.

19. Haukilahti MA, Eranti A, Kentta T, et al. QRS fragmentation patterns representing myocardial scar need to be separated from benign normal variants: hypotheses and proposal for morphology based classification. Front Physiol 2016;7:653.

20. Yang Y, Connelly KA, Zeidan-Shwiri T, et al. Multicontrast late enhancement CMR determined gray zone and papillary muscle involvement predict appropriate ICD therapy in patients with ischemic heart disease. J Cardiovasc Magn Reson 2013;15:57.

21. Ng AC, Bertini M, Borleffs CJ, et al. Predictors of death and occurrence of appropriate implantable defibrillator therapies in patients with ischemic cardiomyopathy. Am J Cardiol 2010;106(11):1566–73.

22. Fallavollita JA, Heavey BM, Luisi AJ Jr, et al. Regional myocardial sympathetic denervation predicts the risk of sudden cardiac arrest in ischemic cardiomyopathy. J Am Coll Cardiol 2014;63(2):141–9.

23. Jacobson AF, Senior R, Cerqueira MD, et al. Myocardial iodine-123 meta-iodobenzylguanidine imaging and cardiac events in heart failure. Results of the prospective ADMIRE-HF (AdreView Myocardial Imaging for Risk Evaluation in Heart Failure) study. J Am Coll Cardiol 2010;55(20):2212–21.

24. Mikami Y, Jolly U, Heydari B, et al. Right ventricular ejection fraction is incremental to left ventricular ejection fraction for the prediction of future arrhythmic events in patients with systolic dysfunction. Circ Arrhythm Electrophysiol 2017;10(1) [pii: e004067].

25. Desai AS, Fang JC, Maisel WH, et al. Implantable defibrillators for the prevention of mortality in patients with nonischemic cardiomyopathy: a

meta-analysis of randomised controlled trials. JAMA 2004;292(23):2874–9.

26. Kober L, Thune JJ, Nielsen JC, et al. Defibrillator implantation in patients with nonischemic systolic heart failure. N Engl J Med 2016;375(13): 1221–30.

27. Goldberger JJ, Subačius H, Patel T, et al. Sudden cardiac risk stratification in patients with nonischemic dilated cardiomyopathy. J Am Coll Cardiol 2014;63:1879–89.

28. Di Marco A, Anguera I, Schmitt M, et al. Late gadolinium enhancement and the risk for ventricular arrhythmias or sudden death in dilated cardiomyopathy: systematic review and meta-analysis. JACC Heart Fail 2017;5(1):28–38.

29. Assomull RG, Prasad SK, Lyne J, et al. Cardiovascular magnetic resonance, fibrosis, and prognosis in dilated cardiomyopathy. J Am Coll Cardiol 2006; 48(10):1977–85.

30. Gulati A, Jabbour A, Ismail TF, et al. Association of fibrosis with mortality and sudden cardiac death in patients with nonischemic dilated cardiomyopathy. JAMA 2013;309:896–908.

31. Spezzacatene A, Sinagra G, Merlo M, et al. Arrhythmogenic phenotype in dilated cardiomyopathy: natural history and predictors of life-threatening arrhythmias. J Am Heart Assoc 2015; 4(10):e002149.

32. Maron BJ, Olivotto I, Spirito P, et al. Epidemiology of hypertrophic cardiomyopathy-related death: revisited in a large non-referral-based patient population. Circulation 2000;102:858–64.

33. Maron BJ, Maron MS. Contemporary strategies for risk stratification and prevention of sudden death with the implantable defibrillator in hypertrophic cardiomyopathy. Heart Rhythm 2016; 13(5):1155–65.

34. O'Mahony C, Lambiase PD, Rahman SM, et al. The relation of ventricular arrhythmia electrophysiological characteristics to cardiac phenotype and circadian patterns in hypertrophic cardiomyopathy. Europace 2012;14(5):724–33.

35. Cecchi F, Olivotto I, Gistri R, et al. Coronary microvascular dysfunction and prognosis in hypertrophic cardiomyopathy. N Engl J Med 2003;349: 1027–35.

36. Ho CY, López B, Coelho-Filho OR, et al. Myocardial fibrosis as an early manifestation of hypertrophic cardiomyopathy. N Engl J Med 2010;363:552–63.

37. Maron BJ, Spirito P, Shen WK, et al. Implantable cardioverter-defibrillators and prevention of sudden cardiac death in hypertrophic cardiomyopathy. JAMA 2007;298(4):405–12.

38. Reant P, Donal E, Schnell F, et al. Clinical and imaging description of the Maron subtypes of hypertrophic cardiomyopathy. Int J Cardiovasc Imaging 2015;31(1):47–55.

39. Eriksson MJ, Sonnenberg B, Woo A, et al. Long-term outcome in patients with apical hypertrophic cardiomyopathy. J Am Coll Cardiol 2002;39(4): 638–45.

40. Maron MS, Finley JJ, Bos JM, et al. Prevalence, clinical significance, and natural history of left ventricular apical aneurysms in hypertrophic cardiomyopathy. Circulation 2008;118(15):1541–9.

41. Elliott PM, Gimeno JR, Tome MT, et al. Left ventricular outflow tract obstruction and sudden death risk in patients with hypertrophic cardiomyopathy. Eur Heart J 2006;27(16):1933–41.

42. Maron MS, Olivotto I, Betocchi S, et al. Effect of left ventricular outflow tract obstruction on clinical outcome in hypertrophic cardiomyopathy. N Engl J Med 2003;348:295–303.

43. Efthimiadis GK, Parcharidou DG, Giannakoulas G, et al. Left ventricular outflow tract obstruction as a risk factor for sudden cardiac death in hypertrophic cardiomyopathy. Am J Cardiol 2009;104(5): 695–9.

44. Greulich S, Schumm J, Grun S, et al. Incremental value of late gadolinium enhancement for management of patients with hypertrophic cardiomyopathy. Am J Cardiol 2012;110(8):1207–12.

45. Ismail TF, Jabbour A, Gulati A, et al. Role of late gadolinium enhancement cardiovascular magnetic resonance in the risk stratification of hypertrophic cardiomyopathy. Heart 2014;100(23):1851–8.

46. Chan RH, Maron BJ, Olivotto I, et al. Prognostic value of quantitative contrast-enhanced cardiovascular magnetic resonance for the evaluation of sudden death risk in patients with hypertrophic cardiomyopathy. Circulation 2014;130(6): 484–95.

47. O'Hanlon R, Grasso A, Roughton M, et al. Prognostic significance of myocardial fibrosis in hypertrophic cardiomyopathy. J Am Coll Cardiol 2010; 56(11):867–74.

48. Rubinshtein R, Glockner JF, Ommen SR, et al. Characteristics and clinical significance of late gadolinium enhancement by contrast-enhanced magnetic resonance imaging in patients with hypertrophic cardiomyopathy. Circ Heart Fail 2010; 3(1):51–8.

49. Jellis CL, Desai MY. Sudden cardiac death prediction in hypertrophic cardiomyopathy using late gadolinium enhancement: trouble in paradise? Heart 2014;100(23):1821–2.

50. Schelbert EB, Moon JC. Exploiting differences in myocardial compartments with native T1 and extracellular volume fraction for the diagnosis of hypertrophic cardiomyopathy. Circ Cardiovasc Imaging 2015;8(12) [pii:e004232].

51. Moon JC, Messroghli DR, Kellman P, et al. Myocardial T1 mapping and extracellular volume quantification: a Society for Cardiovascular Magnetic

Resonance (SMCR) and CMR working group of the European Society of Cardiology consensus statement. J Cardiovasc Magn Reson 2013;15:92–104.

52. Thiene G, Nava A, Corrado D, et al. Right ventricular cardiomyopathy and sudden death in young people. N Engl J Med 1988;318:129–33.

53. Winkel BG, Holst AG, Theilade J, et al. Nationwide study of sudden cardiac death in persons aged 1-35 years. Eur Heart J 2011;32(8):983–90.

54. Marcus FI, Fontaine GH, Guiraudon G, et al. Right ventricular dysplasia: a report of 24 adult cases. Circulation 1982;65:384–98.

55. Lin CY, Lin YJ, Li CH, et al. Heterogeneous distribution of substrates between the endocardium and epicardium promotes ventricular fibrillation in arrhythmogenic right ventricular dysplasia/cardiomyopathy. Europace 2017. [Epub ahead of print].

56. Zorzi A, Rigato I, Pilichou K, et al. Phenotypic expression is a prerequisite for malignant arrhythmic events and sudden cardiac death in arrhythmogenic right ventricular cardiomyopathy. Europace 2016;18(7):1086–94.

57. Corrado D, Wichter T, Link MS, et al. Treatment of arrhythmogenic right ventricular cardiomyopathy/dysplasia: an international task force consensus statement. Circulation 2015;132(5):441–53.

58. Mazzanti A, Ng K, Faragli A, et al. Arrhythmogenic right ventricular cardiomyopathy: clinical course and predictors of arrhythmic risk. J Am Coll Cardiol 2016;68(23):2540–50.

59. Link MS, Laidlaw D, Polonsky B, et al. Ventricular arrhythmias in the North American multidisciplinary study of ARVC: predictors, characteristics, and treatment. J Am Coll Cardiol 2014; 64(2):119–25.

60. Corrado D, Leoni L, Link MS, et al. Implantable cardioverter-defibrillator therapy for prevention of sudden death in patients with arrhythmogenic right ventricular cardiomyopathy/dysplasia. Circulation 2003;108(25):3084–91.

61. Bhonsale A, James CA, Tichnell C, et al. Incidence and predictors of implantable cardioverter-defibrillator therapy in patients with arrhythmogenic right ventricular dysplasia/cardiomyopathy undergoing implantable cardioverter-defibrillator implantation for primary prevention. J Am Coll Cardiol 2011;58(14):1485–96.

62. Corrado D, Calkins H, Link MS, et al. Prophylactic implantable defibrillator in patients with arrhythmogenic right ventricular cardiomyopathy/dysplasia and no prior ventricular fibrillation or sustained ventricular tachycardia. Circulation 2010;122(12):1144–52.

63. Wichter T, Paul M, Wollmann C, et al. Implantable cardioverter/defibrillator therapy in arrhythmogenic right ventricular cardiomyopathy: single-center experience of long-term follow-up and complications in 60 patients. Circulation 2004;109(12):1503–8.

64. Bhonsale A, James CA, Tichnell C, et al. Risk stratification in arrhythmogenic right ventricular dysplasia/cardiomyopathy-associated desmosomal mutation carriers. Circ Arrhythm Electrophysiol 2013;6(3):569–78.

65. Saguner AM, Ganahl S, Baldinger SH, et al. Usefulness of electrocardiographic parameters for risk prediction in arrhythmogenic right ventricular dysplasia. Am J Cardiol 2014;113(10):1728–34.

66. Rigato I, Bauce B, Rampazzo A, et al. Compound and digenic heterozygosity predicts lifetime arrhythmic outcome and sudden cardiac death in desmosomal gene-related arrhythmogenic right ventricular cardiomyopathy. Circ Cardiovasc Genet 2013;6(6):533–42.

67. Finocchiaro G, Papadakis M, Robertus JL, et al. Etiology of sudden death in sports: insights from a United Kingdom regional registry. J Am Coll Cardiol 2016;67(18):2108–15.

68. James CA, Bhonsale A, Tichnell C, et al. Exercise increases age-related penetrance and arrhythmic risk in arrhythmogenic right ventricular dysplasia/cardiomyopathy-associated desmosomal mutation carriers. J Am Coll Cardiol 2013;62(14):1290–7.

69. Corrado D, Basso C, Pavei A, et al. Trends in sudden cardiovascular death in young competitive athletes after implementation of a preparticipation screening program. JAMA 2006;296(13):1593–601.

70. Maury P, Sacher F, Rollin A, et al. Ventricular arrhythmias and sudden death in Tetralogy of Fallot. Arch Cardiovasc Dis 2017;110(5):354–62.

71. Kapel GFL, Sacher F, Dekkers OM, et al. Arrhythmogenic anatomical isthmuses identified by electroanatomical mapping are the substrate for ventricular tachycardia in repaired Tetralogy of Fallot. Eur Heart J 2017;38:268–76.

72. Gatzoulis MA, Balaji S, Webber SA, et al. Risk factors for arrhythmia and sudden cardiac death late after repair of Tetralogy of Fallot: a multicentre study. Lancet 2000;(356):975–81.

73. Priori SG, Gasparini M, Napolitano C, et al. Risk stratification in Brugada syndrome: results of the PRELUDE (PRogrammed ELectrical stimUlation preDictive valuE) registry. J Am Coll Cardiol 2012; 59(1):37–45.

74. Probst V, Veltmann C, Eckardt L, et al. Long-term prognosis of patients diagnosed with Brugada syndrome: results from the FINGER Brugada Syndrome Registry. Circulation 2010;121(5):635–43.

75. Sieira J, Brugada P. Brugada syndrome: defining the risk in asymptomatic patients. Arrhythm Electrophysiol Rev 2016;5(3):164–9.

76. Nademanee K, Veerakul G, Chandanamattha P, et al. Prevention of ventricular fibrillation episodes in Brugada syndrome by catheter ablation over

the anterior right ventricular outflow tract epicardium. Circulation 2011;123(12):1270–9.

77. Haissaguerre M, Extramiana F, Hocini M, et al. Mapping and ablation of ventricular fibrillation associated with long-QT and Brugada syndromes. Circulation 2003;108(8):925–8.

78. Morita H, Fukushima-Kusano K, Nagase S, et al. Site-specific arrhythmogenesis in patients with Brugada syndrome. J Cardiovasc Electrophysiol 2003; 14:373–9.

79. Nademanee K, Raju H, de Noronha SV, et al. Fibrosis, connexin-43, and conduction abnormalities in the brugada syndrome. J Am Coll Cardiol 2015;66(18):1976–86.

80. Hoogendijk MG, Opthof T, Postema PG, et al. The Brugada ECG pattern: a marker of channelopathy, structural heart disease, or neither? Toward a unifying mechanism of the Brugada syndrome. Circ Arrhythm Electrophysiol 2010;3(3):283–90.

81. Brugada P. Brugada syndrome: more than 20 years of scientific excitement. J Cardiol 2016;67(3): 215–20.

82. Calvo D, Florez JP, Valverde I, et al. Surveillance after cardiac arrest in patients with Brugada syndrome without an implantable defibrillator: an alarm effect of the previous syncope. Int J Cardiol 2016;218:69–74.

83. Benito B, Sarkozy A, Mont L, et al. Gender differences in clinical manifestations of Brugada syndrome. J Am Coll Cardiol 2008;52(19):1567–73.

84. Conte G, Sieira J, Ciconte G, et al. Implantable cardioverter-defibrillator therapy in Brugada syndrome: a 20-year single-center experience. J Am Coll Cardiol 2015;65(9):879–88.

85. Kamakura S, Ohe T, Nakazawa K, et al. Long-term prognosis of probands with Brugada-pattern ST-elevation in leads V1-V3. Circ Arrhythm Electrophysiol 2009;2(5):495–503.

86. Priori SG, Napolitano C, Gasparini M, et al. Natural history of Brugada syndrome: insights for risk stratification and management. Circulation 2002;105: 1342–7.

87. Mizusawa Y, Morita H, Adler A, et al. Prognostic significance of fever-induced Brugada syndrome. Heart Rhythm 2016;13(7):1515–20.

88. Morita H, Kusano KF, Miura D, et al. Fragmented QRS as a marker of conduction abnormality and a predictor of prognosis of Brugada syndrome. Circulation 2008;118(17):1697–704.

89. Calo L, Giustetto C, Martino A, et al. A new electrocardiographic marker of sudden death in Brugada syndrome: the S-wave in lead I. J Am Coll Cardiol 2016;67(12):1427–40.

90. Sommariva E, Pappone C, Martinelli Boneschi F, et al. Genetics can contribute to the prognosis of Brugada syndrome: a pilot model for risk stratification. Eur J Hum Genet 2013;21(9):911–7.

91. Meregalli PG, Tan HL, Probst V, et al. Type of SCN5A mutation determines clinical severity and degree of conduction slowing in loss-of-function sodium channelopathies. Heart Rhythm 2009;6(3): 341–8.

92. Brugada R, Brugada J, Antzelevitch C, et al. Sodium channel blockers identify risk for sudden death with ST-segment elevation and right bundle branch block but structurally normal hearts. Circulation 2000;101:510–5.

93. Ikeda T, Abe A, Yusu S, et al. The full stomach test as a novel diagnostic technique for identifying patients at risk of Brugada syndrome. J Cardiovasc Electrophysiol 2006;17(6):602–7.

94. Takigawa M, Noda T, Shimizu W, et al. Seasonal and circadian distributions of ventricular fibrillation in patients with Brugada syndrome. Heart Rhythm 2008;5(11):1523–7.

95. Casado-Arroyo R, Berne P, Rao JY, et al. Long-term trends in newly diagnosed Brugada syndrome: implications for risk stratification. J Am Coll Cardiol 2016;68(6):614–23.

96. Glukhov AV, Fedorov VV, Lou Q, et al. Transmural dispersion of repolarization in failing and nonfailing human ventricle. Circ Res 2010;106(5):981–91.

97. Vijayakumar R, Silva JN, Desouza KA, et al. Electrophysiologic substrate in congenital long QT syndrome: noninvasive mapping with electrocardiographic imaging (ECGI). Circulation 2014; 130(22):1936–43.

98. Vyas H, Hejlik J, Ackerman MJ. Epinephrine QT stress testing in the evaluation of congenital long-QT syndrome: diagnostic accuracy of the paradoxical QT response. Circulation 2006;113(11): 1385–92.

99. Schwartz PJ, Priori SG, Spazzolini C, et al. Genotype-phenotype correlation in the long-QT syndrome: gene-specific triggers for life-threatening arrhythmias. Circulation 2001;103:89–95.

100. Wilde AA, Jongbloed RJE, Doevendans PA, et al. Auditory stimuli as a trigger for arrhythmic events differentiate HERG-related (LQTS2) patients from KVLQT1-related patients (LQTS1). J Am Coll Cardiol 1999;33:327–32.

101. Goldenberg I, Moss AJ, Peterson DR, et al. Risk factors for aborted cardiac arrest and sudden cardiac death in children with the congenital long-QT syndrome. Circulation 2008;117(17): 2184–91.

102. Hobbs JB, Peterson DR, Moss AJ, et al. Risk of aborted cardiac arrest or sudden cardiac death during adolescence in the long-QT syndrome. JAMA 2006;296:1249–54.

103. Priori SG, Schwartz PJ, Napolitano C, et al. Risk stratification in the long-QT syndrome. N Engl J Med 2003;348:1866–74.

104. Frommeyer G, Eckardt L. Drug-induced proarrhythmia: risk factors and electrophysiological
mechanisms. Nat Rev Cardiol 2016;13(1):36–47.

105. Priori SG, Wilde AA, Horie M, et al. Executive summary: HRS/EHRA/APHRS expert consensus statement on the diagnosis and management of
patients with inherited primary arrhythmia syndromes. Europace 2013;15(10):1389–406.

106. Mazzanti A, Kanthan A, Monteforte N, et al. Novel
insight into the natural history of short QT syndrome. J Am Coll Cardiol 2014;63(13):1300–8.

107. Bellocq C, van Ginneken AC, Bezzina CR, et al.
Mutation in the KCNQ1 gene leading to the short
QT-interval syndrome. Circulation 2004;109(20):
2394–7.

108. Brugada R, Hong K, Dumaine R, et al. Sudden
death associated with short-QT syndrome linked
to mutations in HERG. Circulation 2004;109(1):
30–5.

109. Priori SG, Pandit SV, Rivolta I, et al. A novel form of
short QT syndrome (SQT3) is caused by a mutation
in the KCNJ2 gene. Circ Res 2005;96(7):800–7.

110. Anttonen O, Junttila MJ, Rissanen H, et al. Prevalence and prognostic significance of short QT interval in a middle-aged Finnish population. Circulation
2007;116(7):714–20.

111. Gallagher MM, Magliano G, Yap YG, et al. Distribution and prognostic significance of QT intervals in
the lowest half centile in 12,012 apparently healthy
persons. Am J Cardiol 2006;98(7):933–5.

112. Nielsen JB, Graff C, Rasmussen PV, et al. Risk prediction of cardiovascular death based on the QTc
interval: evaluating age and gender differences in
a large primary care population. Eur Heart J
2014;35(20):1335–44.

113. Leenhardt A, Lucet V, Denjoy I, et al. Catecholaminergic polymorphic ventricular tachycardia in
children. A 7-year follow-up of 21 patients. Circulation 1995;91(5):1512–9.

114. Priori SG, Napolitano C, Memmi M, et al. Clinical
and molecular characterization of patients with
catecholaminergic polymorphic ventricular tachycardia. Circulation 2002;106:69–74.

115. Sumitomo N, Harada K, Nagashima M, et al. Catecholaminergic polymorphic ventricular tachycardia:
electrocardiographic characteristics and optimal
therapeutic strategies to prevent sudden death.
Heart 2003;89:66–70.

116. Gussak I, Antzelevitch C. Early repolarization syndrome: clinical characteristics and possible cellular
and ionic mechanisms. J Electrocardiol 2000;33(4):
299–309.

117. Haïssaguerre M, Derval N, Sacher F, et al. Sudden
cardiac arrest associated with early repolarization.
N Engl J Med 2008;358:2016–23.

118. Pelliccia A, Di Paolo FM, Quattrini FM, et al. Outcomes in athletes with marked ECG repolarization
abnormalities. N Engl J Med 2008;358:152–61.

119. Tikkanen JT, Junttila MJ, Anttonen O, et al. Early
repolarization: electrocardiographic phenotypes
associated with favorable long-term outcome. Circulation 2011;123(23):2666–73.

120. Takagi M, Aihara N, Takaki H, et al. Clinical characteristics of patients with spontaneous or inducible
ventricular fibrillation without apparent heart disease presenting with J wave and ST segment
elevation in inferior leads. J Cardiovasc Electrophysiol 2000;11:844–8.

121. Wu SH, Lin XX, Cheng YJ, et al. Early repolarization
pattern and risk for arrhythmia death: a meta-analysis. J Am Coll Cardiol 2013;61(6):645–50.

122. Shimizu W. Arrhythmias originating from the right
ventricular outflow tract: how to distinguish "malignant" from "benign"? Heart Rhythm 2009;6(10):
1507–11.

123. Haïssaguerre M, Shah DC, Jaïs P, et al. Role of Purkinje conducting system in triggering of idiopathic
ventricular fibrillation. Lancet 2002;359:677–8.

124. Sutherland GR. Sudden cardiac death: the proarrhythmic interaction of an acute loading with an
underlying substrate. Eur Heart J 2017. [Epub
ahead of print].

125. Ajijola OA, Lux RL, Khahera A, et al. Sympathetic
modulation of electrical activation in normal and
infarcted myocardium: implications for arrhythmogenesis. Am J Physiol Heart Circ Physiol 2017;
312(3):H608–21.

Heart Failure and Sudden Cardiac Death

Basil Saour, MD[1], Bryan Smith, MD[1], Clyde W. Yancy, MD, Msc*

KEYWORDS

- Sudden cardiac death • Heart failure • Ventricular fibrillation • Ventricular tachycardia

KEY POINTS

- Risk stratification tools outside of left ventricular function have focused on markers of left ventricular depolarization and impulse dispersion and propagation.
- The wearable cardioverter defibrillator device provides a theoretic tool for bridging high-risk patients to undergo permanent implantable cardioverter-defibrillator implantation.
- Ventricular tachycardia is common in patients with heart failure regardless of substrate.

INTRODUCTION

Currently, the Centers for Diseases Control and Prevention estimates that 5.7 million adults in the United States suffer from heart failure and 1 in 9 deaths in 2009 cited heart failure as a contributing cause.[1] This statistic is concerning, given that almost 50% of patients who are diagnosed with heart failure die within 5 years of the diagnosis and 7% of all cardiovascular deaths are due to heart failure.[1] Cardiovascular disease continues to be the leading cause of death in the United States and remains a public health burden, costing US$30.7 billion per year.[2] The prognosis of patients with heart failure has improved significantly in the past few decades as a result of advancements in medical and device therapies.[3–23] However, the risk for death remains high. In prototypical reduced ejection fraction (EF) heart failure, causes of death are mostly limited to progressive pump failure or sudden cardiac death. For heart failure with preserved EF, causes of death are more protean but sudden cardiac death is a surprisingly frequent mode of exit. Thus, managing sudden death risk and intervening appropriately with primary or secondary prevention strategies are of paramount importance.

Sudden cardiac death (SCD) in heart failure is typically due to ventricular arrhythmias, electromechanical dissociation, or asystole owing to cataclysmic cardiovascular collapse as the consequence of pump failure. Clinical trials to define sudden cardiac death in patients with heart failure have used many different definitions,[6,11,24–27] but the definition of sudden cardiac death as "a natural death due to cardiac causes, heralded by abrupt loss of consciousness"[28] is most appropriate for this review. The annual incidence and rate of sudden cardiac death is estimated to be 325,000 in the United States accounting for 15% to 20% of all-cause mortality and for more than 50% of all coronary heart disease–related mortality.

Guidelines for risk stratification to identify patients at high risk for sudden cardiac death have been limited to heart failure with reduced EF and depend on New York Heart Association (NYHA) functional class and especially left ventricular (LV) EF (LVEF).[17–19,29,30] In large part this has been due to the lack of trials that support other

Disclosures: Authors have no financial disclosures or conflict of interest pertinent to the subject of the article.
Department of Internal Medicine, Division of Cardiology, Northwestern University, Feinberg School of Medicine, 420 E Superior Street, Chicago, IL 60611, USA
[1] Both authors contributed equally and are considered co first authors.
* Corresponding author. Northwestern University, Arkes Family Pavilion Suite 600, 676 North Saint Clair, Chicago, IL 60611.
E-mail address: cyancy@nm.org

cardiacEP.theclinics.com

risk stratification parameters and/or the absence of rigorous trials done in other heart failure cohorts, including heart failure with preserved EF, heart failure with improved EF, and especially new-onset heart failure. Even for patients with heart failure with reduced EF, there is wide variability in annual mortality rates and deaths attributable to sudden cardiac death.[18,29,31] The wide variability indicates the heterogeneity of the underlying ventricular substrate, specifically ischemic etiologies versus nonischemic, inherited cardiomyopathies, and concomitant other comorbidities, all of which may exacerbate the risk for sudden cardiac death. A better suite of risk prediction tools for high-risk patients with all iterations of heart failure is needed, but the search for more precise risk prediction tools has been empty. There are also heart failure patient populations that are not suitable for inclusion in clinical trials, but have a known risk for sudden cardiac death and very little data to help with risk stratification. This group includes patients with heart failure and end-stage renal disease, sarcoidosis, amyloidosis, and various laminopathies.[32]

RISK STRATIFICATION: BEYOND THE LEFT VENTRICULAR EJECTION FRACTION

The goal standard variable to assess the risk for sudden cardiac death in heart failure is the EF. The threshold of an LVEF of less than 0.35 represents an agreed upon threshold where the risk is sufficiently high that primary prevention strategies are indicated. The search for other variables has largely focused on nuanced evidence of abnormalities in ventricular depolarization or impulse propagation.

T wave alternans (TWA) is defined as the beat-to-beat variation in T wave morphology and patterns. It was first described in 1908, at a time when only macroscopic changes could be detected and were associated with increased risk of ventricular fibrillation (VF). This limitation yielded to a focus on microvolt TWA. TWA has been shown to be increased in elevated heart rates, coronary artery occlusion and reperfusion, mental stress, adrenergic stimulation, and premature ventricular contractions.[33–36]

There is a body of evidence showing a correlation between TWA and recurrent lethal arrhythmias, with the majority of that work being done on patients with ischemic heart disease.[35–44] It has been shown that a TWA of greater than 60 μV during exercise testing or on ambulatory electrocardiographic (ECG) monitors indicated a significantly elevated risk for sudden cardiac death as well as death from all cardiac causes.[45–50] In the periinfarction window, a TWA of greater than 47 μV has predicted sudden cardiac death. Leino and colleagues[46] also demonstrated a more than 50% increase risk of cardiovascular and sudden death per 20 μV increase in TWA.

TWA has been evaluated in patients who would have met MADIT II criteria (Multicenter Automatic Defibrillator Implantation Trial) for implantation of an ICD (ie, ischemic cardiomyopathies with an LVEF of <30%). In these studies, endpoints of all-cause mortality or ventricular tachycardia (VT)/VF occurred in only 2% to 3% of patients with negative TWA test results.[44,51] TWA has also been shown to help risk stratify MADIT II–type patients for all-cause mortality, but was unable to predict sudden cardiac death or appropriate ICD discharge in the MASTER (Microvolt T Wave Alternans Testing for Risk Stratification of Post-Myocardial Infarction Patients) trial.[52] Furthermore, in the SCD-HEFT (Sudden Cardiac Death in Heart Failure Trial) TWA substudy, TWA was unable to predict sudden cardiac death, ventricular arrhythmias, or appropriate ICD discharges.[53] At this time, there is not enough evidence to support the use of TWA to help screen patients who may not benefit from ICD implantation.

The T peak–T end (TpTe) interval is an ECG marker of arrhythmogenesis that reflects the degree of heterogeneity in repolarization of the myocardium. In the general population, a prolonged TpTe is associated with a 2-fold higher risk of sudden cardiac death.[54] Furthermore, prolonged TpTe or prolonged TpTe/QT intervals have demonstrated potential usefulness for the prediction of sudden cardiac death in patients with hypertrophic obstructive cardiomyopathy, long QT syndrome, and those undergoing percutaneous coronary intervention.[55–57]

The TpTe interval represents the speed of dispersion of the repolarization potential from the epicardium to the endocardium.[58,59] A delay in this interval allows for the possibility of preexcitation and induction of arrhythmias.[60] This measure has been demonstrated in cardiac resynchronization therapy (CRT) patients to predict nonsustained VT and ICD firing.[61] TpTe has also been shown to predict overall mortality and VT/VF in patients with systolic dysfunction and ICD implantation for primary prevention.[61,62] Although a difference in electric potentials (ie, dispersion) between cell lines will always be present, increases in the dispersion have been linked with worse outcomes in disease states.[55,56,63]

The upper limit of normal has been well-accepted to be 110 ms.[54,56,58,62,64] Clinical trials are limited and results regarding the predictive accuracy of a prolonged TpTe segment have been inconsistent.[62,65] The largest of these trials was conducted by Rosenthal and colleagues.[62] In this trial, 305 patients who had primary prevention ICDs implanted with LVEF measurements of less than 35% had their baseline ECGs analyzed for TpTe. Endpoints were VT/VF, death, and a combined endpoint of VT/VF and death. The average corrected TpTe was 107 ± 22 ms. The follow-up period for device check was 31 ± 23 months and 49 ± 21 months for mortality follow-up. During these follow-up periods, 82 patients (27%) had appropriate ICD therapy and 91 patients (30%) died. Univariate analysis showed that for every 10-ms increase in corrected TpTe, there was a 20% increase risk of VT/VF (hazard ratio [HR], 1.20; 95% CI, 1.08–1.33; $P = .001$) and a 12% increase in overall mortality risk (HR, 1.12; 95% CI, 1.02–1.23; $P = .02$). When the endpoints of VT/VF and overall mortality were combined, for every 10-ms increase in corrected TpTe there was a 16% increase in risk of an event occurring (HR, 1.16; 95% CI, 1.07–1.25; $P = .001$). The corrected TpTe interval remained significantly predictive of ICD therapy, all-cause mortality, and the combined endpoint with multivariate analysis ($P = .009, .050,$ and $.001$, respectively). The authors concluded that a corrected TpTe segment was helpful in being predictive for which patients will suffer from VT/VF or death.

Further research is required before TpTe can become routinely used as a reliable method for risk stratification of patients. Although Rosenthal and colleagues showed the predictive power of TpTe, even in patients in the lowest tertile (corrected TpTe < 98.5 ms), a 10% VT/VF event rate, 18% death rate, and a more than 20% combined endpoint rate were noted. These findings would make the use of TpTe as a tool to exclude patients from ICD implantation very difficult. However, further refinement of TpTe in the future may yield a tool that can be used to help identify patients who would benefit most from ICD implantation.

QRS dispersion (QRS-D) is the maximum difference between QRS duration between the right and left precordial leads. QRS-D has been shown to predict mortality and sudden cardiac death in patients with advanced congestive heart failure.[66] QRS-D has also been compared against Qt dispersion, syncope, and negative T waves beyond V1 in a population of patients with arrhythmogenic right ventricular cardiomyopathy and was found to be significantly superior in predicting sudden cardiac death.[67,68] Research is needed to determine if QRS-D is a reliable ECG marker to predict future VT/VF or death in patients whom require risk stratification for ICD implantation.

Additional small studies have explored other novel ECG markers for predicting sudden cardiac death. Novel repolarization indices include JT peak/JT, TpTe/JT peak and T peak/JT.[67] Novel markers being investigated that represent repolarization and conduction abnormalities include the index of cardiac electrophysiologic balance, TpTe/QRS-D, and TpTe/(QT × QRSd).[67]

MRI: DELAYED ENHANCEMENT: METAIODOBENZYLGUANIDINE

Risk stratification tools outside of LV function have focused on markers of LV depolarization and impulse dispersion and propagation. To date, LVEF measurements remain the gold standard, but emerging novel ECG parameters and perhaps delayed enhancement on MRI studies may offer the hope for better discrimination of sudden cardiac death risk.

MEDICAL THERAPIES FOR REDUCTION OF MORTALITY IN PATIENTS WITH HEART FAILURE

There are a number of guideline-directed heart failure therapies that have been shown to reduce the risk of sudden cardiac death in patients with a reduced EF (Table 1). Despite a robust evidence base demonstrating mortality advantages for angiotensin-converting enzyme inhibitors and angiotensin receptor antagonists, including CONSENSUS (Cooperative North Scandinavian Enalapril Survival Study), SOLVD trial (Studies of Left Ventricular Dysfunction), SAVE trial (Survival and Ventricular Enlargement), and the set of CHARM studies (Candesartan in Heart failure Assessment of Reduction in Mortality and morbidity), there are few data to substantiate a sudden cardiac death advantage for angiotensin-converting enzyme inhibitor and angiotensin receptor blocker therapies.

Multiple clinical trials have however demonstrated that beta-blockers have a significant effect on reducing the risk of sudden cardiac death in heart failure. In the CIBIS II trial (The Cardiac Insufficiency Bisoprolol Study), patients with NYHA functional class III or IV and an LVEF of 35% or less, already on optimal medical therapy, were randomized to receive either bisoprolol or placebo. Bisoprolol was shown to have a significant effect on reducing all-cause mortality (HR, 0.66; 95% CI, 0.54–0.81; $P<.0001$).[4] In MERIT-HF (metoprolol CR/XL randomised intervention trial in congestive heart failure), patients with NYHA functional class II to IV disease and an LVEF of less than 40% were randomized to receive either

Table 1
Medical therapies proven to reduce SCD in heart failure

Agent	Mechanism of Action	Evidence Base	Impact on Morbidity/Mortality	Impact on SCD
ACE inhibitor	RAAS inhibition	CONSENSUS SAVE SOLVD		Uncertain
Angiotensin receptor antagonist	Angiotensin II type I receptor antagonist	CHARM		Uncertain
Mineralocorticoid antagonist	Inhibition of aldosterone	RALES EPHESUS EMPHASIS		Yes
Beta-blockers	SNS inhibition	US Carvedilol Trials MERIT HF CIBIS		Yes
Valsartan/Sacubitrl	Neprilysin inhibition	PARADIGM HF		Yes

Abbreviations: ACE, angiotensin-converting enzyme; RAAS, renin–angiotensin–aldosterone system; SCD, sudden cardiac death; SNS, sympathetic nervous system.

metoprolol succinate or placebo with a primary outcome of all-cause mortality. In this study, all-cause mortality was significantly lower in the metoprolol succinate group than in the placebo group (relative risk [RR], 0.66; 95% CI, 0.53–0.81; $P = .00009$). In addition, there were fewer sudden deaths in the metoprolol succinate group than in the placebo group (RR, 0.59; 95% CI, 0.45–0.78; $P = .0002$).[5] This benefit was noted most in those with minimally symptomatic heart failure and justifies today's concern that the risk for sudden cardiac death in heart failure is separate and distinct from the symptom burden and is greatest in mild to moderate heart failure. The mortality benefit of carvedilol was highlighted in 2 landmark clinical trials. In CAPRICORN (Carvedilol Post-Infarct Survival Control in Left Ventricular Dysfunction), patients with a previous myocardial infarction and an LVEF of less than 40% were randomly assigned to receive carvedilol or placebo with primary endpoint of all-cause mortality or hospital admission for cardiovascular causes. This study found that there was a significant reduction in all-cause mortality in the carvedilol group compared with placebo (HR, 0.77; 95% CI, 0.60–0.98; $P = .03$).[69] In the COPERNICUS study (Carvedilol Prospective Randomized Cumulative Survival), symptomatic patients with heart failure with an LVEF of 25% or less were assigned randomly to receive either carvedilol or placebo. Patients treated with carvedilol had a 35% decrease in the risk of death when compared with placebo (95% CI, 19%–48%,; $P = .00013$) and patients treated with carvedilol were less likely to have an episode of sudden death ($P = .016$).[70,71]

Mineralocorticoid antagonists have also been shown to have a significant effect on mortality and sudden cardiac death. In the RALES trial (Randomized Aldactone Evaluation Study), patients with NYHA functional class III and IV symptomatic heart failure and an LVEF of 35% or less were assigned randomly to receive spironolactone or placebo. Spironolactone resulted in a significant reduction in all-cause mortality (RR, 0.70; 95% CI, 0.60–0.82). This 30% reduction in mortality was attributed to a lower risk of death from progressive heart failure and sudden death from cardiac causes ($P<.01$).[72] In the EPHESUS trial (Eplerenone Post–Acute Myocardial Infarction Heart Failure Efficacy and Survival Study), mineralocorticoid antagonists were studied in a population of patients after acute myocardial infarction complicated by LV dysfunction with an LVEF of 40% or less. Patients were assigned randomly to receive either eplerenone or placebo in addition to optimal medical therapy with a primary endpoint of all-cause mortality or death from cardiovascular causes. There were significantly fewer deaths in the eplerenone group (RR, 0.85; 95% CI, 0.75–0.96; $P = .008$) as well as a significant decrease in death from cardiovascular causes or hospitalization for cardiovascular events (RR, 0.87; 95% CI, 0.79–0.95; $P = .002$). Specifically, there was also an important reduction in the rate of sudden death from cardiovascular causes (RR, 0.79; 95% CI, 0.64–0.97; $P = .03$).[12] In the EMPHASIS-HF trial (Eplerenone in Mild Patients Hospitalization and Survival Study in Heart Failure), patients with an LVEF of 35% or less, NYHA functional class II, and already on guideline-directed medical therapy were randomly assigned to receive either eplerenone or placebo with a primary outcome of a composite of death from cardiovascular causes or hospitalization for heart failure. In this study, eplerenone resulted in a significant reduction in all-cause mortality (HR, 0.76; 95% CI, 0.62–0.93; P<.001) and a significant reduction in deaths from cardiovascular causes (HR, 0.76; 95% CI, 0.61–0.94; P = .01). However, this study also found that eplerenone did not have a significant effect on sudden cardiac death (HR, adjusted; 95% CI, 0.54–1.07; P = .12).[31]

Valsartan/sacubitril is a novel combination therapy with dramatically proven survival advantages in heart failure. In PARADIGM-HF (A Multicenter, Randomized, Double-blind, Parallel Group, Active-controlled Study to Evaluate the Efficacy and Safety of LCZ696 Compared to Enalapril on Morbidity and Mortality in Patients With Chronic Heart Failure and Reduced Ejection Fraction), 8442 patients with NYHA functional class II to IV heart failure symptoms and an EF of 40% or less received valsartan/sacubitril or enalapril twice daily in addition to recommended therapy. The primary outcome was a composite of death from cardiovascular causes or a first hospitalization for heart failure. Death from cardiovascular causes or hospitalization for heart failure occurred in 914 patients (21.8%) in the valsartan/sacubitril group and 1117 patients (26.5%) in the enalapril group (HR, 0.80; 95% CI, 0.73–0.87; P<.01). All-cause mortality was also reduced in the valsartan/sacubitril group in which 711 patients died (17.0%) versus 835 in the enalapril group (19.8%; HR, 0.84; 95% CI, 0.76–0.93; P<.001). Importantly, death owing to sudden cardiac events was similarly affected by the use of valsartan/sacubitril, thus adding to the armamentarium of evidence-based medical therapies proven to reduce the incidence of sudden cardiac death in reduced EF heart failure.[73]

DEVICE AND ABLATIVE STRATEGIES FOR REDUCTION OF MORTALITY IN PATIENTS WITH HEART FAILURE

The mainstay of prevention for sudden cardiac death in patients with heart failure on goal-directed optimal therapy is implantation of an ICD, either for primary or secondary prevention.[17,18,21,22,29]

Primary Prevention Implantable Cardioverter-Defibrillator Trial Data

Moss and colleagues[17] in 1996 published the MADIT trial. Patients with NYHA functional class I to III disease (n = 196) secondary to an ischemic cardiomyopathy with an EF of less than 35% who had a documented episode of asymptomatic nonsustained VT and inducible sustained VT on an electrophysiology study (EPS) were assigned randomly to ICD implantation versus conventional medical therapy. The final endpoint of the trial was all-cause mortality. There were a total of 15 deaths in the defibrillator group and 39 deaths in the medical therapy arm. The HR for overall mortality was 0.46 (95% CI, 0.26–0.82; P = .009). Based on this trial, the investigators concluded that prophylactic therapy with an ICD improves survival as compared with medical therapy in patients who are at high risk of VT/VF after prior myocardial infarction.

Buxton and colleagues[21] in 1999 published the MUST trial results (Multicenter Unsustained Tachycardia trial). The authors looked to evaluate if EPS-guided antiarrhythmic therapy or ICD implantation would reduce the risk of sudden death in patients with ischemic cardiomyopathy with an EF of less than 40% who were found to have asymptomatic nonsustained ventricular tachycardia. They randomized 704 patients. The 5-year estimated all-cause mortality was 42% in patients who received antiarrhythmic therapy and 48% in patients who had no antiarrhythmic therapy (RR, 0.8; 95% CI, 0.64–1.01). However, the authors found that patients who were treated with defibrillators had a significant reduction in cardiac arrest or death from arrhythmia (RR, 0.24; 95% CI, 0.13–0.45; P≤.001). The authors subsequently concluded that EPS-guided implantation of ICDs in patients with ischemic cardiomyopathy with an EF of less than 40% and asymptomatic nonsustained ventricular tachycardia reduced the risk of sudden cardiac death.

Moss and colleagues[18] in 2002 published the MADIT II trial, which evaluated 1232 patients with a history of ischemic cardiomyopathy and an EF of less than 30%. Participants were randomized in a 3:2 fashion to having an ICD implanted versus conventional medical therapy. Of note, EPS was not required for enrollment into the trial, nor was the presence of nonsustained ventricular tachycardia. The primary endpoint was all-cause mortality. Mortality rates over an average follow-up period of 20 months in the defibrillator arm were 14.2% compared with 19.8% in the medical therapy arm. The HR for risk of death between the 2 groups was 0.69 (95% CI, 0.51–0.93; P = .16). The authors concluded that the prophylactic implantation of an ICD in patients with severe LV dysfunction improves survival.

Bardy and colleagues[29] in 2005 published the Sudden Cardiac Death in Heart failure trial (SCD-HeFT). The investigators enrolled 2521 patients with NYHA functional class II or III congestive heart failure and an EF of less than 35% (both ischemic and nonischemic patients were included) and randomized them to either conventional therapy plus placebo or conventional therapy plus amiodarone or conventional therapy plus ICD implantation. The primary endpoint was all-cause mortality. The median follow-up was 45.5 months. The authors recorded 244 deaths (29%) in the placebo group, 240 deaths (28%) in the amiodarone group, and 182 deaths (22%) in the ICD group. When compared with the placebo group treatment with amiodarone had no effect on all-cause mortality (HR, 1.06; 97.5% CI, 0.86–1.30; P = .53). ICD therapy, however, was associated with a decreased risk of death when compared with the placebo arm (RR, 0.77; 97.5% CI, 0.62–0.96; P = .007). These results did not vary according to cause of LV dysfunction. The authors concluded that patients with severe LV dysfunction, regardless of etiology, had a significant increase in survival if an ICD was implanted, but found no benefit to routine amiodarone therapy.

Kober and colleagues[74] in 2016 published the DANISH trial (Defibrillator Implantation in patients with nonischemic systolic heart failure). The randomized enrolled 1116 patients with an EF of less than 35% not caused by coronary artery disease in a 1:1 fashion to receive an ICD versus medical therapy. In both groups, 58% of patients received CRT along with a very high exposure to mineralocorticoid antagonists. The primary outcome was death from any cause. After a mean follow-up on 67 months there were 120 deaths (21.6%) in the ICD arm and 131 deaths (23.4%) in the non ICD arm (HR, 0.87; 95% CI, 0.68–1.12; P = .28). Interestingly, sudden cardiac death occurred in 24 patients (4.3%) in the ICD arm compared with 46 (8.3%) in the control arm (HR, 0.50; 95% CI, 0.31–0.82; P = .005). The authors concluded that, in patients with nonischemic cardiomyopathy and an EF of less than 35%, prophylactic ICD implantation has no added all-cause mortality benefit, but the impact of ICD therapy on the risk of sudden cardiac death was nevertheless clear.

Landmark Primary Prevention Cardiac Resynchronization Therapy Trial Data

Bristow and colleagues[75] in 2004 published the COMPANION trial (Cardiac-Resynchronization Therapy with or without an Implantable Defibrillator in Advanced Chronic Heart Failure), which evaluated the effect of CRT pacemaker (CRT-P) versus cardiac resynchronization therapy

defibrillator (CRT-D) in patients with chronic heart failure with ischemic or nonischemic cardiomyopathies and an EF of less than 35% (**Table 2**). Patients were required to have a QRS of greater than 120 ms, a PR of greater than 150 ms, and had to be hospitalized for heart failure within the last 12 months. This was a 3-arm study that included 1520 patients who were randomized in a 1:2:2 fashion to goal-directed medical therapy versus goal-directed medical therapy plus CRT-P versus goal-directed medical therapy plus CRT-D, respectively. The primary endpoint was a composite of time to death or hospitalization for any cause. Death from any cause was a predefined secondary endpoint. Goal-directed medical therapy plus CRT-P versus goal-directed medical therapy showed a significant reduction in the primary endpoint (HR, 0.81; 95% CI, 0.69–0.96; P = .014), as did goal-directed medical therapy plus CRT-D versus goal-directed medical therapy (HR, 0.80; 95% CI, 0.68–0.95; P = .01). Goal-directed medical therapy plus CRT-P versus goal-directed medical therapy showed a strong trend to decreasing all-cause mortality (HR, 0.76; 95% CI, 0.58–1.01; P = .059), whereas goal-directed medical therapy plus CRT-D showed a significant reduction in all-cause mortality compared with goal-directed medical therapy alone (HR, 0.64; 95% CI, 0.48–0.86; P = .003). The authors concluded that, in patients with severe LV dysfunction and a prolonged QRS (>120 ms), CRT-P provides a significant decrease in the combined risk of death or hospitalization and, when combined with a defibrillator, significantly reduces mortality as well.

Cleland and colleagues[76] in 2005 published the CARE HF trial (Cardiac resynchronization on morbidity and mortality in Heart Failure), which evaluated whether cardiac resynchronization affected morbidity and mortality in patients who had been on guideline-directed medical therapy and had persistent NYHA functional class III of IV disease, an EF of less than 35%, a left ventricular end-diastolic diameter of 30 mm, and a QRS of greater than 120 ms. In patients who had QRS 120 to 149 ms, enrollment into the trial required they had 2 or 3 additional criteria for dyssynchrony (ie, an aortic preejection delay of >140 ms, an interventricular mechanical delay of >40 ms, or delayed activation of the posterolateral LV wall). Ischemic and nonischemic causes of LV dysfunction were included in the trial. Overall, 813 patients were enrolled in the trial and were randomized in a 1:1 fashion to medical therapy or medical therapy plus CRT. The primary endpoint was a composite of all-cause mortality of unplanned hospitalization for a major cardiovascular event,

Table 2
Primary prevention and CRT trial data summarized

Trial Name	EF Cutoff	NYHA Functional Class Evaluated	Ischemic or Nonischemic Population	Other Inclusion Criteria	Results
MADIT	<35%	I–III	Ischemic	Asymptomatic nonsustained VT and inducible sustained VT on EPS	ICD improves survival as compared with medical therapy in patients who are at high risk of VT/VF after prior myocardial infarction.
MUST	<40%	II–III	Ischemic	Asymptomatic NSVT	EPS-guided implantation of ICDs in patients with ischemic cardiomyopathy with an EF <40% and asymptomatic NSVT reduced the risk of SCD.
MADIT II	<30%	I–III	Ischemic	None	Implantation of an ICD in patients with severe LV dysfunction improves survival.
SCD HEFT	<35%	II–III	Both	None	ICD improved survival in patients with severe LV dysfunction and amiodarone did not.
DANISH	<35%	II–III	Nonischemic	None	In patients with NICM and EF <35% prophylactic ICD implantation has no added all-cause mortality benefit.
COMPANION	<35%	II–III	Both	QRS >120 ms plus PR >150 ms plus hospitalized for heart failure within the last 12 mo	In patients with severe LV dysfunction and a prolonged QRS >120 ms CRT-P provides a significant decrease in the combined risk of death or hospitalization and when combined with a defibrillator significantly reduces mortality as well.
CARE HF	<35%	III–IV	Both	LVEDD of 30 mm plus QRS of >120 ms	CRT-P implantation on top of guideline directed medical therapy provided a mortality benefit to patients with severe LV dysfunction; NYHA functional class III/IV and QRS >120 ms.
MADIT CRT	<30%	I–II	Both	QRS >130 ms	CRT-D decreased the risk of recurrent heart failure events in relatively asymptomatic patients with severe LV dysfunction and a QRS >130 ms.

Abbreviations: CRT, cardiac resynchronization therapy; CRT-D, cardiac resynchronization therapy defibrillator; CRT-P, cardiac resynchronization therapy pacemaker; EF, ejection fraction; EPS, electrophysiology study; ICD, implantable cardioverter-defibrillator; LV, left ventricular; LVEDD, left ventricular end-diastolic diameter; NICM, nonischemic cardiomyopathy; NSVT, nonsustained ventricular tachycardia; NYHA, New York Heart Association; VF, ventricular fibrillation; VT, ventricular tachycardia.

whichever came first. The mean duration of follow-up was 29.4 months. Interestingly, the median QRS duration was approximately 160 ms in both arms. The primary endpoint was reached in 159 patients (39%) in the CRT-P group compared with 224 patients (55%) in the medical therapy arm (HR, 0.63; 95% CI, 0.51–0.77; $P = .001$). All-cause mortality was analyzed as an independent variable and found to be significantly lower in the CRT-P arm (20% vs 30%; HR, 0.64; 95% CI, 0.48–0.85; $P<.002$). The authors concluded that CRT-P implantation on top of guideline-directed medical therapy provided a mortality benefit to patients with severe LV dysfunction; NYHA functional class III or IV disease, and a QRS of longer than 120 ms.

Moss and colleagues[23] in 2009 published the MADIT-CRT trial (Multicenter Automatic Defibrillator Implantation With Cardiac Resynchronization Therapy), which investigated whether the addition of a CRT system to standard ICD implantation offered a mortality benefit in patients with either ischemic or nonischemic cardiomyopathy, an EF of less than 30%, and a QRS of greater than 130 ms with NYHA functional class I or II symptoms. The investigators randomized 1820 patients in a 3:2 fashion to having a CRT-D system or an ICD alone. The primary endpoint was all-cause mortality or nonfatal heart failure event (whichever came first). Of note, approximately 70% of patients had left bundle branch block with approximately 65% of patients having a QRS of greater than 150 ms. The average follow-up was 2.4 years. The primary endpoint occurred in 187 patients (17.2%) in the CRT-D arm and 185 patients (25.3%) in the ICD-only group (HR, 0.66; 95% CI, 0.52–0.84; $P = .001$). The benefit did not differ significantly between ischemic and nonischemic patients. There was no difference in death rates between the 2 groups. The superiority of CRT was driven by a significant 41% reduction in heart failure events. The authors concluded that CRT-D decreased the risk of recurrent heart failure events in relatively asymptomatic patients with severe LV dysfunction and a QRS of greater than 130 ms.

Summary

There are substantial clinical data to support the use of ICDs in patients with reduced EF heart failure (LVEF <35%).[17,18,21,23,29] There are no data, however, to show a mortality benefit in patients who have heart failure with midrange LVEF, that is, 40% to 50% or heart failure with preserved EF. These cohorts merit de novo clinical trials as the question of sudden cardiac death prevention is of equal importance in all patients with heart

failure. However, care should be taken so as to not implant patients less than 40 days after an acute myocardial event, given that there seems to be no significant all-cause mortality benefit to this strategy.[77,78] Nor should an ICD be implanted before optimization of evidence-based medical therapy for reduced EF heart failure, typically allowing at least 90 days of exposure to goal-directed medical therapy before proceeding with ICD implantation. Some investigators have argued, in the absence of data, that these obligatory waiting periods expose patients to untoward risk and for this reason a novel technology has emerged. The wearable cardioverter defibrillator (WCD) was introduced to address this issue.

WEARABLE CARDIOVERTER DEFIBRILLATOR

The WCD received US Food and Drug Administration approval more than a decade ago but, remarkably, there are no randomized controlled data to refute or confirm the potential benefit to reduce sudden cardiac death events. There have, however, been registries that capture observational data regarding the use of WCD devices. Chung and colleagues[79] in 2010 evaluated 3569 patients who were given a WCD. In this analysis, patients with new ischemic cardiomyopathy as well and nonischemic cardiomyopathy were included, as well as patients who had to have ICD extraction with delayed reimplantation secondary to ICD infections. The average daily use of the WCD was 19.9 hours. Ultimately, 14.2% of patients stopped wearing the WCD owing to comfort issues. The mean amount of time that the WCD was worn for was 53 days. Fifty-nine patients (1.7%) received an appropriate shock. First shock success was 100% for unconscious VT/VF and 79.8% for all VT/VF. Survival after successful cardioversion was 89.5%. A further 17 patients died from asystole, 2 from pulseless electrical activity, and 3 from respiratory arrest, representing a total of 24.5% of sudden cardiac deaths. Inappropriate shocks occurred in 67 patients (1.9%). The major reasons for inappropriate shocks were noise artifact (72%) and supraventricular tachycardia (25.5%).

Epstein and colleagues[80] in 2013 published the largest series of patients that were identified via the WCD medical order registry. They identified 8453 patients who had an acute myocardial infarction and an EF of less than 35% or who had suffered an acute myocardial infarction and given a WCD. Sixty-two percent of patients in this registry underwent complete revascularization. The median daily use by patients was 21.8 hours. The authors evaluated rates of WCD discharge at 30 days after myocardial infarction and 3 months after myocardial infarction. A total of 133 patients (1.6%) received 309 appropriate shocks; 106 patients (79.6%) received an appropriate shock and had an LVEF of less than 30%, 17 (12.7%) had an LVEF of 30% to 35%, and 8 (6%) had an LVEF of greater than 36%. The median time to therapy was 16 days and 75% of patients who received therapy did so within the first month after their index event. Interestingly, the authors also noted that 34 additional deaths (0.4%) occurred owing to bradycardia or asystole. Inappropriate shocks were also infrequent, but not at a substantially lower rate than appropriate shocks. There were 99 patients (1.1%) who received a total of 114 inappropriate shocks. The cause of inappropriate shocks was found to be from noise artifact,[62] supraventricular tachycardia,[21] electrical oversensing,[15] and nonsustained ventricular tachycardia.[3,80]

Zishiri and colleagues[81] evaluated patients from the Cleveland Clinic who had undergone either surgical or percutaneous intervention with an EF of less than 35% and compared them with the 809 patients in the WCD postmarket US database. The 90-day mortality rates were higher in patients who did not received a WCD in both patients after coronary artery bypass grafting (no WCD 7% vs WCD 3%) and after percutaneous coronary intervention (no WCD 10% vs WCD 2%). Inappropriate therapies accounted for 42% of total therapies delivered. However, only 1.3% of patients with an ECD received an appropriate therapy and the authors thus concluded that the mortality difference seen between the 2 groups cannot be explained entirely by prevention of sudden cardiac death.

In 2008, the VEST trial (Prevention of Early Sudden Death) and VEST Registry were started. The estimated completion of the trial is December 2017. The aim of this study is to provide prospective acquired evidence to evaluate if wearing a WCD device for 90 days reduces early mortality in patients who have had an acute myocardial infarction with an EF of less than 35%. We hope that an answer is forthcoming.

Summary

The WCD device provides a theoretic tool for bridging high-risk patients to undergo permanent ICD implantation. However, these devices are unproven and not without important limitations. Currently, no prospective, randomized trial data exist. Ongoing concerns of inappropriate shock rates and failure to detect and treat bradyarrhythmias or asystole may represent insurmountable obstacles. Yet, for those patients at risk for sudden
cardiac death early after the onset of heart failure, this technology may be of value. As the decision to proceed with use of a WCD is contemplated, the benefit of evidence-based medical therapy to reduce the incidence of sudden cardiac death in heart failure should not be discounted.

ANTIARRHYTHMIC DRUGS AND ABLATION FOR VENTRICULAR TACHYCARDIA IN HEART PATIENTS WITH FAILURE

VT is not uncommon in patients with heart failure, with up to 20% of patients developing an episode of VT 3 to 5 years after a primary prevention ICD has been placed.[82–84] It has also been recognized that recurrent ICD shocks reduce qualify of life and are associated with an increased mortality rate.[82–84]

Initial management regimens have traditionally relied on the use of antiarrhythmic drug (AAD) therapies. Amiodarone and sotalol are the drugs of choice, but often yield suboptimal results and generate side effect profiles that are not insignificant.[82] Celivarone (an inhibitor of sodium, calcium and potassium channels) and azimilide (a class III antiarrhythmic) have also been studied to evaluate attenuation of VT episodes; however, these trials to date were negative.[85,86] Connolly and colleagues[82] evaluated 412 patients who had received an ICD for spontaneous VT or VF. Patients were randomized in a 1:1:1 fashion to beta-blockers alone, sotalol alone, or amiodarone and beta-blocker therapy. Amiodarone plus beta-blocker therapy significantly reduced the risk for recurrent shocks compared with beta-blocker therapy alone (HR, 0.27; 95% CI, 0.14–0.52; $P<.001$) or sotalol therapy (HR, 0.43; 95% CI, 0.22–0.85; $P<.02$). Sotalol showed a strong trend to reduce shocks compared with beta-blocker therapy alone (HR, 0.61; 95% CI, 0.37–1.01; $P = .055$). Unfortunately, rates of drug discontinuation after 1 year were very high in the AAD arms, with an 18.2% discontinuation rate for amiodarone and a 23.5% discontinuation rate for sotalol. Combination therapy with amiodarone plus mexiletine or sotalol plus procainamide or quinidine have been evaluated in cohort studies and showed significant reductions in ventricular events,[87,88] but these multidrug regimens are not well-tolerated by most patients with heart failure. Importantly, most AAD therapies are negative inotropes that may worsen heart failure. The rates of drug discontinuation, suboptimal results, and side effect profiles of AADs have made catheter ablation increasingly used as an intervention to treat VT.

A recent metaanalysis published by Santangeli and colleagues comparing AAD with catheter ablation as initial strategies demonstrated that there was no difference in outcomes; thus, the best approach for persistent VT is based on a shared decision making discussion with the patient where risks and benefits for each approach are reviewed. This approach is endorsed by recent society statements.[89,90]

Catheter ablation in patients with recurrent and refractory VT can be lifesaving when VT is incessant.[30,91–93] Furthermore, VT ablation has been shown to dramatically reduce VT events; however, overall mortality benefits could not be demonstrated in these underpowered trials.[94,95] Sapp and colleagues[96] in 2016 compared escalating AAD therapy versus catheter ablation in patients with NYHA functional class I to III heart failure owing to ischemic heart disease complicated by refractory VT who already had an ICD implanted. Patients (n = 259) were enrolled and randomized in a 1:1 fashion to either catheter ablation or escalating AAD therapy. The primary endpoint was a composite of all cause death, VT storm, or appropriate ICD shock. Prespecified secondary outcomes were the individual components of the primary outcome. The average EF of patients included in both arms was 31%. In both groups, approximately 50% of patients were NYHA functional class II and approximately 25% were NYHA functional class I and NYHA functional class III. The primary endpoint occurred in 78 of 132 patients (59.1%) in the ablation group and in 87 of 127 patients (68.5%) randomized to escalating medical therapy. There was a statistically significant decrease in events in favor of ablation (HR, 0.72; 95% CI, 0.53–0.98; $P = .04$). Of the prespecified secondary outcomes, there was no significant difference in all-cause mortality or appropriate ICD shock between the groups ($P = .86$ and .19, respectively). However, there was a strong trend to reduce episodes of VT storm in the ablation arm (HR, 0.66; 95% CI, 0.42–1.05; $P = .08$). Adverse event rates were comparable between the 2 groups, with the increase in procedural complications in the ablation arm being offset by increased episodes of drug toxicity and adverse events in the escalating drug therapy arm. The authors concluded that, in patients with reduced EF heart failure owing to ischemic heart disease complicated by recurrent VT despite AAD therapy, catheter ablation should be considered over escalating AAD therapy to improve outcomes.

NONISCHEMIC CARDIOMYOPATHIES
Dilated Cardiomyopathy

Monomorphic VT is far less common in nonischemic patients then in those who have ischemic cardiomyopathies. This distinction is important because the initial onset of polymorphic VT is not easily localized despite contemporary mapping technology. When monomorphic VT does occur, it is either due to the presence of a scar related reentry circuit and bundle branch reentry or from a focal origin.[93,97–99] Epicardial ablation is required in more than one-third of cases and ablation is often more difficult than in patients with ischemic cardiomyopathies. Success rates for persistent suppression of VT in dilated cardiomyopathies approaches 60%.

Right Ventricular Cardiomyopathies

Most commonly, right ventricular VTs are seen in patients who suffer from cardiac sarcoidosis, arrhythmogenic right ventricular cardiomyopathy, or idiopathic cardiomyopathies.[93,100–104] All forms of VT can occur in these patients ranging from reentry circuits, focal breakthroughs, as well as epicardial circuits. Although initial ablation often suppresses the presenting VT, recurrence is common and is believed to be a manifestation of progression of the patients underlying disease state.[93]

Summary

VT is common in patients with heart failure, regardless of substrate. It is important to consider the clinical situation of the patient when evaluating candidacy for VT ablation. Unstable VT requires substrate modification and may need hemodynamic support. Stable VT can be mapped and successfully targeted with limited radiofrequency ablation. At this time, there is no consensus in the EP community regarding which approach (clinical VT ablation vs substrate modification) is superior; small studies suggest that substrate modification improves the rate of hospitalization and recurrence of VT, but not mortality.

VT ablation can improve outcomes in patients with heart failure who are refractory to AAD therapy; however, recurrence is common and long-term mortality has not been proven to be dramatically altered. VT ablation can, however, offer a mechanism whereby quality of life can be increased and frequency of ICD shocks may be reduced with potential improvements in morbidity and mortality.

Further advancements in technology to help guide VT ablation are required to help improve outcomes. Using imaging modalities like MRI and PET/computed tomography scanning may identify scar and possible new targets for ablation.[105–109] Fahmy and colleagues[107] have shown that cardiac PET/computed tomography with electroanatomical mapping is a feasible and accurate way to target VT sites for ablation. Currently, the Magnetic-VT trial (Comparison of VT Ablation Outcomes Using Remote MAGNETIC Navigation Versus Manual Approach in a Low LVEF Population) is underway to evaluate if the routine use of a remote magnetic navigation-guided ablation strategy provides superior outcomes compared with a manual approach in patients with ischemic cardiomyopathies.[110] New techniques including transcoronary ethanol ablation, bipolar ablation, intramyocardial needle mapping, and gamma knife ablation are promising new approaches to providing improved ablation strategies.

END-OF-LIFE CARE

In patients with advanced heart failure and recurrent hospitalizations, goals of care should be addressed. A shared decision making conversation is helpful to establish if more aggressive therapy is to be considered, for example, mechanical circulatory support or heart transplantation; palliation, for example, home–inotropes or hospice care. Especially for palliative and hospice care, it may be appropriate to turn off the defibrillator function of implanted devices. For this reason, establishing a healthy rapport with patients is important, because these can sometimes become very challenging decisions that involve extended family, clergy, and even ethicists. If a palliative care route or hospice option is selected, care should be focused on relief of symptoms and comfort for those patients involved. Palliative care teams are best equipped to manage patients who wish to enroll into hospice or palliative care and their expertise should be enlisted early with involvement in the decision making process.[111]

REFERENCES

1. Writing Group Members, Mozaffarian D, Benjamin EJ, Go AS, et al. Executive summary: heart disease and stroke statistics–2016 update: a report from the American Heart Association. Circulation 2016;133(4):447–54.
2. Kochanek KD, Xu J, Murphy SL, et al. Deaths: final data for 2009. Natl Vital Stat Rep 2011;60(3):1–116.
3. Beta-Blocker Evaluation of Survival Trial Investigators, Eichhorn EJ, Domanski MJ, Krause-Steinrauf H, et al. A trial of the beta-blocker bucindolol in patients with advanced chronic heart failure. N Engl J Med 2001;344(22):1659–67.
4. Committees C-IIa. The cardiac insufficiency bisoprolol study II (CIBIS-II): a randomised trial. Lancet 1999;353(9146):9–13.
5. MERIT-HF Study Group. Effect of metoprolol CR/XL in chronic heart failure: metoprolol CR/XL randomised intervention trial in congestive heart failure (MERIT-HF). Lancet 1999;353(9169):2001–7.
6. Desai AS, McMurray JJ, Packer M, et al. Effect of the angiotensin-receptor-neprilysin inhibitor LCZ696 compared with enalapril on mode of death in heart failure patients. Eur Heart J 2015;36(30):1990–7.
7. CONSENSUS Trial Study Group. Effects of enalapril on mortality in severe congestive heart failure. Results of the Cooperative North Scandinavian Enalapril Survival Study (CONSENSUS). N Engl J Med 1987;316(23):1429–35.
8. SOLVD Investigators, Yusuf S, Pitt B, Davis CE, et al. Effect of enalapril on survival in patients with reduced left ventricular ejection fractions and congestive heart failure. N Engl J Med 1991;325(5):293–302.
9. Packer M, Bristow MR, Cohn JN, et al. The effect of carvedilol on morbidity and mortality in patients with chronic heart failure. U.S. Carvedilol Heart Failure Study Group. N Engl J Med 1996;334(21):1349–55.
10. Pfeffer MA, Braunwald E, Moye LA, et al. Effect of captopril on mortality and morbidity in patients with left ventricular dysfunction after myocardial infarction. Results of the survival and ventricular enlargement trial. The SAVE Investigators. N Engl J Med 1992;327(10):669–77.
11. Pitt B, Pfeffer MA, Assmann SF, et al. Spironolactone for heart failure with preserved ejection fraction. N Engl J Med 2014;370(15):1383–92.
12. Pitt B, Remme W, Zannad F, et al. Eplerenone, a selective aldosterone blocker, in patients with left ventricular dysfunction after myocardial infarction. N Engl J Med 2003;348(14):1309–21.
13. Taylor AL, Ziesche S, Yancy C, et al. Combination of isosorbide dinitrate and hydralazine in blacks with heart failure. N Engl J Med 2004;351(20):2049–57.
14. Waagstein F, Hjalmarson A, Varnauskas E, et al. Effect of chronic beta-adrenergic receptor blockade in congestive cardiomyopathy. Br Heart J 1975;37(10):1022–36.
15. Woodley SL, Gilbert EM, Anderson JL, et al. Beta-blockade with bucindolol in heart failure caused by ischemic versus idiopathic dilated cardiomyopathy. Circulation 1991;84(6):2426–41.
16. Writing Committee Members, Yancy CW, Jessup M, Bozkurt B, et al. 2013 ACCF/AHA guideline for the management of heart failure: a report of the American College of Cardiology Foundation/American Heart Association Task Force on practice guidelines. Circulation 2013;128(16):e240–327.
17. Moss AJ, Hall WJ, Cannom DS, et al. Improved survival with an implanted defibrillator in patients with

coronary disease at high risk for ventricular arrhythmia. Multicenter Automatic Defibrillator Implantation Trial Investigators. N Engl J Med 1996; 335(26):1933–40.

18. Moss AJ, Zareba W, Hall WJ, et al. Prophylactic implantation of a defibrillator in patients with myocardial infarction and reduced ejection fraction. N Engl J Med 2002;346(12):877–83.

19. Priori SG, Aliot E, Blomstrom-Lundqvist C, et al. Task Force on sudden cardiac death, European Society of Cardiology. Europace 2002;4(1):3–18.

20. Antiarrhythmics versus Implantable Defibrillators (AVID) Investigators. A comparison of antiarrhythmic-drug therapy with implantable defibrillators in patients resuscitated from near-fatal ventricular arrhythmias. N Engl J Med 1997; 337(22):1576–83.

21. Buxton AE, Lee KL, DiCarlo L, et al. Electrophysiologic testing to identify patients with coronary artery disease who are at risk for sudden death. Multicenter Unsustained Tachycardia Trial Investigators. N Engl J Med 2000;342(26):1937–45.

22. Kadish A, Dyer A, Daubert JP, et al. Prophylactic defibrillator implantation in patients with nonischemic dilated cardiomyopathy. N Engl J Med 2004; 350(21):2151–8.

23. Moss AJ, Hall WJ, Cannom DS, et al. Cardiac-resynchronization therapy for the prevention of heart-failure events. N Engl J Med 2009;361(14): 1329–38.

24. Ahmed A, Rich MW, Fleg JL, et al. Effects of digoxin on morbidity and mortality in diastolic heart failure: the ancillary digitalis investigation group trial. Circulation 2006;114(5):397–403.

25. Rickenbacher P, Pfisterer M, Burkard T, et al. Why and how do elderly patients with heart failure die? Insights from the TIME-CHF study. Eur J Heart Fail 2012;14(11):1218–29.

26. Solomon SD, Wang D, Finn P, et al. Effect of candesartan on cause-specific mortality in heart failure patients: the Candesartan in Heart failure Assessment of Reduction in Mortality and morbidity (CHARM) program. Circulation 2004;110(15): 2180–3.

27. Zile MR, Gaasch WH, Anand IS, et al. Mode of death in patients with heart failure and a preserved ejection fraction: results from the Irbesartan in heart failure with Preserved Ejection Fraction Study (I-Preserve) trial. Circulation 2010;121(12):1393–405.

28. Buxton AE, Calkins H, Callans DJ, et al. ACC/AHA/HRS 2006 key data elements and definitions for electrophysiological studies and procedures: a report of the American College of Cardiology/American Heart Association Task Force on Clinical Data Standards (ACC/AHA/HRS Writing Committee to Develop Data Standards on Electrophysiology). J Am Coll Cardiol 2006;48(11):2360–96.

29. Bardy GH, Lee KL, Mark DB, et al. Amiodarone or an implantable cardioverter-defibrillator for congestive heart failure. N Engl J Med 2005; 352(3):225–37.

30. European Heart Rhythm Association, Heart Rhythm Society, Zipes DP, Camm AJ, Borggrefe M, et al. ACC/AHA/ESC 2006 guidelines for management of patients with ventricular arrhythmias and the prevention of sudden cardiac death: a report of the American College of Cardiology/American Heart Association Task Force and the European Society of Cardiology Committee for Practice Guidelines (Writing Committee to Develop Guidelines for Management of Patients with ventricular arrhythmias and the prevention of sudden cardiac death). J Am Coll Cardiol 2006;48(5):e247–346.

31. Zannad F, McMurray JJ, Krum H, et al. Eplerenone in patients with systolic heart failure and mild symptoms. N Engl J Med 2011;364(1):11–21.

32. Kusumoto FM, Calkins H, Boehmer J, et al. HRS/ACC/AHA expert consensus statement on the use of implantable cardioverter-defibrillator therapy in patients who are not included or not well represented in clinical trials. Circulation 2014;130(1): 94–125.

33. Kaufman ES, Mackall JA, Julka B, et al. Influence of heart rate and sympathetic stimulation on arrhythmogenic T wave alternans. Am J Physiol Heart Circ Physiol 2000;279(3):H1248–55.

34. Narayan SM, Lindsay BD, Smith JM. Demonstration of the proarrhythmic preconditioning of single premature extrastimuli by use of the magnitude, phase, and distribution of repolarization alternans. Circulation 1999;100(18):1887–93.

35. Nearing BD, Huang AH, Verrier RL. Dynamic tracking of cardiac vulnerability by complex demodulation of the T wave. Science 1991; 252(5004):437–40.

36. Nearing BD, Oesterle SN, Verrier RL. Quantification of ischaemia induced vulnerability by precordial T wave alternans analysis in dog and human. Cardiovasc Res 1994;28(9):1440–9.

37. El-Sherif N, Turitto G, Pedalino RP, et al. T-wave alternans and arrhythmia risk stratification. Ann Noninvasive Electrocardiol 2001;6(4):323–32.

38. Konta T, Ikeda K, Yamaki M, et al. Significance of discordant ST alternans in ventricular fibrillation. Circulation 1990;82(6):2185–9.

39. Pastore JM, Girouard SD, Laurita KR, et al. Mechanism linking T-wave alternans to the genesis of cardiac fibrillation. Circulation 1999;99(10):1385–94.

40. Rosenbaum DS, Jackson LE, Smith JM, et al. Electrical alternans and vulnerability to ventricular arrhythmias. N Engl J Med 1994;330(4):235–41.

41. Smith JM, Clancy EA, Valeri CR, et al. Electrical alternans and cardiac electrical instability. Circulation 1988;77(1):110–21.

42. Surawicz B, Fisch C. Cardiac alternans: diverse mechanisms and clinical manifestations. J Am Coll Cardiol 1992;20(2):483–99.

43. Verrier RL, Nearing BD. Electrophysiologic basis for T wave alternans as an index of vulnerability to ventricular fibrillation. J Cardiovasc Electrophysiol 1994;5(5):445–61.

44. Verrier RL, Klingenheben T, Malik M, et al. Microvolt T-wave alternans physiological basis, methods of measurement, and clinical utility–consensus guideline by International Society for Holter and Noninvasive Electrocardiology. J Am Coll Cardiol 2011; 58(13):1309–24.

45. Leino J, Minkkinen M, Nieminen T, et al. Combined assessment of heart rate recovery and T-wave alternans during routine exercise testing improves prediction of total and cardiovascular mortality: the Finnish Cardiovascular Study. Heart Rhythm 2009;6(12):1765–71.

46. Leino J, Verrier RL, Minkkinen M, et al. Importance of regional specificity of T-wave alternans in assessing risk for cardiovascular mortality and sudden cardiac death during routine exercise testing. Heart Rhythm 2011;8(3):385–90.

47. Minkkinen M, Kahonen M, Viik J, et al. Enhanced predictive power of quantitative TWA during routine exercise testing in the Finnish Cardiovascular Study. J Cardiovasc Electrophysiol 2009;20(4): 408–15.

48. Nieminen T, Lehtimaki T, Viik J, et al. T-wave alternans predicts mortality in a population undergoing a clinically indicated exercise test. Eur Heart J 2007;28(19):2332–7.

49. Stein PK, Sanghavi D, Domitrovich PP, et al. Ambulatory ECG-based T-wave alternans predicts sudden cardiac death in high-risk post-MI patients with left ventricular dysfunction in the EPHESUS study. J Cardiovasc Electrophysiol 2008;19(10): 1037–42.

50. Stein PK, Sanghavi D, Sotoodehnia N, et al. Association of Holter-based measures including T-wave alternans with risk of sudden cardiac death in the community-dwelling elderly: the Cardiovascular Health Study. J Electrocardiol 2010;43(3):251–9.

51. Bloomfield DM, Steinman RC, Namerow PB, et al. Microvolt T-wave alternans distinguishes between patients likely and patients not likely to benefit from implanted cardiac defibrillator therapy: a solution to the Multicenter Automatic Defibrillator Implantation Trial (MADIT) II conundrum. Circulation 2004;110(14):1885–9.

52. Chow T, Kereiakes DJ, Onufer J, et al. Does microvolt T-wave alternans testing predict ventricular tachyarrhythmias in patients with ischemic cardiomyopathy and prophylactic defibrillators? The MASTER (Microvolt T Wave Alternans Testing for Risk Stratification of Post-Myocardial Infarction

Patients) trial. J Am Coll Cardiol 2008;52(20): 1607–15.

53. Gold MR, Ip JH, Costantini O, et al. Role of microvolt T-wave alternans in assessment of arrhythmia vulnerability among patients with heart failure and systolic dysfunction: primary results from the T-wave alternans sudden cardiac death in heart failure trial substudy. Circulation 2008; 118(20):2022–8.

54. Antzelevitch C. Role of spatial dispersion of repolarization in inherited and acquired sudden cardiac death syndromes. Am J Physiol Heart Circ Physiol 2007;293(4):H2024–38.

55. Haarmark C, Hansen PR, Vedel-Larsen E, et al. The prognostic value of the Tpeak-Tend interval in patients undergoing primary percutaneous coronary intervention for ST-segment elevation myocardial infarction. J Electrocardiol 2009;42(6):555–60.

56. Panikkath R, Reinier K, Uy-Evanado A, et al. Prolonged Tpeak-to-tend interval on the resting ECG is associated with increased risk of sudden cardiac death. Circ Arrhythm Electrophysiol 2011; 4(4):441–7.

57. Shimizu M, Ino H, Okeie K, et al. T-peak to T-end interval may be a better predictor of high-risk patients with hypertrophic cardiomyopathy associated with a cardiac troponin I mutation than QT dispersion. Clin Cardiol 2002;25(7):335–9.

58. Antzelevitch C, Sicouri S, Di Diego JM, et al. Does Tpeak-Tend provide an index of transmural dispersion of repolarization? Heart Rhythm 2007;4(8): 1114–6 [author reply: 6–9].

59. Kalantzi K, Gouva C, Letsas KP, et al. The impact of hemodialysis on the dispersion of ventricular repolarization. Pacing Clin Electrophysiol 2013;36(3): 322–7.

60. Akar FG, Yan GX, Antzelevitch C, et al. Unique topographical distribution of M cells underlies reentrant mechanism of torsade de pointes in the long-QT syndrome. Circulation 2002;105(10): 1247–53.

61. Barbhaiya C, Po JR, Hanon S, et al. Tpeak - Tend and Tpeak - Tend /QT ratio as markers of ventricular arrhythmia risk in cardiac resynchronization therapy patients. Pacing Clin Electrophysiol 2013; 36(1):103–8.

62. Rosenthal TM, Stahls PF 3rd, Abi Samra FM, et al. T-peak to T-end interval for prediction of ventricular tachyarrhythmia and mortality in a primary prevention population with systolic cardiomyopathy. Heart Rhythm 2015;12(8):1789–97.

63. Topilski I, Rogowski O, Rosso R, et al. The morphology of the QT interval predicts torsade de pointes during acquired bradyarrhythmias. J Am Coll Cardiol 2007;49(3):320–8.

64. Antzelevitch C, Yan GX, Shimizu W. Transmural dispersion of repolarization and arrhythmogenicity:

the Brugada syndrome versus the long QT syndrome. J Electrocardiol 1999;32(Suppl):158–65.

65. Porthan K, Viitasalo M, Toivonen L, et al. Predictive value of electrocardiographic T-wave morphology parameters and T-wave peak to T-wave end interval for sudden cardiac death in the general population. Circ Arrhythm Electrophysiol 2013;6(4):690–6.

66. Anastasiou-Nana MI, Nanas JN, Karagounis LA, et al. Relation of dispersion of QRS and QT in patients with advanced congestive heart failure to cardiac and sudden death mortality. Am J Cardiol 2000;85(10):1212–7.

67. Tse G, Yan BP. Traditional and novel electrocardiographic conduction and repolarization markers of sudden cardiac death. Europace 2017;19(5): 712–21.

68. Turrini P, Corrado D, Basso C, et al. Dispersion of ventricular depolarization-repolarization: a noninvasive marker for risk stratification in arrhythmogenic right ventricular cardiomyopathy. Circulation 2001;103(25):3075–80.

69. Dargie HJ. Effect of carvedilol on outcome after myocardial infarction in patients with left-ventricular dysfunction: the CAPRICORN randomised trial. Lancet 2001;357(9266):1385–90.

70. Packer M, Coats AJ, Fowler MB, et al. Effect of carvedilol on survival in severe chronic heart failure. N Engl J Med 2001;344(22):1651–8.

71. Packer M, Fowler MB, Roecker EB, et al. Effect of carvedilol on the morbidity of patients with severe chronic heart failure: results of the carvedilol prospective randomized cumulative survival (COPERNICUS) study. Circulation 2002;106(17):2194–9.

72. Pitt B, Zannad F, Remme WJ, et al. The effect of spironolactone on morbidity and mortality in patients with severe heart failure. Randomized Aldactone Evaluation Study Investigators. N Engl J Med 1999;341(10):709–17.

73. McMurray JJ, Packer M, Desai AS, et al. Angiotensin-neprilysin inhibition versus enalapril in heart failure. N Engl J Med 2014;371(11):993–1004.

74. Kober L, Thune JJ, Nielsen JC, et al. Defibrillator implantation in patients with nonischemic systolic heart failure. N Engl J Med 2016;375(13): 1221–30.

75. Bristow MR, Saxon LA, Boehmer J, et al. Cardiac-resynchronization therapy with or without an implantable defibrillator in advanced chronic heart failure. N Engl J Med 2004;350(21):2140–50.

76. Cleland JG, Daubert JC, Erdmann E, et al. The effect of cardiac resynchronization on morbidity and mortality in heart failure. N Engl J Med 2005; 352(15):1539–49.

77. Hohnloser SH, Kuck KH, Dorian P, et al. Prophylactic use of an implantable cardioverter-defibrillator after acute myocardial infarction. N Engl J Med 2004;351(24):2481–8.

78. Steinbeck G, Andresen D, Seidl K, et al. Defibrillator implantation early after myocardial infarction. N Engl J Med 2009;361(15):1427–36.

79. Chung MK, Szymkiewicz SJ, Shao M, et al. Aggregate national experience with the wearable cardioverter-defibrillator: event rates, compliance, and survival. J Am Coll Cardiol 2010;56(3):194–203.

80. Epstein AE, Abraham WT, Bianco NR, et al. Wearable cardioverter-defibrillator use in patients perceived to be at high risk early post-myocardial infarction. J Am Coll Cardiol 2013;62(21):2000–7.

81. Zishiri ET, Williams S, Cronin EM, et al. Early risk of mortality after coronary artery revascularization in patients with left ventricular dysfunction and potential role of the wearable cardioverter defibrillator. Circ Arrhythm Electrophysiol 2013;6(1): 117–28.

82. Connolly SJ, Dorian P, Roberts RS, et al. Comparison of beta-blockers, amiodarone plus beta-blockers, or sotalol for prevention of shocks from implantable cardioverter defibrillators: the OPTIC Study: a randomized trial. JAMA 2006;295(2): 165–71.

83. Moss AJ, Greenberg H, Case RB, et al. Long-term clinical course of patients after termination of ventricular tachyarrhythmia by an implanted defibrillator. Circulation 2004;110(25):3760–5.

84. Schron EB, Exner DV, Yao Q, et al. Quality of life in the antiarrhythmics versus implantable defibrillators trial: impact of therapy and influence of adverse symptoms and defibrillator shocks. Circulation 2002;105(5):589–94.

85. Dorian P, Borggrefe M, Al-Khalidi HR, et al. Placebo-controlled, randomized clinical trial of azimilide for prevention of ventricular tachyarrhythmias in patients with an implantable cardioverter defibrillator. Circulation 2004;110(24):3646–54.

86. Kowey PR, Crijns HJ, Aliot EM, et al. Efficacy and safety of celivarone, with amiodarone as calibrator, in patients with an implantable cardioverter-defibrillator for prevention of implantable cardioverter-defibrillator interventions or death: the ALPHEE study. Circulation 2011;124(24):2649–60.

87. Gao D, Van Herendael H, Alshengeiti L, et al. Mexiletine as an adjunctive therapy to amiodarone reduces the frequency of ventricular tachyarrhythmia events in patients with an implantable defibrillator. J Cardiovasc Pharmacol 2013;62(2):199–204.

88. Lee SD, Newman D, Ham M, et al. Electrophysiologic mechanisms of antiarrhythmic efficacy of a sotalol and class Ia drug combination: elimination of reverse use dependence. J Am Coll Cardiol 1997;29(1):100–5.

89. Pedersen CT, Kay GN, Kalman J, et al. EHRA/HRS/APHRS expert consensus on ventricular arrhythmias. Heart Rhythm 2014;11(10):e166–96.

90. Santangeli P, Muser D, Maeda S, et al. Comparative effectiveness of antiarrhythmic drugs and catheter ablation for the prevention of recurrent ventricular tachycardia in patients with implantable cardioverter-defibrillators: a systematic review and metaanalysis of randomized controlled trials. Heart Rhythm 2016;13(7):1552–9.

91. Bansch D, Oyang F, Antz M, et al. Successful catheter ablation of electrical storm after myocardial infarction. Circulation 2003;108(24):3011–6.

92. Brugada J, Berruezo A, Cuesta A, et al. Nonsurgical transthoracic epicardial radiofrequency ablation: an alternative in incessant ventricular tachycardia. J Am Coll Cardiol 2003;41(11):2036–43.

93. Stevenson WG, Soejima K. Catheter ablation for ventricular tachycardia. Circulation 2007;115(21):2750–60.

94. Kuck KH, Tilz RR, Deneke T, et al. Impact of substrate modification by catheter ablation on implantable cardioverter-defibrillator interventions in patients with unstable ventricular arrhythmias and coronary artery disease: results from the multicenter randomized controlled SMS (Substrate Modification Study). Circ Arrhythm Electrophysiol 2017;10(3) [pii:e004422].

95. Reddy VY, Reynolds MR, Neuzil P, et al. Prophylactic catheter ablation for the prevention of defibrillator therapy. N Engl J Med 2007;357(26):2657–65.

96. Sapp JL, Wells GA, Parkash R, et al. Ventricular tachycardia ablation versus escalation of antiarrhythmic drugs. N Engl J Med 2016;375(2):111–21.

97. Nazarian S, Bluemke DA, Lardo AC, et al. Magnetic resonance assessment of the substrate for inducible ventricular tachycardia in nonischemic cardiomyopathy. Circulation 2005;112(18):2821–5.

98. Soejima K, Stevenson WG, Sapp JL, et al. Endocardial and epicardial radiofrequency ablation of ventricular tachycardia associated with dilated cardiomyopathy: the importance of low-voltage scars. J Am Coll Cardiol 2004;43(10):1834–42.

99. Sosa E, Scanavacca M. Images in cardiovascular medicine. Percutaneous pericardial access for mapping and ablation of epicardial ventricular tachycardias. Circulation 2007;115(21):e542–4.

100. Borger van der Burg AE, de Groot NM, van Erven L, et al. Long-term follow-up after radiofrequency catheter ablation of ventricular tachycardia: a successful approach? J Cardiovasc Electrophysiol 2002;13(5):417–23.

101. Koplan BA, Soejima K, Baughman K, et al. Refractory ventricular tachycardia secondary to cardiac sarcoid: electrophysiologic characteristics, mapping, and ablation. Heart Rhythm 2006;3(8):924–9.

102. Marchlinski FE, Zado E, Dixit S, et al. Electroanatomic substrate and outcome of catheter ablative therapy for ventricular tachycardia in setting of right ventricular cardiomyopathy. Circulation 2004;110(16):2293–8.

103. Satomi K, Kurita T, Suyama K, et al. Catheter ablation of stable and unstable ventricular tachycardias in patients with arrhythmogenic right ventricular dysplasia. J Cardiovasc Electrophysiol 2006;17(5):469–76.

104. Verma A, Kilicaslan F, Schweikert RA, et al. Short- and long-term success of substrate-based mapping and ablation of ventricular tachycardia in arrhythmogenic right ventricular dysplasia. Circulation 2005;111(24):3209–16.

105. Dickfeld T, Tian J, Ahmad G, et al. MRI-Guided ventricular tachycardia ablation: integration of late gadolinium-enhanced 3D scar in patients with implantable cardioverter-defibrillators. Circ Arrhythm Electrophysiol 2011;4(2):172–84.

106. Estner HL, Zviman MM, Herzka D, et al. The critical isthmus sites of ischemic ventricular tachycardia are in zones of tissue heterogeneity, visualized by magnetic resonance imaging. Heart Rhythm 2011;8(12):1942–9.

107. Fahmy TS, Wazni OM, Jaber WA, et al. Integration of positron emission tomography/computed tomography with electroanatomical mapping: a novel approach for ablation of scar-related ventricular tachycardia. Heart Rhythm 2008;5(11):1538–45.

108. Fernandez-Armenta J, Berruezo A, Andreu D, et al. Three-dimensional architecture of scar and conducting channels based on high resolution ce-CMR: insights for ventricular tachycardia ablation. Circ Arrhythm Electrophysiol 2013;6(3):528–37.

109. Tao Q, Milles J, VAN Huls VAN Taxis C, et al. Toward magnetic resonance-guided electroanatomical voltage mapping for catheter ablation of scar-related ventricular tachycardia: a comparison of registration methods. J Cardiovasc Electrophysiol 2012;23(1):74–80.

110. Briceno DF, Romero J, Gianni C, et al. Substrate ablation of ventricular tachycardia: late potentials, scar dechanneling, local abnormal ventricular activities, core isolation, and homogenization. Card Electrophysiol Clin 2017;9(1):81–91.

111. Goodlin SJ. Palliative care in congestive heart failure. J Am Coll Cardiol 2009;54(5):386–96.

Sudden Cardiac Death in Acute Coronary Syndromes

Nikolaos Dagres, MD*, Gerhard Hindricks, MD

KEYWORDS

- Acute coronary syndrome • Sudden cardiac death • Ventricular fibrillation

KEY POINTS

- Sudden cardiac death due to ventricular tachyarrhythmias is a major threat in patients with acute coronary syndromes despite a decline in the incidence as a result of contemporary management.
- Acute treatment of life-threatening ventricular tachyarrhythmias consists of electrical defibrillation and coronary revascularization.
- Apart from beta-blockers and amiodarone, the role of other antiarrhythmic drugs is marginal. Catheter ablation may be very effective in selected patients.

INTRODUCTION

Sudden cardiac death is a major cause of mortality in acute coronary syndromes, mostly caused by complex ventricular arrhythmias, in particular, ventricular fibrillation (VF). This article focuses on sudden cardiac death and complex ventricular arrhythmias occurring in the acute phase of coronary syndromes and not in the long-term phase after such an episode. For the latter, abundant literature exists.[1-4]

SUDDEN CARDIAC ARREST AS INITIAL MANIFESTATION OF AN ACUTE CORONARY SYNDROME

Complex ventricular arrhythmias and VF are frequent in the setting of acute myocardial ischemia. In contrast to the chronic phase of coronary artery disease, in which monomorphic ventricular tachycardia (VT) occurs based on myocardial substrate, acute ischemia predominantly leads to VF and not monomorphic tachycardia. In a substantial number of cases, sudden cardiac arrest caused by VF may represent the initial manifestation of the acute coronary syndrome. Thus, in a recent study with a large number of subjects admitted to the hospital for ST-segment elevation myocardial infarction (STEMI), 7.0% had out-of-hospital cardiac arrest; that is, a sudden cardiac arrest as an initial manifestation of the acute ischemic episode.[5]

IN-HOSPITAL COMPLEX VENTRICULAR ARRHYTHMIAS

Following admission, the risk of VF and sudden cardiac death in patients with acute coronary syndromes is highest in the early phase. The incidence of in-hospital VF has been reported in numerous studies. As a result of advances in the management of patients with episodes of acute myocardial ischemia, the incidence of VF in this setting seems to be declining and is currently mostly reported in the range of 2% to 7%. Thus, in the Global Use of Strategies To Open coronary arteries (GUSTO) V trial, 4.4% of the subjects

Conflict of Interest Declaration: The authors have no conflict of interest in relation to this particular work. Research grants are provided to the institution (Heart Center Leipzig) from St. Jude Medical, Boston Scientific, and Biotronik; however, the authors report no personal fees.
Department of Electrophysiology, University Leipzig - Heart Center, Strümpellstr. 39, Leipzig 04289, Germany
* Corresponding author.
E-mail address: nikolaosdagres@yahoo.de

cardiacEP.theclinics.com

with STEMI developed early VT or VF (VT/VF) occurring within 48 hours after admission.[6] This rate was lower in the Acute Coronary Syndrome Israeli Survey in a large population including both subjects with STEMI and subjects with non-STEMI (NSTEMI). Ventricular tachyarrhythmias occurred in 3.8% of subjects with 2.1% occurring within the first 48 hours and 1.7% after the first 48 hours.[7] Similarly, more recent investigations, such as the Early Glycoprotein IIb/IIIa Inhibition in Non-ST Segment Elevation Acute Coronary Syndrome (EARLY ACS) reported a considerably lower rate of VT/VF of 1.5% in subjects with NSTEMI with a similar distribution between the early and late phase (before and after the first 48 hours).[8] In contrast, a considerably higher incidence of VT/VF was reported in other populations with NSTEMI. In a report of NSTEMI subjects undergoing cardiac catheterization within 48 hours, the rate of VT/VF was 7.6% with 60% of the life-threatening ventricular tachyarrhythmic episodes occurring in the first 48 hours after admission.[9]

PROGNOSTIC SIGNIFICANCE OF IN-HOSPITAL COMPLEX VENTRICULAR ARRHYTHMIAS

Thus, VF/VT is still relatively common in the setting of an acute episode of myocardial ischemia (particularly in the first 48 hours), and represents a major threat to the patient's life. Obviously, a successful acute management of these arrhythmic episodes is mandatory, but the short-term and long-term prognostic significance is still debated.

For episodes occurring after the early phase, which is mostly defined as the first 48 hours after the beginning of symptoms, there is general agreement that they are associated with impaired prognosis.[7] This is different for episodes occurring in the early phase of an acute ischemic episode; that is, within the first 48 hours. Although some investigators have reported a considerably worse prognosis of subjects with acute coronary syndromes suffering episodes of VF in the early phase of the syndrome, others did not confirm this association. Thus, in a large series of patients with STEMI and NSTEMI, VTs in both the early (within 48 hours) and in the late (later than 48 hours) phase were significantly associated with in-hospital death; however, only episodes in the late phase were associated with increased 30-day mortality.[7] In an older study of subjects with acute myocardial infarction, in-hospital mortality during the initial hospitalization was higher for subjects in whom VT/VF occurred (27% vs 7%, P<.001); however, long-term mortality of hospital survivors showed no difference.[10] Similarly, in a more recent series of STEMI subjects, a large cohort of subjects

with VF episodes in the first 48 hours had a higher in-hospital mortality. The long-term prognosis of those discharged was similar in subjects who did not experience VF during the acute episode.[11] Recently, in a large series of STEMI subjects treated predominantly by fibrinolysis, VF occurring before admission to the intensive care unit was an independent predictor of in-hospital mortality. This was not the case for subjects treated with primary angioplasty.[12] In contrast, in the GUSTO V study, VT/VF occurring in the first 48 hours of myocardial infarction was associated with a significant and marked increase of 30-day mortality (22% vs 5%, P<.001).[6]

Overall, the occurrence of VT/VF within the first 48 hours is associated with a significantly increased in-hospital mortality. Doubt remains whether the increased risk also applies to long-term mortality, provided, of course, that the tachyarrhythmia episode is successfully acutely treated. Conversely, VT/VF occurring in the late phase of the syndrome; that is, 48 hours from the start of the ischemic episode, is associated with an impairment of both short-term and long-term prognosis.

ACUTE TREATMENT OF VENTRICULAR TACHYARRHYTHMIAS IN THE SETTING OF ACUTE CORONARY SYNDROMES

VF/VT occurring in the setting of an acute coronary syndrome must be immediately terminated in the same way as episodes occurring outside of this setting.[13] Electrical defibrillation is obviously the cornerstone of management and should be performed without any delay. Rapid detection of the episode is of major importance and, in this particular setting, has been greatly facilitated by the introduction of coronary care units in which subjects are continuously monitored. Indeed, coronary care units have revolutionized the management of patients with acute coronary syndromes and have significantly contributed to the considerable reduction of mortality observed in the last decade.[14]

In contrast, the role of antiarrhythmic drugs is much less clear. Beta-blockers are an established treatment in acute coronary syndromes and have a beneficial effect for relief of ischemia. Recent evidence suggests that early application of beta-blockers may also reduce the incidence of in-hospital ventricular tachyarrhythmic episodes in patients with acute coronary syndromes.[15] This was confirmed by Global Registry of Acute Coronary Events (GRACE), in which oral beta-blockers were associated with a decrease in the risk of ventricular arrhythmias.[16] However, early administration of beta-blockers was associated with an increase in hospital mortality in this particular registry.[16] Results from other registries, such as the VALsartan In Acute myocardial iNfarcTion trial (VALIANT) registry, also confirmed the value of beta-blockers in this setting, with early beta blocker use leading to a decrease of early mortality.[17] For these reasons, the current guidelines of the European Society of Cardiology (ESC) recommend prophylactic treatment with beta-blockers.[2]

The role of conventional antiarrhythmic drugs in this setting is much more controversial. Apart from beta-blockers, amiodarone is, in principle, the only antiarrhythmic drug with an acceptable risk profile in these patients and has been indeed used for many years in patients with acute myocardial ischemia for suppression of ventricular arrhythmias.[18] However, it is well known that amiodarone has a variety of significant adverse effects that significantly limits its use.[19] More importantly, a beneficial effect of the drug in this setting is questionable. An analysis in subjects with STEMI and sustained VT/VF in Global Use of Strategies to Open Occluded Coronary Arteries in Acute Coronary Syndromes (GUSTO) IIB and GUSTO III showed that amiodarone use was associated with an increased risk of death.[20]

Lidocaine has traditionally been used for many years in STEMI patients for suppression of ventricular arrhythmias. However, adverse effects of lidocaine and a potential increase in mortality have been reported.[21] Later trials confirmed that lidocaine may suppress VF in the setting of acute myocardial infarction but may also adversely affect mortality rates.[22] A recent Cochrane review reported that prophylactic lidocaine had very little or no effect on mortality or VF in patients with acute myocardial infarction, and the safety profile was found to be unclear.[23] For these reasons, prophylactic administration of lidocaine is not recommended.

Use of other class I antiarrhythmic drugs, such as propafenone in acute coronary syndromes, has been previously reported[24] but was abandoned after the Cardiac Arrhythmia Suppression Trial, which reported a significantly increased mortality in postmyocardial infarction subjects receiving encainide or flecainide.[25]

Considering this, the current ESC guidelines discourage prophylactic treatment with antiarrhythmic drugs other than beta-blockers in patients with acute coronary syndromes and recommend the use of beta-blockers and intravenous amiodarone for recurrent polymorphic VT.[2] Lidocaine may be considered in patients with recurrent sustained VT/VF not responsive to beta-blockers and amiodarone.[2]

OTHER MEASURES FOR MANAGEMENT OF VENTRICULAR TACHYARRHYTHMIAS IN PATIENTS WITH ACUTE CORONARY SYNDROMES

Coronary revascularization is currently the cornerstone of treatment of patients with acute coronary syndromes. Immediate coronary revascularization is also an effective means for suppression of malignant ventricular arrhythmias and should be performed whenever possible and as completely as possible if recurrent episodes of VF/VT occur.[2,26]

Other general measures, such as correction of electrolyte abnormalities, may also be beneficial. Deep sedation may reduce the arrhythmic burden by reducing sympathetic activity. Although no sufficient data to support deep sedation in this setting exist, it is applied with success in selected cases in clinical routine.

CATHETER ABLATION IN THE ACUTE SETTING

Catheter ablation has emerged as an important treatment modality for patients with VT.[27] It is mostly preserved for high-risk patients due to the complexity of the procedure.[28] VF in the setting of acute myocardial ischemia may be triggered by premature ventricular contractions arising from injured Purkinje fibers. In these patients, catheter ablation can be performed in the acute setting with good success and can be life-saving for the patient (**Fig. 1**).[29,30] Because these are, in most cases, severely compromised patients, the procedure has a considerable risk and should be performed in high-volume centers by operators with great experience in VT ablation who are able to manage acute complications.

IMPLANTABLE CARDIOVERTER-DEFIBRILLATOR

Despite the increased risk of sudden cardiac death in the early phase after an acute myocardial infarction, the implantation of a cardioverter-defibrillator in the first 40 days after myocardial infarction did not show any benefit in 2 randomized trials. The Defibrillator in Acute Myocardial Infarction Trial compared defibrillator therapy versus no defibrillator therapy in subjects 6 to 40 days after myocardial infarctions.[31] The Immediate Risk Stratification Improves Survival (IRIS) trial enrolled subjects 5 to 31 days after myocardial infarction.[32] In both trials, arrhythmic mortality was reduced but there was no significant effect on all-cause death that was obviously due to competing risks of death. Therefore, defibrillator implantation in the first 40 days after myocardial infarction is not recommended. Nevertheless, defibrillator implantation

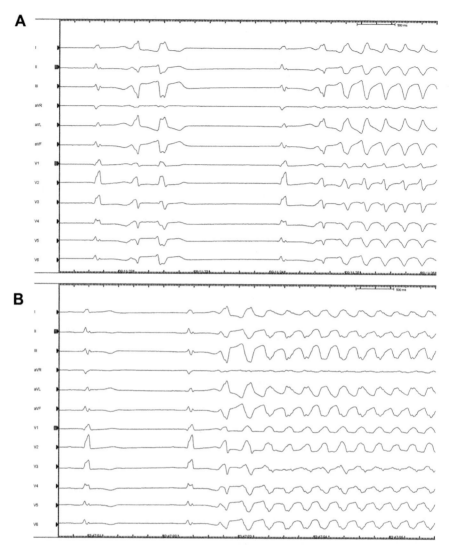

Fig. 1. (*A, B*) Monomorphic ventricular premature contractions triggering multiple episodes of ventricular tachycardia and ventricular fibrillation in a 73-year-old patient with acute coronary syndrome and coronary 3-vessel disease. The patient was successfully treated with catheter ablation of the premature ventricular contractions and the electrical storm was terminated.

may be indicated in selected subjects such as those with pre-existing left ventricular dysfunction, incomplete revascularization, and occurrence of VT/VF after the first 48 hours of the event.[2]

SUMMARY

In conclusion, the incidence of life-threatening episodes of ventricular arrhythmias in the setting of acute coronary syndromes has fallen as a result of contemporary patient management but still poses a threat for a considerable number of patients. Treatment consists of immediate termination by electrical cardioversion and coronary revascularization for relief of ischemia. Beta-blockers have

a protective effect and should be administered prophylactically. For recurrent episodes of VT/VF, pharmacologic treatment consists of beta-blockers and amiodarone or, in nonresponsive patients, lidocaine. Other antiarrhythmic drugs do not play a role due to their adverse effects. Catheter ablation can be very effective in patients with recurrent episodes of VT/VF triggered by premature ventricular contractions; however, it should be performed in qualified centers.

REFERENCES

1. Dagres N, Hindricks G. Risk stratification after myocardial infarction: is left ventricular ejection

fraction enough to prevent sudden cardiac death? Eur Heart J 2013;34(26):1964–71.

2. Priori SG, Blomström-Lundqvist C, Mazzanti A, et al. 2015 ESC guidelines for the management of patients with ventricular arrhythmias and the prevention of sudden cardiac death. Europace 2015; 17(11):euv319.

3. Amara N, Boveda S, Defaye P, et al. Implantable cardioverter-defibrillator therapy among patients with non-ischaemic vs. ischaemic cardiomyopathy for primary prevention of sudden cardiac death. Europace 2017 [pii:euw379].

4. van der Heijden AC, van Rees JB, Levy WC, et al. Application and comparison of the FADES, MADIT, and SHFM-D risk models for risk stratification of prophylactic implantable cardioverter-defibrillator treatment. Europace 2017;19(1):72–80.

5. Demirel F, Rasoul S, Elvan A, et al. Impact of out-of-hospital cardiac arrest due to ventricular fibrillation in patients with ST-elevation myocardial infarction admitted for primary percutaneous coronary intervention: impact of ventricular fibrillation in STEMI patients. Eur Heart J Acute Cardiovasc Care 2015;4(1): 16–23.

6. Askari AT, Shishehbor MH, Kaminski MA, et al. The association between early ventricular arrhythmias, renin-angiotensin-aldosterone system antagonism, and mortality in patients with ST-segment-elevation myocardial infarction: Insights from Global Use of Strategies to Open coronary arteries (GUSTO) V. Am Heart J 2009;158(2):238–43.

7. Orvin K, Eisen A, Goldenberg I, et al. Outcome of contemporary acute coronary syndrome complicated by ventricular tachyarrhythmias. Europace 2016;18(2):219–26.

8. Piccini JP, White JA, Mehta RH, et al. Sustained ventricular tachycardia and ventricular fibrillation complicating non-ST-segment-elevation acute coronary syndromes. Circulation 2012;126(1):41–9.

9. Gupta S, Pressman GS, Figueredo VM. Incidence of, predictors for, and mortality associated with malignant ventricular arrhythmias in non-ST elevation myocardial infarction patients. Coron Artery Dis 2010;21(8):460–5.

10. Tofler GH, Stone PH, Muller JE, et al. Prognosis after cardiac arrest due to ventricular tachycardia or ventricular fibrillation associated with acute myocardial infarction (the MILIS Study). Multicenter Investigation of the Limitation of Infarct Size. Am J Cardiol 1987;60(10):755–61.

11. Demidova MM, Smith JG, Höijer C-J, et al. Prognostic impact of early ventricular fibrillation in patients with ST-elevation myocardial infarction treated with primary PCI. Eur Heart J Acute Cardiovasc Care 2012;1(4):302–11.

12. Medina-Rodríguez KE, Almendro-Delia M, García-Alcántara Á, et al. Prognostic implication of early ventricular fibrillation among patients with ST elevation myocardial infarction. Coron Artery Dis 2017. [Epub ahead of print].

13. Monsieurs KG, Nolan JP, Bossaert LL, et al. European resuscitation council guidelines for resuscitation 2015: section 1. Executive summary. Resuscitation 2015;95:1–80.

14. Karlson BW, Herlitz J, Wiklund O, et al. Characteristics and prognosis of patients with acute myocardial infarction in relation to whether they were treated in the coronary care unit or in another ward. Cardiology 1992;81(2–3):134–44.

15. Maclean E, Zheng S, Nabeebaccus A, et al. Effect of early bisoprolol administration on ventricular arrhythmia and cardiac death in patients with non-ST elevation myocardial infarction. Heart Asia 2015;7(2):46–51.

16. Park KL, Goldberg RJ, Anderson FA, et al. Beta-blocker use in ST-segment elevation myocardial infarction in the reperfusion era (GRACE). Am J Med 2014;127(6):503–11.

17. Piccini JP, Hranitzky PM, Kilaru R, et al. Relation of mortality to failure to prescribe beta blockers acutely in patients with sustained ventricular tachycardia and ventricular fibrillation following acute myocardial infarction (from the VALsartan in Acute myocardial iNfarcTion trial [VALIANT] registry). Am J Cardiol 2008;102(11):1427–32.

18. Hockings BE, George T, Mahrous F, et al. Effectiveness of amiodarone on ventricular arrhythmias during and after acute myocardial infarction. Am J Cardiol 1987;60(13):967–70.

19. Doyle JF, Ho KM. Benefits and risks of long-term amiodarone therapy for persistent atrial fibrillation: a meta-analysis. Mayo Clin Proc 2009;84(3):234–42.

20. Piccini JP, Schulte PJ, Pieper KS, et al. Antiarrhythmic drug therapy for sustained ventricular arrhythmias complicating acute myocardial infarction. Crit Care Med 2011;39(1):78–83.

21. Dunn HM, McComb JM, Kinney CD, et al. Prophylactic lidocaine in the early phase of suspected myocardial infarction. Am Heart J 1985;110(2): 353–62.

22. Sadowski ZP, Alexander JH, Skrabucha B, et al. Multicenter randomized trial and a systematic overview of lidocaine in acute myocardial infarction. Am Heart J 1999;137(5):792–8.

23. Martí-Carvajal AJ, Simancas-Racines D, Anand V, et al. Prophylactic lidocaine for myocardial infarction. Cochrane Database Syst Rev 2015;(8): CD008553.

24. Rehnqvist N, Ericsson CG, Eriksson S, et al. Comparative investigation of the antiarrhythmic effect of propafenone (Rytmonorm) and lidocaine in patients with ventricular arrhythmias during acute myocardial infarction. Acta Med Scand 1984; 216(5):525–30.

25. Echt DS, Liebson PR, Mitchell LB, et al. Mortality and morbidity in patients receiving encainide, flecainide, or placebo. N Engl J Med 1991;324(12):781–8.

26. Roffi M, Patrono C, Collet J-P, et al. 2015 ESC guidelines for the management of acute coronary syndromes in patients presenting without persistent ST-segment elevation. Eur Heart J 2016;37(3):267–315.

27. Briceño DF, Romero J, Villablanca PA, et al. Long-term outcomes of different ablation strategies for ventricular tachycardia in patients with structural heart disease: systematic review and meta-analysis. Europace 2017. [Epub ahead of print].

28. Chen J, Todd DM, Proclemer A, et al. Management of patients with ventricular tachycardia in Europe: results of the European Heart Rhythm Association Survey. Europace 2015;17(8):1294–9.

29. Enjoji Y, Mizobuchi M, Muranishi H, et al. Catheter ablation of fatal ventricular tachyarrhythmias storm in acute coronary syndrome—role of Purkinje fiber network. J Interv Card Electrophysiol 2009;26(3):207–15.

30. Bode K, Hindricks G, Piorkowski C, et al. Ablation of polymorphic ventricular tachycardias in patients with structural heart disease. Pacing Clin Electrophysiol 2008;31(12):1585–91.

31. Hohnloser SH, Kuck KH, Dorian P, et al. Prophylactic use of an implantable cardioverter–defibrillator after acute myocardial infarction. N Engl J Med 2004;351(24):2481–8.

32. Steinbeck G, Andresen D, Seidl K, et al. Defibrillator implantation early after myocardial infarction. N Engl J Med 2009;361(15):1427–36.

Neuromuscular Disease
Cardiac Manifestations and Sudden Death Risk

Worawan Limipitikul, BS[a], Chin Siang Ong, MBBS[b],
Gordon F. Tomaselli, MD[c],*

KEYWORDS

- Muscular dystrophy • Arrhythmia • Conduction block • Sudden death • Pacemaker
- Implantable cardioverter-defibrillator (ICD)

KEY POINTS

- Neuromuscular diseases, including the most common muscular dystrophies, affect the heart.
- Conduction system disease is common when the heart is involved.
- Pacemakers and defibrillators can be life-saving in selected patients.

INTRODUCTION AND GENERAL PRINCIPLES

Neurologic diseases often affect the heart and vascular system, and in many cases cardiovascular disease limits life expectancy in these patients. Many neuromuscular diseases (NMD) have been associated with myocardial impairment, significant arrhythmia, and sudden cardiac death (SCD). This review focuses on the muscular dystrophies exhibiting prominent cardiac manifestations, including myotonic dystrophy, Duchenne (DMD), Becker (BMD), Emery-Dreifuss (EDMD), and limb-girdle (LGMD) muscular dystrophies. In each disease, recognition and treatment of cardiac involvement can prolong and improve the quality of life.

Muscular dystrophies are a group of complex multisystem disorders that commonly and prominently affect striated muscle. Several NMDs significantly impact function of the heart and in some cases cardiac disease is the cause of mortality. The spectrum of cardiovascular manifestations of NMDs range from asymptomatic incidental findings to life-threatening arrhythmias. NMDs often produce conduction system disorders[1] with resulting bradyarrhythmias and tachyarrhythmias, cardiac dilation, hypertrophy, hypertrabeculation, and cardiomyopathy (**Table 1**).

The cardiovascular presentation and management of patients with an NMD is dependent on the specific type of disease. To optimize the care of these patients, a team of practitioners is required, often with the neurologist or internist taking the lead. The treatment of patients with NMDs is likely to require input from neurologists, pulmonary specialists, gastroenterologists, cardiologists, endocrinologists, orthopedists, and general surgeons.[2] The treatment of cardiac manifestations occurs in the context of other potentially life-limiting comorbidities. Often the main concern is the risk of a serious cardiac arrhythmia.[3]

MUSCULAR DYSTROPHIES, CARDIAC ARRHYTHMIAS, AND SUDDEN CARDIAC DEATH

The NMDs may be classified on the basis of their clinical features, molecular genetics, or pathophysiological consequences. In this group of

The authors have no relevant disclosures relevant to this work.
[a] Department of Biomedical Engineering, Johns Hopkins University, Baltimore, MD, USA; [b] Department of Medicine, Division of Cardiology, Johns Hopkins University School of Medicine, Baltimore, MD, USA; [c] Department of Medicine, Division of Cardiology, Johns Hopkins University School of Medicine, Johns Hopkins University, Baltimore, MD 21205, USA
* Corresponding author.
E-mail address: gtomasel@jhmi.edu

Table 1
Cardiovascular complications of muscular dystrophies

Disease	DCM	Conduction Abnormality	Ventricular Arrhythmia	Atrial Arrhythmia
DM1	Rare	+++	+	++
DM2	Rare	+	+	+
DMD	++	+	+	+
BMD	++	+	+	+
FSHMD (AD)	Rare	Rare	Rare	Rare
EDMD	++	+++	Rare	Rare
KSS	+	+++	Rare	+

Abbreviations: AD, autosomal dominant; BMD, Becker muscular dystrophy; DCM, dilated cardiomyopathy; DMD, Duchenne muscular dystrophy; EDMD, Emery-Dreifuss muscular dystrophy; FSHMD, facioscapulohumeral muscular dystrophy; KSS, Kearns-Sayre Syndrome.

disorders are nucleotide repeat diseases (myotonic dystrophies, Friedrich ataxia), laminopathies, desminopathies, dystrophinopathies, sarcoglycanopathies, and mitochondrial disorders. The latter includes mitochondrial encephalomyopathy lactic acidosis and strokelike episodes, myoclonic epilepsy with ragged-red fibers, Kearns-Sayre syndrome, beta oxidation defects, primary carnitine deficiency, carnitine-palmitoyl-transferase deficiency, medium chain acyl CoA deficiency, and Barth syndrome.

Mutations in cytoskeletal proteins that link to the extracellular matrix with the structural muscle proteins are associated with skeletal and cardiac myopathies. For example, the dystrophin-glycoprotein membrane complex is composed of laminin-2, dystroglycans, sarcoglycans, syntrophins, and dystrophins. Mutations in dystrophin cause DMD and BMD, sarcoglycan mutations have been associated with LGMD, and mutations in lamins have been demonstrated in EDMD, LGMD, and dilated cardiomyopathy (DCM) **(Table 2)**.

Myotonic Dystrophy

Myotonic dystrophy is the most common neuromuscular disorder presenting in adulthood and often affects the heart. These are multisystem disorders with protean manifestations, but 2 prominent features: myotonia and muscular dystrophy. The cardiac manifestations include conduction system disorders, atrial fibrillation (AF), and cardiomyopathy.[1,4,5]

Genetics and molecular pathogenesis
There are 2 major genetic types of myotonic dystrophy that are transmitted in autosomal dominant fashion. Dystrophia myotonia type 1 (DM1, Steiner disease, Online Mendelian Inheritance in Man [OMIM]#160900) is due to a triplet nucleotide

(CTG) expansion in the 3' untranslated region *DMPK* and immediately upstream to the promoter region of the transcription factor SIX5 on chromosome 19. DM type 2 (DM2, proximal myotonic myopathy) is due to a tetranucleotide repeat (CCTG, OMIM #602668) in intron 1 of ZNF9 (CNBP) on chromosome 3.[6]

Genetic anticipation, which is an increase in the number of repeats in subsequent generations, was first described in DM1.[7] Short tandem repeats are found in healthy individuals (up to 37 in the DM1 locus in healthy individuals); however, when the expansion size gets too long, it becomes unstable and prone to further expansion because of wobble in the DNA replication machinery. The increase in expansion size leads to earlier onset and increased severity of disease in subsequent generations. In addition to vertical (through generations) instability in the nucleotide repeat expansion size, there is somatic instability with different tissues exhibiting differences in repeat expansion. Studies have shown that skeletal muscle and neurons harbor more repeats than white blood cells (WBCs).[8] Somatic instability has a prominent role in disease severity and age of onset of symptoms in DM1. This instability is a heritable trait suggesting a role for transcriptional disease modifiers that may be therapeutic targets.[9] There is a maternal transmission bias, particularly in congenital forms of DM1, disproportionately affected infants are born to mothers with disease or repeat expansions in the premutation (38–50 CTG) range. The mechanism of the gender bias is unknown; speculation includes unstable repeat expansion during oogenesis or failure of sperm with large repeat expansions to survive.

There is a general association between disease onset and severity with repeat expansion size; however, it is not an exact correlation and it is

Table 2
Muscular dystrophies

Type (#OMIM)	Inheritance	Chromosome	Abnormality	Incidence	Onset	Prognosis
Duchenne #310200	X-linked	Xp21.2	Absent dystrophin	1/3000–5000	2nd–3rd y	Rapidly progressive
Becker #300376	X-linked	Xp21.2	Abnormal dystrophin	1/30,000	1st–4th decade	Ambulatory into teens
EDMD1 #310300	X-linked	Xp28	Emerin	1/100,000	Childhood	Ambulatory 3rd decade, SCD
EDMD2 #181350	AD	1q21.2	Lamin A/C			
EDMD3 #604929	AR	1q21.2	Lamin A/C			
FSHMD	AD	4q35	Homeobox gene	1/20,000	Childhood –young adult	Normal life expectancy
LGMD	AR, AD	Multiple	Sarcoglycans, calpain, cav-3, lamin A/C	1/25,000	Childhood –adulthood	Variable
DM1 #160900	AD	19q13.3	DMPK (CTG in 3'UTR)	1/7500	Variable, anticipation	Middle age, premature death
DM2/PROMM #602668	AD	3q13.3	ZNF-9 (CCTG intron-1)	1/200,000	3rd–4th decade	Near normal life expectancy

Abbreviations: AD, autosomal dominant; AR, autosomal recessive; EDMD, Emery-Dreifuss muscular dystrophy; FSHMD, facioscapulohumeral muscular dystrophy; LGMD, limb-girdle muscular dystrophy; OMIM, Online Mendelian Inheritance in Man; PROMM, proximal myotonic myopathy; UTR, untranslated region.

very difficult to predict disease severity when the repeat size is large (>100 CTG) and expansions are particularly unstable.[10] It is important to note that genetic testing typically measures expansion size in WBCs and somatic mosaicism may limit the ability of testing to predict the severity of specific features of DM1. DM1 and DM2 share clinical features but differ dramatically in the number of nucleotide repeats. In DM2, the number of repeats can be in the 11,000 range (average ~5000) despite a milder clinical phenotype and there are no reports of a congenital onset. In DM2, phenotypic features have been reported to cosegregate with mutations in *CLCN1*, *SCN4A*.[11,12]

The molecular pathogenesis and understanding of the multisystem nature of myotonic dystrophy have been clarified over the past 15 years. The consensus is that a toxic gain of function driven by aberrant RNA accounts for the pathogenesis of DM1 and DM2. Pre-mRNA is transcribed from DNA containing the nucleotide repeats, which forms hairpin loops, aggregates in the nucleus, and sequesters several proteins important in RNA processing and translation accounting for the multisystem manifestations of myotonic dystrophies. In particular, splicing defects in RNA transcripts, such as those encoding the insulin receptor, cardiac troponin T, voltage-dependent Na ($Na_V1.5$)[13] and Ca channels ($Ca_V1.1$),[14] ryanodine receptor, and sarcoplasmic reticulum Ca^{2+} ATPases may contribute to the cardiac phenotype.[15,16]

Epidemiology and clinical features

The combined prevalence of types 1 and 2 myotonic dystrophy is estimated to be 1 in 8000. There is a wide variability in prevalence in different populations. There is higher prevalence of DM1 in Northern Europe, Quebec, and the Basque region of Spain; it is less common in Japan; is rare in India and the Middle East; and is exceedingly rare in Africa. DM2 is most common in people of Northern European extraction.

The onset and clinical classification of DM1 is varied from antenatal onset to diagnosis of minimally symptomatic parents of affected children. The congenital form (>1000 CTG repeats) is the most severe type of DM1 with an incompletely understood maternal transmission. Congenital DM1 presents at birth with hypotonia and cardiopulmonary failure. For children who survive, mental retardation is typical. Childhood-onset DM1 (usually >100 CTG repeats) is characterized by mild cognitive impairment, muscular weakness, and cardiac conduction system abnormalities. Typical adult-onset disease is a multisystem disorder with a spectrum of neuromuscular symptoms, including myotonia, weakness, and fatigue. Characteristically, the eyes, heart, endocrine system, and integument may be affected. Repeat expansion size may vary from 50 to 1000 CTGs. Late adult onset is commonly diagnosed in parents of affected children and muscular symptoms, often atrophy, is mild. In general, DM1 is associated with more disability due to muscle disease than DM2, and patients with DM1 have a shortened life expectancy. DM2 does not exhibit clinical subclasses.

Weakness and myotonia are common presenting neuromuscular features. In myotonic dystrophy, flexor muscles are affected more than extensors, distinguishing this from facioscapulohumeral muscular dystrophy. Central/midline musculature is prominently involved, resulting in ptosis, open mouth, and neck flexion, producing the classic "hatchet" facies. The flexors of forearm, thumb and fingers, hip and shoulder girdle also are frequently affected in myotonic dystrophy. Myotonia is almost always present in DM1 but not as severe as myotonia congenita. Myotonia in DM1 may exhibit warm up; however, cold-induced contractures like those seen in paramyotonias are absent. Myotonia is more variable in DM2 and may not be observed clinically, but electrical myotonia is invariably present in both DM1 and DM2. Weakness in DM1 is usually significantly greater than in DM2; deep tendon reflexes are reduced or absent in DM1 but are normal or brisk in DM2 (**Table 3**). Alveolar hypoventilation secondary to weakness of respiratory muscles and aspiration associated with dysphagia may lead to chronic pulmonary disease and right heart impairment in DM1; there is relative sparing of respiratory function in DM2. Smooth muscle also may be affected, and gastrointestinal dysfunction is frequent and occasionally disabling in patients with DM1. Patients exhibit dysphagia, diarrhea, constipation, and incontinence. Reduction in gastrointestinal motility can lead to obstruction and megacolon.

Central nervous system features may accompany more severe forms of myotonic dystrophy. DM1 has been associated with behavioral and personality disorders, mental retardation, and dementia. More subtle disturbances of executive function may occur in DM1 and DM2.

Daytime somnolence and fatigue are prominent in DM1, along with several sleep disorders, such as central and obstructive apnea, hypnogogic hallucination, muscle pain with awakening, and excessive sleep duration. In DM2, sleep hygiene is often impaired by frequent awakening due to muscle pain, but daytime somnolence is less

Table 3
Clinical characteristics of myotonic dystrophies

Feature	DM1	DM2
Myotonia	+++	++
Cataracts	+	+
Muscle weakness	++ distal	++ proximal
Muscle pain	−	++
Deep tendon reflexes	Reduced or absent	Normal or increased
Arrhythmia	++	+
Muscle enzymes	Increased	Increased
Cognitive function	Impaired	± impaired
Inheritance	Autosomal dominant	Autosomal dominant
Chromosome	19q13.3	3q21.3
Genetic abnormality	$(CTG)_n$	$(CCTG)_n$
Congenital form	Present	Absent

Abbreviations: DM1, Dystrophia myotonia type 1; DM2, DM type 2; +, relative severity; −, not present.

pronounced. The deficits in sleep hygiene may contribute to the frequency of arrhythmias, such as atrial fibrillation (AF) in myotonic dystrophy. Neurons in the limbic system and brain stem of patients with DM1 and DM2 have been shown to contain tau-associated neurofibrillary tangles, suggesting a neuropathological process that may link several features of DM, such as somnolence and apathy.[17]

Patients with myotonic dystrophy exhibit a wide array of extramuscular signs and symptoms. A consistent ophthalmologic feature is early onset, posterior subcapsular cataracts whose appearance inspired the description "Christmas tree" cataracts. Hyperinsulinemia, hyperglycemia, and insulin resistance are common in DM1 and variably observed in DM2, with diabetes occurring in both disorders. Other endocrinological manifestations include disorders of the thyroid that are rare but can exacerbate myopathy, testicular failure, and adrenocortical dysregulation in DM1. Male pattern balding, seborrheic dermatitis, and epitheliomas have been observed in DM1 and variably in DM2, and hyperhidrosis of hands and trunk has been described in DM2.[18]

Clinical laboratory abnormalities are common in DM1 and DM2. In addition to endocrinological findings of reduced sex hormone levels and abnormal thyroid function studies, low blood urea nitrogen, creatinine, serum albumin, and calcium have been described. Abnormal liver function tests and an increase in skeletal muscle enzymes, but not to the levels seen in DMD or BMD, are characteristic of myotonic dystrophy. Hyperlipidemia and hypercholesterolemia, particularly in the setting of glucose intolerance or diabetes,

may be associated with the development of atherosclerotic cardiovascular disease. Patients with DM1 and DM2 may exhibit hypogammaglobulinemia with low immunoglobulin (Ig)G and IgM levels. The frequency of autoimmune diseases and presence of autoantibodies, such as antinuclear antibodies and rheumatoid factor, is increased in DM2.[19]

Cardiac involvement: evaluation and management

Histopathologic studies of patients with myotonic dystrophy reveal myocyte loss, hypertrophy, interstitial fibrosis, and fat deposition. There is preferential targeting of the specialized conduction system resulting in early and more consistent development of cardiac arrhythmias.[20] There is a general correlation between the presence of cardiac involvement and the severity of skeletal muscle involvement.

The most common clinical cardiac manifestations of DM are arrhythmias, some severe with an estimated incidence of SCD in DM1 of approximately 15%.[20–25] It is certain that some of these SCDs are the result of bradyarrhythmias. Conduction system disease and block are conspicuous involving the sinoatrial node, atrioventricular (AV) and intraventricular conduction with more than a quarter of patients with DM1 affected.[5,21,23,26] A major concern is the unpredictable course of progression of conduction disease (**Fig. 1**). Early-onset AF is seen in up to a quarter of patients with myotonic dystrophy.[21,23,27,28] Left ventricular (LV) dilation and systolic dysfunction is observed in a significant minority of patients, but clinical heart failure (HF) is rare. LV noncompaction also

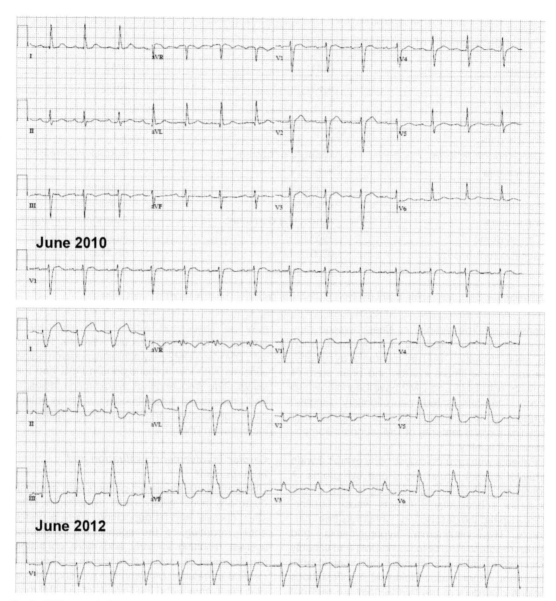

Fig. 1. ECGs recorded 2 years apart in a 40-year-old woman with type 1 myotonic dystrophy with 666 CTG repeats and a normal cardiac MRI.

has been described in patients with myotonic dystrophy.[29,30] The presence of glucose intolerance and diabetes in the setting of dyslipidemia increases the risk of atherosclerotic cardiovascular disease in both DM1 and DM2.

Cardiovascular disease is the second leading cause of death in patients with DM1; thus, the main goal is to identify patients at risk for serious arrhythmias and SCD. A large observational study evaluated patients with DM1 with at least 38 CTG repeats for the presence of "severe" electrocardiogram (ECG) changes, which included a rhythm other than sinus, PR interval

≥240 ms, QRS duration ≥120 ms, or second-degree or third-degree AV block. These findings were present in a quarter of the DM1 population; a severe ECG change (3-fold increased risk) and the presence of an atrial tachycardia (5-fold) were independent risk factors for SCD over approximately 6 years of follow-up. Notably, almost 10% of all deaths were sudden and presumed arrhythmic, some occurring in patients who had permanent pacemakers.[23] In the absence of randomized trial data, the evaluation of patients with myotonic dystrophy may be informed by these findings (**Fig. 2**).

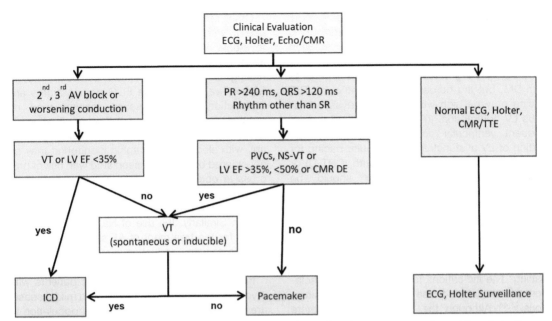

Fig. 2. Algorithm for evaluation of patients with myotonic dystrophy. The same approach would apply to the cardiac evaluation of other NMDs. Echo, echocardiogram; LVEF, left ventricular ejection fraction; SR, sinus rhythm; TTE, transthoracic echocardiogram.

The cardiac evaluation of patients with DM is aimed at determining the presence and assessing the risk of the development or progression of cardiovascular disease. The history is informative but may be confounded by significant skeletal muscle involvement. For example, many patients will complain of fatigue at rest or with exertion that is muscular in nature. The presence of exercise intolerance, chest discomfort, and shortness of breath or palpitations may be an indication of cardiac involvement that should be further evaluated. Syncope should prompt an aggressive and if necessary an invasive evaluation for risk of SCD and advanced conduction block. The cardiovascular physical examination may reveal the presence of a cardiac arrhythmia, pulmonary disease, and/or right or left heart dysfunction. Resting and ambulatory electrocardiography are especially important in evaluating patients for the presence of significant cardiac arrhythmias. For patients who are able, exercise testing may be useful to assess chronotropic competence. It is recommended that the ambulatory ECG recording be repeated every 2 to 3 years in patients with a stable resting ECG. In general, conduction disease warrants pacing, but in patients with conduction system involvement that are not paced or who have concerning symptoms, long-term ECG recording should be repeated more frequently. Electrophysiological study to assess AV conduction (HV interval) and arrhythmia inducibility is useful for risk

stratification. In view of the frequency of conduction system disease that requires pacing, the role of implanted loop recorders may be limited in this population.

Cardiac function may be assessed with one of several imaging modalities. Transthoracic echocardiography allows for assessment of heart chamber size, systolic and diastolic function, and regional wall motion. Early changes in longitudinal strain have been identified in patients with DM1 with preserved overall LV systolic function.[31,32] Notably, the frequency of mitral valve prolapse is increased in patients with DM1.[33–36] Contrast-enhanced cardiac MRI (CMR) and T1 mapping are useful modalities for identifying intramural scar. In some circumstances, the presence of scar is not predicted by ECG and echocardiographic evaluation.[37–40]

Patients with significant sinus node dysfunction or AV or intraventricular conduction defects who are candidates for pacemaker implantation should be evaluated for their risk of ventricular arrhythmias. If the CMR reveals scar or if LV dysfunction is present, programmed stimulation of the ventricle may be appropriate. If a ventricular tachyarrhythmia is inducible with a nonaggressive protocol (double extrastimuli or less), an implantable cardioverter-defibrillator (ICD) may be the preferred cardiac rhythm management device. The combination of conduction slowing and preservation of LV function in myotonic dystrophy is an ideal electrophysiological substrate for bundle branch reentry ventricular tachycardia (VT) (**Fig. 3**) in which radiofrequency catheter ablation may be appropriate.

Cardiac pacing can be life-saving for patients with DM, but the burden of right ventricular (RV) pacing may be high with attendant dyssynchronous LV contraction. In patients who will require frequent ventricular pacing, particularly in the setting of LV dysfunction, biventricular pacing for cardiac resynchronization (CRT) with (CRT-D) or without (CRT-P) a defibrillator should be considered.[41,42]

AF in the DM population is managed in a manner similar to that in other patients. A few considerations include the presence of conduction system disease that may limit the spectrum of antiarrhythmic drugs that can be used without backup pacing. The indications for pulmonary vein isolation are similar to those in other clinical situations.[43,44] Although the data are limited, there has been a suggestion that patients with myotonic dystrophy may be more prone to thromboembolism,[45] thus anticoagulation should be considered in these patients.

Other management considerations include the use of Na channel blocking drugs (mexiletine) for myotonia, weakness, and muscle pain.[46] In the absence of cardiac involvement and a normal resting ECG, mexiletine can be used without further evaluation. If the ECG demonstrates any conduction system disease, pacing may be required to safely use mexiletine. In situations in which pacing is not possible, instituting drug therapy with electrocardiographic monitoring may be considered but may be associated with risk of progressive conduction system disease and should be avoided in any patient with advanced AV or intraventricular conduction block without a pacemaker. Similarly, the use of Na channel blocking drugs for the treatment of AF should be avoided in patients with conduction system disease in the absence of a pacemaker.

In is important to recognize that patients with myotonic dystrophy, even those with mild disease, are far more likely than the general population to have adverse reactions to anesthesia and analgesia. The possible complications include arrhythmias and the development of conduction defects. Hypoventilation and inability to protect the airway

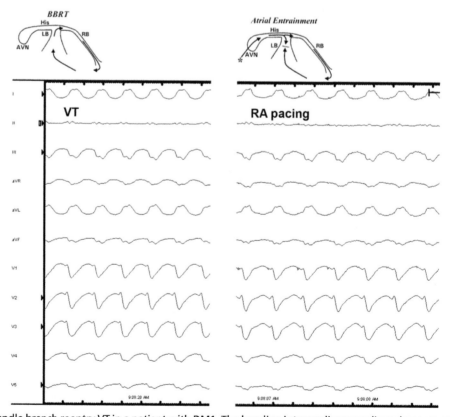

Fig. 3. Bundle branch reentry VT in a patient with DM1. The baseline intracardiac recordings demonstrated a prolonged HV interval. In VT, a His potential preceded the ventricular electrogram and changes in the H-H interval anticipated changes in the V-V interval. Right atrium pacing (*right*) generated a QRS identical to that in VT.

and decreased gastrointestinal motility are recognized anesthetic complications. Patients have unpredictable responses to neuromuscular blockers, such as succinylcholine, including masseter spasm and hyperkalemia; as such, these drugs should be avoided.

Muscular Dystrophies: Duchenne and Becker

Epidemiology and genetics

DMD is the commonest of the inherited muscular dystrophies, affecting approximately 1 in 5000 live male births. The disease is X-linked, with 30% of cases being sporadic. DMD is a dystrophinopathy with the complete absence of dystrophin. In X-linked BMD, dystrophin is not absent but dysfunctional; BMD exhibits a more benign course than DMD. Women who are carriers of dystrophin mutations may exhibit skeletal muscle and cardiac symptoms.[47] The absence or abnormalities of dystrophin (or other proteins in the dystrophin-associated membrane complex) render muscle cells susceptible to membrane damage and destruction in both skeletal muscle and the heart.[48,49]

Clinical manifestations and progression

Typically, boys are healthy at delivery and asymptomatic very early in childhood. Affected children exhibit symmetric central (pelvic girdle, neck) weakness and muscle wasting followed by contractures. Physical signs include pseudohypertrophy of the calves due to fat and connective tissue replacement of muscles. Gowers' sign, a waddling or Trendelenburg gait, and lordosis result from the loss of pelvic and paraspinous muscles. The weakness is progressive, moving from the pelvis to more distal muscles, with patients losing the ability to walk by late childhood or early adolescence, ultimately affecting respiratory muscles, with respiratory failure typically with death in the second to third decade of life.[50]

The evaluation of patients reveals creatine kinase (CK) levels that can be 50-fold to 100-fold greater than normal even in the preclinical stages; in fact, mild elevations in CK are inconsistent with the diagnosis except late in the course of the disease. The electromyogram is characterized by a "myopathic" pattern with low-amplitude polyphasic potentials mimicking myotonia. Muscle biopsy in DMD shows hypervariable muscle fiber calibers with hypertrophy, cellular infiltrates, and regenerating fibers. In the later stages of disease, fibrofatty replacement of muscle is observed.[47]

Dystrophin is expressed in skeletal, cardiac, and smooth muscles, and to a lesser extent in the brain. It is not surprising that patients with DMD exhibit gastrointestinal symptoms, such as impaired peristalsis, gastric distension, and intestinal pseudo-obstruction. Cognitive impairment and mental retardation is observed in some cases.

Cardiovascular manifestations and management

DMD and BMD prominently affect the heart. More than 90% of patients with DMD develop cardiomyopathy, which is a significant cause of mortality.[49,50] Cardiomyopathy may be life-limiting in BMD, and is present in nearly half of female carriers of mutant dystrophin.[51] The electrophysiological abnormalities in DMD and BMD are a consequence of the associated cardiomyopathy. In light of the frequency of cardiomyopathy, regular echocardiographic screening is recommended beginning in childhood.[49,50] The development of late gadolinium enhancement on cardiac MRI heralds the onset of decline in LV function.[52,53] Atrial and ventricular arrhythmias, as well as SCD, are not uncommon in DMD, BMD, and in female carriers (see **Table 1**). In BMD, arrhythmias reflect the severity of structural cardiac involvement.[1] The characteristic findings on ECG include intraventricular conduction delays (prolonged QRS), R/S >1 V1, and a pseudo-infarction pattern in the lateral leads. Sinus tachycardia and short PR intervals also have been observed. In more advanced disease, AF, VT, and QT prolongation can be seen. Incomplete right bundle branch block may be observed in BMD and may signal RV involvement (**Fig. 4**). Ventricular arrhythmias, most frequently premature ventricular contractions (PVCs), occur in up to one-third of patients with DMD, and SCD occurs most often in the setting of end-stage muscle disease and the etiology is uncertain.

There is no specific treatment for DMD or its cardiac manifestations. Corticosteroids and angiotensin receptor blockers have been used to treat skeletal muscle disease and may delay the progression the associated cardiomyopathy.[54] Treatment of cardiovascular disease typically involves the treatment of the cardiomyopathy, including standard pharmacotherapy that includes angiotensin converting enzyme inhibitors (ACEIs) or angiotensin II receptor blockers (ARBs), beta blockers, and diuretics for congestion.[55] The addition of aldosterone antagonists may provide benefit if used early.[56] Antiarrhythmic drug therapy is complicated by the presence of structural heart disease and heightened proarrhythmic liability. Most often, specific arrhythmic complications of DMD are managed by device implantation, either pacemakers or ICDs. In patients with DMD or BMD and female carriers with cardiomyopathy and dyssynchronous contraction, CRT should be

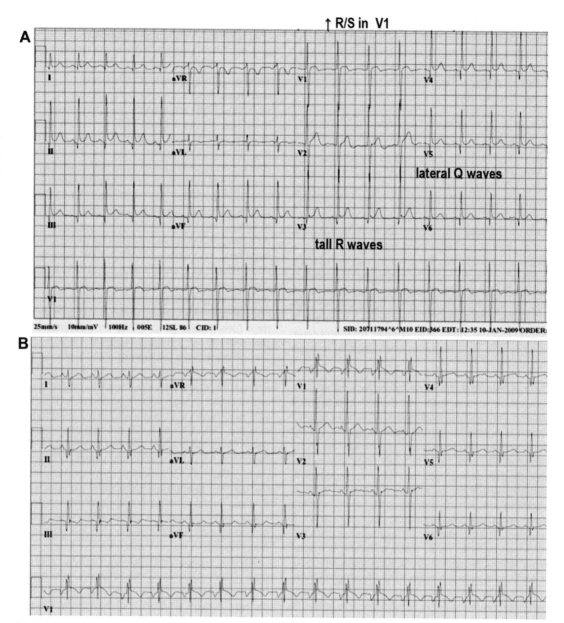

Fig. 4. (*A*) ECG recorded in a 15-year-old boy with DMD demonstrating characteristic features including sinus tachycardia, an increase in the R wave amplitude in lead V1 and lateral Q waves. (*B*) ECG recorded in a 26-year-old man with BMD. An RV conduction delay is present suggesting the presence of RV cardiomyopathic changes.

considered.[57,58] The use of ICD treatment should be individualized based on the patient's condition and desires.

There are several experimental therapies that have been tested in DMD or models of the disease, including gene replacement (micro or mini-dystrophins), exon-skipping oligonucleotides, genome editing, cell therapy, and plasma membrane stabilizers (poloxamer 188).[59,60]

Emery-Dreifuss Muscular Dystrophy and Associated Disorders

Genetics and cardiac pathology

EDMD is an X-linked early-onset muscular dystrophy with cardiac involvement in virtually all cases.[61,62] EDMD1 is inherited as an X-linked (Xq28) recessive trait with heterogeneity of transmission within families. EDMD1 is caused by a mutation in *EMD (STA)*, which encodes the nuclear membrane protein emerin. In EDMD1, emerin is absent not only in muscle cells, but also in other cell types (blood, skin). The spectrum of associated disorders include autosomal dominant (EDMD2) and recessive (EDMD3) variants due to mutations in the nuclear proteins lamin A and C on chromosome 1, respectively,[63] autosomal dominant DCM with conduction disease,[64] and lipodystrophy with associated cardiac abnormalities.[1]

Lamins are intermediate filament proteins that form the meshwork inner nuclear lamina that interact with emerin, as well as the cytoskeleton through the multiprotein linker of nucleoskeleton and cytoskeleton complex. Lamins are important for maintenance of the structural integrity of the nucleus and are involved in chromatin regulation and nucleic acid replication and processing. Mutations in lamins have been identified in up to 6% of patients with DCM[65] and 33% of those patients presenting with conduction defects.[66]

Clinical presentation

The muscular features of EDMD1 include limited range of motion and flexor contractures of the elbow, ankle, and posterior cervical muscles with progressive muscle weakness and atrophy, especially in humeroperoneal muscles. The onset is typically in childhood and characterized by an inability to straighten the upper limb, toe walking, pes equinus, and frequent falls. A diagnosis of EDMD1 is made in the absence of emerin in buccal smears, skin, or muscle biopsy in a male individual with an elevated CK. In lamin-associated EDMD, emerin expression is normal, and the diagnosis is made by genetic testing. At times, cardiac manifestations including SCD may precede significant skeletal muscle involvement. The autosomal forms exhibit more variable muscular phenotypes and a variant of the autosomal dominant form is associated with lipodystrophy exhibiting a marked loss of subcutaneous fat, diabetes, and dyslipidemia.[67]

Cardiovascular manifestations and management

Patients with EDMD1 exhibit sinus node dysfunction, conduction system disease with associated arrhythmias, such as AF, and less commonly DCM. In the X-linked recessive variant ECGs are abnormal by the third decade of life, commonly showing first-degree AV block. The conduction disease is progressive, with pacing required in most patients before age 40.[68] Mutations in emerin are rarely the cause of idiopathic conduction disturbances in young men.[69] Typically atria are affected before the ventricles, most commonly atrial standstill with a junctional escape rhythm,

although AF and atrial flutter with thromboembolic complications have also been observed. Less commonly, VT and ventricular fibrillation have been described. Arrhythmias are the earliest and most common manifestations of cardiac involvement in EMDM1; however, DCM can occur, particularly in patients who have undergone cardiac device implantation. Skeletal muscle disease does not occur in female carriers of X-linked recessive EDMD, but cardiac disease including conduction abnormalities and sudden death have been observed.[70]

In patients with lamin A and C mutations, early-onset DCM is a more prominent feature, and conduction disease, and atrial and ventricular arrhythmias tend to occur later in this context.[71] Skeletal muscle disease may not be present. Patients are at risk for SCD and progression to end-stage cardiomyopathy requiring heart transplantation or mechanical hemodynamic support has been described. Heart block and bradyarrhythmias require pacing; the presence of DCM and the increased risk of ventricular arrhythmias generally mandates the placement of an ICD, as SCD is the most common mode of death in both the emerin-associated and lamin-associated forms of EDMD.[72,73]

It is appropriate to screen all patients with EDMD as well as female carriers of emerin mutations for electrophysiological as well as structural cardiac involvement. Regular assessment of LV function should be performed. Transthoracic echocardiography is most readily available, but cardiac MR may be useful to examine tissue characteristics in patients with preserved ventricular function. Patients should be monitored for development of electrocardiographic conduction abnormalities and arrhythmias. AV block can occur with anesthesia, and sudden death has been observed in patients with pacemakers. The presence of even first-degree AV conduction block should prompt an investigation for more advanced conduction system disease with ambulatory monitoring or intracardiac recording. Pacing should be considered in any patient with EDMD with conduction system disease given the unpredictable rate of progression of disease. The use of biventricular pacing (CRT) should be considered in patients who require ventricular pacing, particularly those with LV systolic dysfunction.

Sinus node dysfunction and atrial standstill are associated with AF often before the development of bradyarrhythmias. AF is associated with a relatively high frequency of embolic stroke, even in the absence of ventricular dysfunction; therefore, anticoagulation should be considered in patients with EDMD with atrial standstill or AF.[74]

SCD risk prediction is imperfect, and primary prevention ICD placement has been advocated in patients with EDMD in whom pacing is being considered. In a European cohort study of lamin A/C mutation carriers, nearly 20% of patients experienced SCD or potentially lethal ventricular arrhythmias in less than 4 years of follow-up. The independent risk factors for SCD or malignant ventricular arrhythmias were the presence of nonsustained VT, male gender, LV ejection fraction less than 45%, and nonsense mutations in lamin A/C.[72]

Patients with LV dysfunction should be managed with guideline-recommended medical therapies, including ACEIs or ARBs, beta blockers, and diuretics. Advanced HF treatment, including mechanical cardiac support (ventricular assist devices) and heart transplantation should be considered in appropriate patients. Skeletal muscle involvement in EDMD is often mild and generally not life-limiting. The prognosis is determined by the type and course of cardiac involvement. Aggressive evaluation and treatment of cardiac manifestations of EDMD can improve longevity and quality of life.

Limb-Girdle Muscular Dystrophy

Epidemiology and genetics

LGMD is a group of more than 25 muscle diseases. The naming convention is based on the mode of genetic transmission, with LGMD1 being inherited as autosomal dominant traits and LGMD2 as autosomal recessive. Within each class, there are subclasses of LGMDs identified by a letter designation. There are 6 prevalent LGMDs, several with cardiac manifestations. In the autosomal dominant group, LGMD1B results from mutations in lamin A/C analogous to EDMD2 and 3. Several of the autosomal recessive forms of LGMD are more prevalent than LGMD1B, such as LGMD2A due to mutations in calpain (CAPN3), LGMD2B resulting from mutations in dysferlin (DYSF), LGMD2C-F with mutations in sarcoglycans (SGCG), and LGMD2I due to mutations in Fukutin-related protein (FKRP).[75] Of these, only patients with LGMD2C-F, 2I, and 1B exhibit related cardiac disease.[76]

The dystrophin-glycoprotein membrane complex is composed of dystrophin, sarcospan, dystroglycans, and sarcoglycans (α, β, γ, δ). This complex links sarcomeres and cytoskeleton to the extracellular matrix through the cell membrane and is involved in signaling and trafficking of proteins. LGMD2C-F results from mutations in γ-, α-, β-, and δ-sarcoglycan, respectively. The LGMDs resulting from mutations in the different sarcoglycans produce a similar spectrum of muscle and cardiac disease.[77]

FKRP is homologous to a group of proteins that modify cell surface glycoproteins and lipids. FKRP is highly expressed in striated muscle and modifies dystroglycans. Mutations in FKRP can produce more severe congenital muscular dystrophy (MDC1C) and later-onset LGMD2I, the latter characterized by recurrent myoglobinuria, elevated serum CK, and DCM.[78]

Mutations in LMNA produce a wide spectrum of allelic human disorders, including skeletal myopathies, such as LGMD1B, EDMD2 and 3, congenital muscular dystrophy, and autosomal dominant DCM with conduction block (CMD1A).[79] Among the nonmuscle disorders are familial forms of partial lipodystrophy, Charcot-Marie Tooth (autosomal dominant and autosomal recessive variants)[80] and Hutchinson-Gilford progeria form of premature aging.[81] DCM without skeletal muscle disease is also caused by LMNA mutations.[64]

Clinical features

Symptom is LGMD like several other muscular diseases include weakness in the hip girdle, thighs, shoulders, and arms proximally. LGMD2C-F, I, 1B can present from childhood to early adulthood, typically well before approximately 25 years of age. Sarcoglycan-associated LGMDs more prominently affect flexor muscle groups and exhibit a rapidly progressive course with wheelchair confinement within a decade.[82] CK levels can be dramatically elevated more than 100 times the upper limits of normal. Muscle biopsies with staining for individual sarcoglycans can be used, but the diagnosis is typically made by genetic testing. The onset of LGMD2I is usually in the second decade of life; pelvic and femoral weakness may exhibit a stuttering course, with patients often able to walk into the fourth decade of life. Ultimately, weakness spreads to the lower extremities, calf hypertrophy and lumbar lordosis may mimic BMD.[83] Patients with LGMD2I may exhibit exertional myoglobinuria.[84] LGMD1B presents over a wide range of ages; there is a congenital form and descriptions of presentations as late as the 40s.[85] Weakness is prominent in humeroperoneal (biceps and lower leg) and limb-girdle muscle groups. Independent of the onset of skeletal muscle disease, cardiac manifestations are usually apparent by the second or third decade of life.[86]

Cardiac manifestations and management

Cardiac involvement in the form of myopathy and significant arrhythmia is the rule in sarcoglycan-associated forms of LGMD. In a recent long-term follow-up study of 34 patients with LGMD2C and 2D, median age 30 years, nearly 40% of patients had a reduced ejection fraction at the time of diagnosis. Over 6 years of follow-up, 14% of patients experienced either HF or a serious arrhythmia.[77] Other studies have suggested more extensive cardiac involvement with a number of ECG abnormalities including AF, sinus tachycardia, LV hypertrophy, PVCs, nonspecific T-wave changes, and, as has been described in DMD and BMD, R > S wave amplitude in lead V1.[87,88] In up to 50% of patients, echocardiographic abnormalities, including reduced systolic function, abnormal diastolic function, and chamber enlargement have also been described.[1,89,90] There may some variability in cardiac involvement in the sarcoglycanopathies that depends on the specific sarcoglycan and the particular mutation.[87,91] Importantly, the severity of cardiac involvement may not be correlated with the degree of skeletal muscle impairment.

The other autosomal recessive LGMD that exhibits significant cardiac involvement is LGMD2I, often due to a common mutation in *FKRP* (C826A). Most of these patients have a reduced LV ejection fraction, with a significant minority developing HF. Cardiac MR was abnormal in most patients, with a high prevalence of regional functional abnormalities, fibrosis, and fatty replacement of the myocardium.[78,84,92]

As is the case with laminopathies causing EDMD, LGMD1B is often associated with progressive conduction system disease and cardiomyopathy.[1,81,93–95] In patients with EDMD and LGMD1B with lamin mutations, cardiac involvement may precede the development of skeletal muscle disease. In a large series of LMNA-associated myopathies (~50% LGMD1B and 20% EDMD2), cardiac involvement serious enough to require pacemaker or ICD implantation was present in more than 50% of patients, and over the period of observation, more than 10% of patients were transplanted and a similar number died.[96]

The frequency and severity of cardiac involvement in LGMD and in particular the laminopathies, mandates an aggressive approach to evaluation and management. This is particularly relevant in view of the often milder skeletal muscle disease in these patients. There are no data that inform the frequency of cardiac functional and electrical evaluation, but all patients should be seen by a cardiologist once the diagnosis is made. In addition to a thorough cardiovascular history and physical examination, the recommended evaluation includes resting and ambulatory ECGs, echocardiography, and, in cases in which there is any suggestion of cardiac involvement, cardiac MR with contrast. Treatment of LV dysfunction even in the absence of clinical HF is appropriate and should include ACEIs or ARBs and beta blockers in the absence

of contraindications.[87] The lack of predictability of the course of conduction system disease in these and other patients with NMDs suggests the early use of permanent pacemaking. The presence of a substrate for ventricular tachyarrhythmias, either structural cardiac involvement or a history of spontaneous or induced ventricular arrhythmias, generally requires treatment with an ICD.[1]

SUMMARY/FUTURE DIRECTIONS

NMDs frequently involve the heart and disproportionately the cardiac conduction system. Cardiomyopathy and sudden death are common causes of morbidity and mortality. Patients with NMDs should be carefully and frequently evaluated for the presence of bradycardia, heart block, and tachyarrhythmias. Preemptive treatment with permanent pacemakers is appropriate in patients with conduction system disease. Patients, even those with pacemakers, should undergo regular evaluation for risk of SCD, and a defibrillator should be implanted in patients with a substrate for ventricular arrhythmias. Early identification and the outcomes of treatment of patients with NMDs are areas of active investigation.

REFERENCES

1. Groh WJ. Arrhythmias in the muscular dystrophies. Heart Rhythm 2012;9(11):1890–5.
2. Sommerville RB, Vincenti MG, Winborn K, et al. Diagnosis and management of adult hereditary cardio-neuromuscular disorders: a model for the multidisciplinary care of complex genetic disorders. Trends Cardiovasc Med 2017;27(1):51–8.
3. Priori SG, Blomstrom-Lundqvist C, Mazzanti A, et al. 2015 ESC guidelines for the management of patients with ventricular arrhythmias and the prevention of sudden cardiac death: the task force for the management of patients with ventricular arrhythmias and the prevention of sudden cardiac death of the European Society of Cardiology (ESC). Endorsed by: Association for European Paediatric and Congenital Cardiology (AEPC). Eur Heart J 2015;36(41):2793–867.
4. Finsterer J, Stollberger C. Cardiac abnormalities in myotonic dystrophy type 1. Am Heart J 2004;148(6):e33 [author reply: e34].
5. Tanawuttiwat T, Wagner KR, Tomaselli G, et al. Left ventricular dysfunction and conduction disturbances in patients with myotonic muscular dystrophy type I and II. JAMA Cardiol 2017;2(2):225–8.
6. Thornton CA. Myotonic dystrophy. Neurol Clin 2014;32(3):705–19, viii.
7. Howeler CJ, Busch HF, Geraedts JP, et al. Anticipation in myotonic dystrophy: fact or fiction? Brain 1989;112(Pt 3):779–97.

8. Thornton CA, Johnson K, Moxley RT 3rd. Myotonic dystrophy patients have larger CTG expansions in skeletal muscle than in leukocytes. Ann Neurol 1994;35(1):104–7.

9. Morales F, Couto JM, Higham CF, et al. Somatic instability of the expanded CTG triplet repeat in myotonic dystrophy type 1 is a heritable quantitative trait and modifier of disease severity. Hum Mol Genet 2012;21(16):3558–67.

10. Redman JB, Fenwick RG Jr, Fu YH, et al. Relationship between parental trinucleotide GCT repeat length and severity of myotonic dystrophy in offspring. JAMA 1993;269(15):1960–5.

11. Bugiardini E, Rivolta I, Binda A, et al. SCN4A mutation as modifying factor of myotonic dystrophy type 2 phenotype. Neuromuscul Disord 2015;25(4): 301–7.

12. Suominen T, Schoser B, Raheem O, et al. High frequency of co-segregating CLCN1 mutations among myotonic dystrophy type 2 patients from Finland and Germany. J Neurol 2008;255(11):1731–6.

13. Freyermuth F, Rau F, Kokunai Y, et al. Splicing misregulation of SCN5A contributes to cardiac-conduction delay and heart arrhythmia in myotonic dystrophy. Nat Commun 2016;7:11067.

14. Tang ZZ, Yarotskyy V, Wei L, et al. Muscle weakness in myotonic dystrophy associated with misregulated splicing and altered gating of Ca(V)1.1 calcium channel. Hum Mol Genet 2012;21(6):1312–24.

15. Kimura T, Nakamori M, Lueck JD, et al. Altered mRNA splicing of the skeletal muscle ryanodine receptor and sarcoplasmic/endoplasmic reticulum Ca2+-ATPase in myotonic dystrophy type 1. Hum Mol Genet 2005;14(15):2189–200.

16. Santoro M, Piacentini R, Masciullo M, et al. Alternative splicing alterations of Ca2+ handling genes are associated with Ca2+ signal dysregulation in myotonic dystrophy type 1 (DM1) and type 2 (DM2) myotubes. Neuropathol Appl Neurobiol 2014;40(4):464–76.

17. Turner C, Hilton-Jones D. Myotonic dystrophy: diagnosis, management and new therapies. Curr Opin Neurol 2014;27(5):599–606.

18. Meola G, Moxley RT 3rd. Myotonic dystrophy type 2 and related myotonic disorders. J Neurol 2004; 251(10):1173–82.

19. Tieleman AA, den Broeder AA, van de Logt AE, et al. Strong association between myotonic dystrophy type 2 and autoimmune diseases. J Neurol Neurosurg Psychiatry 2009;80(11):1293–5.

20. Schoser BG, Ricker K, Schneider-Gold C, et al. Sudden cardiac death in myotonic dystrophy type 2. Neurology 2004;63(12):2402–4.

21. Benhayon D, Lugo R, Patel R, et al. Long-term arrhythmia follow-up of patients with myotonic dystrophy. J Cardiovasc Electrophysiol 2015;26(3): 305–10.

22. Laurent V, Pellieux S, Corcia P, et al. Mortality in myotonic dystrophy patients in the area of prophylactic pacing devices. Int J Cardiol 2011;150(1):54–8.

23. Groh WJ, Groh MR, Saha C, et al. Electrocardiographic abnormalities and sudden death in myotonic dystrophy type 1. N Engl J Med 2008;358(25): 2688–97.

24. Lazarus A, Varin J, Babuty D, et al. Long-term follow-up of arrhythmias in patients with myotonic dystrophy treated by pacing: a multicenter diagnostic pacemaker study. J Am Coll Cardiol 2002;40(9): 1645–52.

25. Grigg LE, Chan W, Mond HG, et al. Ventricular tachycardia and sudden death in myotonic dystrophy: clinical, electrophysiologic and pathologic features. J Am Coll Cardiol 1985;6(1):254–6.

26. Lund M, Diaz LJ, Ranthe MF, et al. Cardiac involvement in myotonic dystrophy: a nationwide cohort study. Eur Heart J 2014;35(32):2158–64.

27. Petri H, Witting N, Ersboll MK, et al. High prevalence of cardiac involvement in patients with myotonic dystrophy type 1: a cross-sectional study. Int J Cardiol 2014;174(1):31–6.

28. Brembilla-Perrot B, Schwartz J, Huttin O, et al. Atrial flutter or fibrillation is the most frequent and life-threatening arrhythmia in myotonic dystrophy. Pacing Clin Electrophysiol 2014;37(3):329–35.

29. Sa MI, Cabral S, Costa PD, et al. Cardiac involvement in type 1 myotonic dystrophy. Rev Port Cardiol 2007;27(9):829–40.

30. Finsterer J, Stollberger C, Wegmann R, et al. Acquired left ventricular hypertrabeculation/noncompaction in myotonic dystrophy type 1. Int J Cardiol 2009;137(3):310–3.

31. Garcia R, Labarre Q, Degand B, et al. Apical left ventricular myocardial dysfunction is an early feature of cardiac involvement in myotonic dystrophy type 1. Echocardiography 2017;34(2):184–90.

32. Galderisi M, De Stefano F, Santoro C, et al. Early changes of myocardial deformation properties in patients with dystrophia myotonica type 1: a three-dimensional Speckle Tracking echocardiographic study. Int J Cardiol 2014;176(3):1094–6.

33. Streib EW, Meyers DG, Sun SF. Mitral valve prolapse in myotonic dystrophy. Muscle Nerve 1985;8(8):650–3.

34. Winters SJ, Schreiner B, Griggs RC, et al. Familial mitral valve prolapse and myotonic dystrophy. Ann Intern Med 1976;85(1):19–22.

35. Gottdiener JS, Hawley RJ, Gay JA, et al. Left ventricular relaxation, mitral valve prolapse, and intracardiac conduction in myotonia atrophica: assessment by digitized echocardiography and noninvasive His bundle recording. Am Heart J 1982;104(1):77–85.

36. Bhakta D, Lowe MR, Groh WJ. Prevalence of structural cardiac abnormalities in patients with myotonic dystrophy type I. Am Heart J 2004;147(2):224–7.

37. Nazarian S, Bluemke DA, Wagner KR, et al. QRS prolongation in myotonic muscular dystrophy and diffuse fibrosis on cardiac magnetic resonance. Magn Reson Med 2010;64(1):107–14.

38. Turkbey EB, Gai N, Lima JA, et al. Assessment of cardiac involvement in myotonic muscular dystrophy by T1 mapping on magnetic resonance imaging. Heart Rhythm 2012;9(10):1691–7.

39. Petri H, Ahtarovski KA, Vejlstrup N, et al. Myocardial fibrosis in patients with myotonic dystrophy type 1: a cardiovascular magnetic resonance study. J Cardiovasc Magn Reson 2014;16:59.

40. Hermans MC, Faber CG, Bekkers SC, et al. Structural and functional cardiac changes in myotonic dystrophy type 1: a cardiovascular magnetic resonance study. J Cardiovasc Magn Reson 2012;14:48.

41. Kilic T, Vural A, Ural D, et al. Cardiac resynchronization therapy in a case of myotonic dystrophy (Steinert's disease) and dilated cardiomyopathy. Pacing Clin Electrophysiol 2007;30(7):916–20.

42. Epstein AE, DiMarco JP, Ellenbogen KA, et al. ACC/AHA/HRS 2008 guidelines for device-based therapy of cardiac rhythm abnormalities: a report of the American College of Cardiology/American Heart Association Task Force on Practice Guidelines (Writing Committee to Revise the ACC/AHA/NASPE 2002 Guideline Update for Implantation of Cardiac Pacemakers and Antiarrhythmia Devices): developed in collaboration with the American Association for Thoracic Surgery and Society of Thoracic Surgeons. Circulation 2008;117(21):e350–408.

43. Calkins H, Kuck KH, Cappato R, et al. 2012 HRS/EHRA/ECAS expert consensus statement on catheter and surgical ablation of atrial fibrillation: recommendations for patient selection, procedural techniques, patient management and follow-up, definitions, endpoints, and research trial design: a report of the Heart Rhythm Society (HRS) Task Force on Catheter and Surgical Ablation of Atrial Fibrillation. Developed in partnership with the European Heart Rhythm Association (EHRA), a registered branch of the European Society of Cardiology (ESC) and the European Cardiac Arrhythmia Society (ECAS); and in collaboration with the American College of Cardiology (ACC), American Heart Association (AHA), the Asia Pacific Heart Rhythm Society (APHRS), and the Society of Thoracic Surgeons (STS). Endorsed by the governing bodies of the American College of Cardiology Foundation, the American Heart Association, the European Cardiac Arrhythmia Society, the European Heart Rhythm Association, the Society of Thoracic Surgeons, the Asia Pacific Heart Rhythm Society, and the Heart Rhythm Society. Heart Rhythm 2012;9(4):632–96.e21.

44. January CT, Wann LS, Alpert JS, et al. 2014 AHA/ACC/HRS guideline for the management of patients with atrial fibrillation: a report of the American College of Cardiology/American Heart Association Task Force on practice guidelines and the Heart Rhythm Society. Circulation 2014;130(23):e199–267.

45. Wahbi K, Sebag FA, Lellouche N, et al. Atrial flutter in myotonic dystrophy type 1: patient characteristics and clinical outcome. Neuromuscul Disord 2016;26(3):227–33.

46. Logigian EL, Martens WB, Moxley RT 4th, et al. Mexiletine is an effective antimyotonia treatment in myotonic dystrophy type 1. Neurology 2010;74(18):1441–8.

47. Emery AE. The muscular dystrophies. Lancet 2002;359(9307):687–95.

48. Townsend D, Yasuda S, McNally E, et al. Distinct pathophysiological mechanisms of cardiomyopathy in hearts lacking dystrophin or the sarcoglycan complex. FASEB J 2011;25(9):3106–14.

49. McNally EM, Kaltman JR, Benson DW, et al. Contemporary cardiac issues in Duchenne muscular dystrophy. Working Group of the National Heart, Lung, and Blood Institute in collaboration with parent project muscular dystrophy. Circulation 2015;131(18):1590–8.

50. Bushby K, Finkel R, Birnkrant DJ, et al. Diagnosis and management of Duchenne muscular dystrophy, part 1: diagnosis, and pharmacological and psychosocial management. Lancet Neurol 2010;9(1):77–93.

51. McCaffrey T, Guglieri M, Murphy AP, et al. Cardiac involvement in female carriers of Duchenne or Becker muscular dystrophy. Muscle Nerve 2017;55(6):810–8.

52. Tandon A, Villa CR, Hor KN, et al. Myocardial fibrosis burden predicts left ventricular ejection fraction and is associated with age and steroid treatment duration in Duchenne muscular dystrophy. J Am Heart Assoc 2015;4(4) [pii:e001338].

53. Tandon A, Jefferies JL, Villa CR, et al. Dystrophin genotype-cardiac phenotype correlations in Duchenne and Becker muscular dystrophies using cardiac magnetic resonance imaging. Am J Cardiol 2015;115(7):967–71.

54. Schram G, Fournier A, Leduc H, et al. All-cause mortality and cardiovascular outcomes with prophylactic steroid therapy in Duchenne muscular dystrophy. J Am Coll Cardiol 2013;61(9):948–54.

55. Duboc D, Meune C, Lerebours G, et al. Effect of perindopril on the onset and progression of left ventricular dysfunction in Duchenne muscular dystrophy. J Am Coll Cardiol 2005;45(6):855–7.

56. Raman SV, Hor KN, Mazur W, et al. Eplerenone for early cardiomyopathy in Duchenne muscular dystrophy: results of a two-year open-label extension trial. Orphanet J Rare Dis 2017;12(1):39.

57. Stollberger C, Finsterer J. Left ventricular synchronization by biventricular pacing in Becker muscular dystrophy as assessed by tissue Doppler imaging. Heart Lung 2005;34(5):317–20.

58. Fayssoil A, Nardi O, Annane D, et al. Successful cardiac resynchronisation therapy in Duchenne muscular dystrophy: a 5-year follow-up. Presse Med 2014;43(3):330–1.

59. Jarmin S, Kymalainen H, Popplewell L, et al. New developments in the use of gene therapy to treat Duchenne muscular dystrophy. Expert Opin Biol Ther 2014;14(2):209–30.

60. Yue Y, Binalsheikh IM, Leach SB, et al. Prospect of gene therapy for cardiomyopathy in hereditary muscular dystrophy. Expert Opin Orphan Drugs 2016;4(2):169–83.

61. Muchir A, Worman HJ. Emery-Dreifuss muscular dystrophy. Curr Neurol Neurosci Rep 2007;7(1): 78–83.

62. Wessely R, Seidl S, Schomig A. Cardiac involvement in Emery-Dreifuss muscular dystrophy. Clin Genet 2005;67(3):220–3.

63. Raffaele Di Barletta M, Ricci E, Galluzzi G, et al. Different mutations in the LMNA gene cause autosomal dominant and autosomal recessive Emery-Dreifuss muscular dystrophy. Am J Hum Genet 2000;66(4):1407–12.

64. Fatkin D, MacRae C, Sasaki T, et al. Missense mutations in the rod domain of the lamin A/C gene as causes of dilated cardiomyopathy and conduction-system disease. N Engl J Med 1999; 341(23):1715–24.

65. Hershberger RE, Siegfried JD. Update 2011: clinical and genetic issues in familial dilated cardiomyopathy. J Am Coll Cardiol 2011;57(16):1641–9.

66. Arbustini E, Pilotto A, Repetto A, et al. Autosomal dominant dilated cardiomyopathy with atrioventricular block: a lamin A/C defect-related disease. J Am Coll Cardiol 2002;39(6):981–90.

67. Wiltshire KM, Hegele RA, Innes AM, et al. Homozygous lamin A/C familial lipodystrophy R482Q mutation in autosomal recessive Emery Dreifuss muscular dystrophy. Neuromuscul Disord 2013; 23(3):265–8.

68. Karst ML, Herron KJ, Olson TM. X-linked nonsyndromic sinus node dysfunction and atrial fibrillation caused by emerin mutation. J Cardiovasc Electrophysiol 2008;19(5):510–5.

69. Vytopil M, Vohanka S, Vlasinova J, et al. The screening for X-linked Emery-Dreifuss muscular dystrophy amongst young patients with idiopathic heart conduction system disease treated by a pacemaker implant. Eur J Neurol 2004;11(8):531–4.

70. Emery AE. Emery-Dreifuss muscular dystrophy—a 40 year retrospective. Neuromuscul Disord 2000; 10(4–5):228–32.

71. Cattin ME, Muchir A, Bonne G. 'State-of-the-heart' of cardiac laminopathies. Curr Opin Cardiol 2013; 28(3):297–304.

72. van Rijsingen IA, Arbustini E, Elliott PM, et al. Risk factors for malignant ventricular arrhythmias in lamin A/C mutation carriers a European cohort study. J Am Coll Cardiol 2012;59(5):493–500.

73. Sakata K, Shimizu M, Ino H, et al. High incidence of sudden cardiac death with conduction disturbances and atrial cardiomyopathy caused by a nonsense mutation in the STA gene. Circulation 2005; 111(25):3352–8.

74. Boriani G, Gallina M, Merlini L, et al. Clinical relevance of atrial fibrillation/flutter, stroke, pacemaker implant, and heart failure in Emery-Dreifuss muscular dystrophy: a long-term longitudinal study. Stroke 2003;34(4):901–8.

75. Bushby KM, Beckmann JS. The limb-girdle muscular dystrophies–proposal for a new nomenclature. Neuromuscul Disord 1995;5(4):337–43.

76. Wicklund MP, Kissel JT. The limb-girdle muscular dystrophies. Neurol Clin 2014;32(3):729–49, ix.

77. Fayssoil A, Ogna A, Chaffaut C, et al. Natural history of cardiac and respiratory involvement, prognosis and predictive factors for long-term survival in adult patients with limb girdle muscular dystrophies type 2C and 2D. PLoS One 2016;11(4): e0153095.

78. Poppe M, Bourke J, Eagle M, et al. Cardiac and respiratory failure in limb-girdle muscular dystrophy 2I. Ann Neurol 2004;56(5):738–41.

79. Rankin J, Ellard S. The laminopathies: a clinical review. Clin Genet 2006;70(4):261–74.

80. Chaouch M, Allal Y, De Sandre-Giovannoli A, et al. The phenotypic manifestations of autosomal recessive axonal Charcot-Marie-Tooth due to a mutation in Lamin A/C gene. Neuromuscul Disord 2003; 13(1):60–7.

81. Villa F, Maciag A, Spinelli CC, et al. A G613A missense in the Hutchinson's progeria lamin A/C gene causes a lone, autosomal dominant atrioventricular block. Immun Ageing 2014;11(1):19.

82. McNally EM, Passos-Bueno MR, Bonnemann CG, et al. Mild and severe muscular dystrophy caused by a single gamma-sarcoglycan mutation. Am J Hum Genet 1996;59(5):1040–7.

83. Poppe M, Cree L, Bourke J, et al. The phenotype of limb-girdle muscular dystrophy type 2I. Neurology 2003;60(8):1246–51.

84. Wahbi K, Meune C, Hamouda el H, et al. Cardiac assessment of limb-girdle muscular dystrophy 2I patients: an echography, Holter ECG and magnetic resonance imaging study. Neuromuscul Disord 2008;18(8):650–5.

85. Benedetti S, Menditto I, Degano M, et al. Phenotypic clustering of lamin A/C mutations in neuromuscular patients. Neurology 2007;69(12):1285–92.

86. Bonne G, Mercuri E, Muchir A, et al. Clinical and molecular genetic spectrum of autosomal dominant Emery-Dreifuss muscular dystrophy due to mutations of the lamin A/C gene. Ann Neurol 2000; 48(2):170–80.

87. Fanin M, Melacini P, Boito C, et al. LGMD2E patients risk developing dilated cardiomyopathy. Neuromuscul Disord 2003;13(4):303–9.

88. Politano L, Nigro V, Passamano L, et al. Evaluation of cardiac and respiratory involvement in sarcoglycanopathies. Neuromuscul Disord 2001;11(2):178–85.

89. Melacini P, Fanin M, Duggan DJ, et al. Heart involvement in muscular dystrophies due to sarcoglycan gene mutations. Muscle Nerve 1999;22(4):473–9.

90. Petri H, Sveen ML, Thune JJ, et al. Progression of cardiac involvement in patients with limb-girdle type 2 and Becker muscular dystrophies: a 9-year follow-up study. Int J Cardiol 2015;182:403–11.

91. Mascarenhas DA, Spodick DH, Chad DA, et al. Cardiomyopathy of limb-girdle muscular dystrophy. J Am Coll Cardiol 1994;24(5):1328–33.

92. Gaul C, Deschauer M, Tempelmann C, et al. Cardiac involvement in limb-girdle muscular dystrophy 2I: conventional cardiac diagnostic and cardiovascular magnetic resonance. J Neurol 2006;253(10):1317–22.

93. Meune C, Khouzami L, Wahbi K, et al. Blood glutathione decrease in subjects carrying lamin A/C gene mutations is an early marker of cardiac involvement. Neuromuscul Disord 2012;22(3):252–7.

94. Decostre V, Ben Yaou R, Bonne G. Laminopathies affecting skeletal and cardiac muscles: clinical and pathophysiological aspects. Acta Myol 2005;24(2): 104–9.

95. Antoniades L, Eftychiou C, Kyriakides T, et al. Malignant mutation in the lamin A/C gene causing progressive conduction system disease and early sudden death in a family with mild form of limb-girdle muscular dystrophy. J Interv Card Electrophysiol 2007;19(1):1–7.

96. Maggi L, D'Amico A, Pini A, et al. LMNA-associated myopathies: the Italian experience in a large cohort of patients. Neurology 2014;83(18):1634–44.

Sudden Cardiac Death
Lessons Learned from Cardiac Implantable Rhythm Devices

Pasquale Santangeli, MD, PhD*,
Andrew E. Epstein, MD, FHRS

KEYWORDS

- Sudden cardiac death • Implantable rhythm devices • Cardiac arrest • Left ventricular dysfunction
- Left ventricular ejection fraction • Implantable cardioverter-defibrillator

KEY POINTS

- Multiple randomized controlled trials have clearly demonstrated that implantable–cardioverter defibrillators (ICDs) are highly effective in preventing sudden cardiac death (SCD).
- In patients who have suffered a cardiac arrest, there is consistent evidence supporting a benefit of ICDs to reduce mortality owing to recurrent cardiac arrest events.
- Left ventricular dysfunction is currently the only parameter to identify primary prevention populations at higher risk of SCD, in which prophylactic implantation of ICDs may reduce the longitudinal mortality risk.
- Application of current risk stratification approaches based on left ventricular ejection fraction (LVEF) alone has failed to prevent most SCD in the general population without LV dysfunction.
- Future studies should focus on the discovery and validation of newer arrhythmic risk markers, to improve the predictive value of LVEF and improve SCD prevention.

INTRODUCTION

Sudden cardiac death (SCD) accounts for 450,000 deaths yearly in the United States,[1] with similar incidence in Europe. Analyses of disease progression patterns over the last 20 years have consistently shown a decrease in overall cardiovascular mortality, mostly driven by an expanded use of evidence-based medical therapies as well as changes in risk factors and lifestyle modifications.[2–4] Although overall cardiovascular mortality has decreased, the proportion of SCD mortality to overall cardiovascular mortality has remained stable over the years.[5] Despite a large evidence base from randomized, controlled, clinical trials and the tremendous advances with implantable cardioverter–defibrillator (ICD) technologies shown to reduce SCD in high-risk patients, defined solely on the clinical history of prior resuscitated cardiac arrest or based on the degree of left ventricular (left ventricular) dysfunction (indexed as the LV ejection fraction [LVEF]),[6–8] there is increasing recognition that the use of these established criteria as standalone risk factors to define who will benefit from an ICD is insufficient. In this regard, many patients who qualify per current guidelines for an ICD will never experience a major arrhythmic event, thus blunting the potential benefit of ICDs and unnecessarily exposing these patients to risky and costly procedures.[9,10] In addition, the absolute number of SCDs prevented using current guidelines is small when compared to the large number of SCDs that occur in the

Cardiovascular Division, Hospital of the University of Pennsylvania, Philadelphia, PA, USA
* Corresponding author. Electrophysiology Section, Cardiovascular Division, Hospital of the University of Pennsylvania, 9 Founders Pavilion, 3400 Spruce Street, Philadelphia, PA 19104.
E-mail address: Pasquale.Santangeli@uphs.upenn.edu

Card Electrophysiol Clin 9 (2017) 749–759
http://dx.doi.org/10.1016/j.ccep.2017.08.005
1877-9182/17/Published by Elsevier Inc.

general population as the first and last manifestation of subclinical cardiac disease.[11,12] In this context, there remains an unmet need for more effective preventive and treatment strategies to reduce the morbidity and mortality of out-of-hospital cardiac arrest.[13] Survival rates with good neurologic status remain poor, averaging 8.5%. Despite early data suggesting a benefit of antiarrhythmic medications to improve survival in out-of-hospital ventricular tachycardia (VT) and ventricular fibrillation (VF) cardiac arrest that is refractory to cardiopulmonary resuscitation and defibrillation,[14,15] recent data suggest a more limited role of antiarrhythmic medications such as lidocaine or amiodarone in this context.[16]

In this article, we summarize the cumulative evidence on SCD learned from major cardiac implantable rhythm device trials, reviewing the positive and negative lessons learned from these trials and providing a critical overview of the merits and pitfalls of current SCD risk stratification methods.

ESTABLISHMENT OF IMPLANTABLE CARDIOVERTER–DEFIBRILLATOR DEVICES
Secondary Prevention Implantable Cardioverter–Defibrillator Trials

Three major randomized controlled trials, the CASH (Cardiac Arrest Study Hamburg),[17] the AVID (Antiarrhythmics versus Implantable Defibrillators) trial,[18] and the CIDS (Canadian Implantable Defibrillator Study)[19] were consistent in demonstrating a survival benefit from ICD implantation compared with antiarrhythmic drug therapy (primarily amiodarone) for survivors of life-threatening ventricular arrhythmias (**Table 1**).[17–20] The AVID study was the largest of these trials and included 1016 patients. The populations studied in these trials were fairly homogeneous, although some differences were present. In particular, CASH included only patients with previously

documented cardiac arrest owing to VF, whereas CIDS and AVID included patients with either VF or symptomatic sustained VT (and syncope with inducible VT and an LVEF <35% in CIDS). CASH compared ICD with propafenone, metoprolol, and amiodarone therapy, whereas CIDS compared ICD treatment with amiodarone, and AVID compared it with class III antiarrhythmic drugs, although amiodarone was used primarily. The combined results of these trials were summarized in an excellent metaanalysis by Connolly and colleagues.[20] After a mean duration of follow-up of 2.33 ± 1.89 years, ICD therapy was associated with a significant reduction in death from any cause compared with amiodarone (hazard ratio [HR], 0.72; 95% CI, 0.60–0.87; P = .0006). Based on these results, current guidelines give a class I indications for ICD therapy for the secondary prevention of SCD in survivors of cardiac arrest, unstable VT, and sustained VT that occurs in the setting of structural heart disease, either stable or unstable.[21] However, it is important to emphasize that, in these trials, the treatment effect with ICD therapy was not homogeneous across all the subgroups of patients. In particular, subgroup analyses showed that the survival benefit from ICD therapy was largely driven by a positive effect in patients with severe LV dysfunction (LVEF ≤35%), whereas no conclusive benefit was found for patients with an LVEF of greater than 35%.[20,22] Although this heterogeneous treatment effect did not translate in specific treatment recommendations by device guidelines, it constituted one of the major drivers for further clinical studies testing ICDs in broader primary prevention populations.

Primary Prevention Implantable Cardioverter–Defibrillator Trials

Table 2 shows a summary of major primary prevention ICD trials. The first randomized study that tested the ICD in primary prevention of SCD was

Table 1
Clinical trials evaluating implantable cardioverter–defibrillators for the secondary prevention of sudden cardiac death

Study[Ref#]	Year	No. of Patients	Medical Treatment	Clinical Presentation for Inclusion	Follow-up (mo)
AVID[18]	1997	1016	Amiodarone/sotalol	Cardiac arrest, VF, VT	18
CASH[17]	2000	191	Amiodarone/propafenone/ metoprolol	Cardiac arrest, VF	54
CIDS[19]	2000	659	Amiodarone	Cardiac arrest, VF, VT, syncope	36

Abbreviations: AVID, The Antiarrhythmics versus Implantable Defibrillators; CASH, Cardiac Arrest Study Hamburg; CIDS, Canadian Implantable Defibrillator Study; VF, ventricular fibrillation; VT, ventricular tachycardia.
   Follow-up represents mean value.

Table 2
Summary of major randomized trials evaluating ICD implantation for the primary prevention of sudden cardiac death

Characteristics	MADIT-I[7]	MADIT-II[8]	DINAMIT[37]	DEFINITE[25]	SCD-HeFT[6]	IRIS[38]	DANISH[23]
Year	1996	2002	2004	2004	2005	2009	2016
Design of the trial	ICD vs Medical Rx	ICD vs Medical Rx	ICD vs Medical Rx	ICD vs Medical Rx	ICD vs amiodarone vs Medical Rx	ICD vs Medical Rx	ICD vs Medical Rx
Clinical scenario	LVEF ≤35%, prior MI, NSVT, inducible nonsuppressible VT at PES	LVEF ≤30%, prior MI	LVEF ≤35%, recent MI, depressed HRV	LVEF <36%, nonischemic etiology, PVCs or NSVT	LVEF ≤35%, prior MI and nonischemic etiology	LVEF ≤40%, recent MI, HR ≥90 bpm, NSVT	LVEF ≤35%, nonischemic etiology
Number of patients	196	1232	674	458	2521	898	556
Primary endpoint	Total mortality	Total mortality	Total mortality	Total mortality	Total mortality	Total mortality	Total mortality
Intent-to-treat analysis	Yes	Yes	Yes	Yes	Yes	Yes	Yes
Events committee	Blinded	Blinded	Blinded	Blinded	Blinded	Blinded	Blinded
ICD type	Transvenous	Transvenous	Transvenous	Transvenous	Transvenous	Transvenous	Transvenous
ICD programming	Discretional	Discretional	ATP/shock for VT ≥175 bpm; shock for VF ≥200 bpm	Shock only for VF ≥ 80 bpm	Shock only for VF ≥187 bpm	Shock only for VF ≥200 bpm	Discretional (≥2 zones recommended)
Industry sponsorship	Guidant	Guidant	St. Jude Medical	St. Jude Medical	Medtronic, Wyeth-Ayerst, Knoll	Medtronic, Astra-Zeneca	Medtronic, St. Jude Medical

Abbreviations: ATP, anti-tachycardia pacing; DANISH, Danish ICD study; DEFINITE, Defibrillators in Non-Ischemic Cardiomyopathy Treatment Evaluation; DINAMIT, Defibrillator in Acute Myocardial Infarction trial; HR, heart rate; HRV, heart rate variability; ICD, implantable cardioverter-defibrillator; IRIS, Immediate Risk Stratification Improves Survival; LVEF, left ventricular ejection fraction; MADIT, Multicenter Automatic Defibrillator Implantation trial; Medical Rx, standard medical therapy; MI, myocardial infarction; NS, nonsustained; PES, programmed electrical stimulation; PVCs, premature ventricular complexes; SCD-HeFT, Sudden Cardiac Death in Heart Failure trial; VF, ventricular fibrillation; VT, ventricular tachycardia.

the MADIT I trial (Multicenter Automatic Defibrillator Implantation Trial).[7] Inclusion criteria were an LVEF of less than 35% and prior myocardial infarction with inducible sustained VT not suppressed after the intravenous administration of procainamide (or an equivalent intravenous antiarrhythmic agent if the patient had had a previous reaction to procainamide) according to a prespecified protocol. In the MADIT I trial, 196 patients were randomized to ICD or antiarrhythmic therapy, which consisted mainly of amiodarone. At the 5-year follow-up, there was a 23% reduction in total, all-cause mortality for patients treated with an ICD. The encouraging results of the MADIT I led to the MADIT II. This trial was designed specifically to evaluate the prophylactic benefit of ICD implantation in patients with coronary artery disease and an LVEF of 30% or less who had had at least 1 myocardial infarction; there was no further risk stratification.[8] The study enrolled 1232 patients and demonstrated a 31% reduction in overall mortality compared with conventional therapy over an average follow-up period of 2 years.

Based on the pooled results of the 2 MADIT trials, a class I indication for prophylactic (primary prevention) ICD implantation was given for patients with an ischemic cardiomyopathy and an LVEF of 30% or less. This indication was further extended in 2006 after the publication of the SCD-HeFT trial (Sudden Cardiac Death in Heart Failure Trial), the largest primary prevention ICD trial to date.[6] SCD-HeFT enrolled 2521 patients with class II or III chronic, stable heart failure (52% ischemic and 48% nonischemic) and an LVEF of less than 35%, again with no further risk stratification. Patients were randomized to conventional therapy, amiodarone, or ICD implantation. ICD therapy reduced all-cause mortality compared with placebo (from 29% to 22% at 45 months; $P = .007$). On these premises, current guidelines recommend the implantation of an ICD in all patients with an LVEF of 35% or less, regardless of further risk stratification.[21]

Although the evidence supporting ICD implantation in patients with ischemic cardiomyopathy was consistent across the different trials, the benefit of prophylactic ICD therapy in patients with nonischemic cardiomyopathy is far from conclusive, because it was largely derived from a subgroup analysis of the SCD-HeFT study, which showed only a marginal benefit associated with ICD implantation in these patients, especially those with New York Heart Association functional class II disease.[6] To further our understanding of the role of ICD therapy in nonischemic cardiomyopathy, in the recent DANISH study (Danish Study to Assess the Efficacy of ICDs in Patients with Non-ischemic Systolic Heart Failure on Mortality), 556 patients with symptomatic nonischemic symptomatic heart failure and an LVEF of 35% or less were assigned to receive an ICD, and 560 patients were assigned to receive usual clinical care (control group).[23] In both groups, 58% of the patients received cardiac resynchronization therapy (CRT). After a median follow-up of 67.6 months, the primary outcome of death from any cause occurred in 120 patients (21.6%) in the ICD group and in 131 patients (23.4%) in the control group (HR, 0.87; 95% CI, 0.68–1.12; $P = .28$). The secondary outcome of SCD occurred in 24 patients (4.3%) in the ICD group and in 46 patients (8.2%) in the control group (HR, 0.50; 95% CI, 0.31–0.82; $P = .005$). The authors concluded that primary prevention ICD implantation in patients with nonischemic cardiomyopathy was not associated with a significantly lower long-term rate of death from any cause than was usual clinical care. These results, although unanticipated, were largely in line with prior smaller ICD trials specifically focused on patients with nonischemic cardiomyopathy, such as the CAT trial (Cardiomyopathy Trial)[24] and the DEFINITE trial (Defibrillators in Non-Ischemic Cardiomyopathy Treatment Evaluation).[25] There were at least 2 unique aspects of the DANISH study to explain the neutral result. First, although a metaanalysis of 5 trials in this area showed a 31% reduction in mortality with a control mortality of 7%, in DANISH the mortality in controls was only 3% to 4%.[26] Furthermore, there was a high use of CRT in DANISH (>90% use in left bundle branch block with a QRS duration of ≥150 ms) that likely had a large effect on the outcome by decreasing both overall mortality and the chance that the addition of ICD capability to contribute further. Of note, in the large COMPANION study (Comparison of Medical Therapy, Pacing, and Defibrillation in Heart Failure), the degree of benefit to decrease the primary endpoint of death or hospitalization for heart failure was the same in the CRT-pacemaker and CRT-defibrillator groups (18%) demonstrating the huge benefit of CRT.[27] Other considerations in DANISH deserve mention. In DANISH, as in SCD-HeFT, the survival curves separate at 5 years, suggesting that benefit may be delayed. However, despite the median follow-up in DANISH being more than 5 years, ICD therapy still did not improve survival. Because death rates in nonischemic cardiomyopathy are lower than with ischemic cardiomyopathy, showing a benefit with ICD therapy is more difficult. Finally, guideline-directed medical therapy was outstanding in DANISH, further decreasing the control mortality rate.

THE NEGATIVE LESSONS
Use of Implantable Cardioverter–Defibrillators: Current Trends

Data on use trends and appropriateness of ICD therapy derive from large observational studies or voluntary registries. These studies are affected by substantial limitations related to the quality of data collection and reporting, as well as the lack of appropriate adjustments for clinical features that are not captured in the data collection process. On these premises, available analyses of ICD use rates based on current recommendations have provided mixed results, with evidence of both underuse in potentially eligible patients,[28–30] and possible inappropriate use outside the current guideline recommendations.[31] Evidence for underuse of ICDs for the primary prevention of SCD stems from observational studies showing an overall use rates ranging from 20% to 40% in potentially eligible patients.[28–30] Only a small number of hospitals across the United States have ICD implantation rates of greater than 50% for eligible patients.[30] In contrast, there is also evidence from national insurer registries of possible overuse of ICDs.[31] In this regard, it should be emphasized that the "appropriateness" of a given therapy, including ICD, does not necessarily reflect reimbursement criteria advanced by Medicare and other insurers. Notwithstanding the limitations inherent to these studies, the heterogeneous trends in use of ICD therapy largely reflect the inability of current guideline criteria, which base ICD recommendations primarily on the degree of LV dysfunction, to reliably identify subjects at risk of SCD who may actually benefit from ICD therapy.

Performance of Left Ventricular Ejection Fraction as a Risk Stratification Tool

The results of the 2 MADIT trials and the SCD-HeFT drove the enthusiasm to use LVEF as the only risk factor to identify high-risk patients most likely to benefit from a prophylactic ICD. However, the hypothesis tested in ICD trials was that ICD therapy would be better than conventional therapy in preventing sudden death in a high-risk population; no ICD trial was truly designed as a risk stratification trial. To use any risk stratification test logically, one should be able to demonstrate a causal relationship between the test and SCD. However, a direct "causal" link between LV dysfunction and SCD has never been proven. As mentioned, when SCD is measured in absolute number of events per year, only a minority of events occur in high-risk subgroups studied in clinical trials (**Fig. 1**).[11]

In the ATRAMI study (Autonomic Tone and Reflexes After Myocardial Infarction), La Rovere and colleagues[32] prospectively studied the predictive role of autonomic markers such as heart rate variability and baroreflex sensitivity in patients after myocardial infarction. The study enrolled 1284 patients with a recent myocardial infarction, of whom 49 died suddenly during a mean follow-up of 21 months. Of these, only 22 (44%) had an LVEF of 35% or less, thus

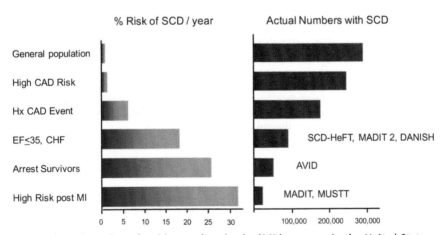

Fig. 1. Incidence and total number of sudden cardiac deaths (SCD) per year in the United States according to different populations of patients. AVID, Antiarrhythmics versus Implantable Defibrillators; CAD, coronary artery disease; CHF, congestive heart failure; DANISH, Danish ICD Study in Patients with Dilated Cardiomyopathy; EF, ejection fraction; Hx, history; MADIT, Multicenter Automatic Defibrillator Implantation trial; MI, myocardial infarction; MUSTT, Multicenter Unsustained Tachycardia Trial; SCD-HeFT, Sudden Cardiac Death in Heart Failure trial. (*Modified from* Myerburg RJ, Kessler KM, Castellanos A. Sudden cardiac death: epidemiology, transient risk, and intervention assessment. Ann Intern Med 1993;119:1187–97.)

suggesting a low sensitivity of LVEF alone to predict SCD. In fact, in ATRAMI, LVEF was significantly associated with major arrhythmic events only when associated with evidence of cardiac autonomic dysfunction. The poor sensitivity of LVEF in predicting SCD was further supported by subsequent data from the Maastricht Circulatory Arrest Registry, which is one of the largest SCD registry to date.[33] Data were collected in the wide Maastricht area, including more than 180,000 inhabitants, during a 4-year period. A total of 492 SCD victims were included, of whom 224 (46%) had a previously known history of cardiac disease and 200 had echocardiographic data on LVEF. Although an increase in SCD was evident at lower LVEFs, indicating a higher risk with worsening LV function, no clinically significant difference in risk of SCD was observed between patients with a severely depressed LVEF ($\leq$30%) compared with those with a moderately depressed LVEF ($\leq$40%), with an incidence of SCD of 7.5% versus 5.1%, respectively. As expected, the absolute number of SCD victims was highest in the normal LVEF category. Also in the subgroup of patients with ischemic heart disease, LVEF was not a good predictor of SCD. Indeed, data on LVEF of 52 SCD cases with coronary artery disease showed that only 25 (48%) of these had an LVEF of 30% or less, with more than 30% actually showing an LVEF of greater than 40% (**Table 3**). Based on this evidence, the sensitivity of LVEF in predicting SCD seems to be less than optimal, and any SCD risk stratification based on LVEF only implies that a substantial proportion of subjects who will die suddenly will not be identified.

With regard to the specificity of LVEF in identifying patients at risk of SCD, data from subgroup analyses of large randomized trials would also suggest an inadequate specificity of LVEF in predicting SCD. Analyzing data from the MUSTT trial (Multicenter Unsustained Tachycardia Trial), Buxton and colleagues[34] assessed the relation of EF to mode of death in 1791 patients with coronary artery disease. Although a low LVEF was associated with higher mortality, the degree of LV dysfunction did not predict the mode of death, because approximately one-half of the deaths occurred suddenly both in patients with an LVEF of less than 30% and in those with an LVEF of 30% or greater (**Fig. 2**). In a separate large observational study, Huikuri and colleagues[35] evaluated the role of different risk variables including nonsustained VT, LVEF, heart rate variability, baroreflex sensitivity, signal-averaged electrocardiogram, QT dispersion, and QRS duration in predicting SCD in a consecutive series of 700 patients with acute myocardial infarction. Over a mean follow-up of 43 $\pm$ 16 months, 22 (3.2%) SCDs and 37 (5.5%) non-SCDs occurred. Notably, the LVEF was lower in patients who died of non-SCD compared with those with SCD (average 37% vs 41%).[35] In conclusion, a low LVEF seems to lack adequate specificity in predicting SCD, because it identifies a subgroup of patients with a higher mortality, but not specifically owing to SCD.

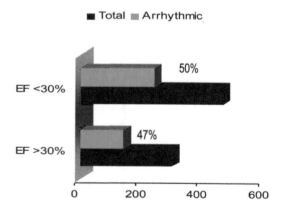

Fig. 2. Relation between left ventricular ejection fraction (EF) and mode of death in patients with coronary artery disease enrolled in the Multicenter Unsustained Tachycardia Trial (MUSTT) study. (*Data from* Buxton AE, Lee KL, Hafley GE, et al. Relation of ejection fraction and inducible ventricular tachycardia to mode of death in patients with coronary artery disease: an analysis of patients enrolled in the multicenter unsustained tachycardia trial. Circulation 2002;106:2466–72.)

Table 3		
Left ventricular ejection fraction data of 52 SCD cases with history of coronary artery disease in the Maastricht Circulatory Arrest Registry		
LVEF (%)	**n**	**SCD (%)**
0–30	25	48
31–40	10	19
41–50	7	13
>50%	10	19

Abbreviations: LVEF, left ventricular ejection fraction; SCD, sudden cardiac death.

From Gorgels AP, Gijsbers C, de Vreede-Swagemakers J, et al. Out-of-hospital cardiac arrest–the relevance of heart failure. The Maastricht Circulatory Arrest Registry. Eur Heart J 2003;24:1204–9.

Value of the Left Ventricular Ejection Fraction Compared with Other Risk Factors and Markers

Although a low LVEF has been repeatedly shown a suboptimal parameter to predict longitudinal risk of SCD, LVEF remains the most useful available tool to give an indication for prophylactic ICD implantation.[21] In fact, there is no convincing evidence that any other proposed risk factor or marker may perform better than LVEF alone in predicting subsequent SCD. Heart rate variability and other measurements of cardiac autonomic dysfunction (ie, heart rate turbulence [HRT] and baroreflex sensitivity) have been shown predictive of total and arrhythmic mortality in earlier studies conducted on patients with acute myocardial infarction.[32,36] However, since modern therapies (ie, percutaneous revascularization, beta-blockers and angiotensin-converting enzyme inhibitors) have become the standard form of treatment in myocardial infarction, there are no convincing data on whether markers of cardiac autonomic dysfunction maintain their prognostic value. In fact, prophylactic ICD therapy failed to improve survival in the DINAMIT trial (Defibrillator in Acute Myocardial Infarction Trial),[37] which included patients with a recent myocardial infarction, LV dysfunction, and depressed heart rate variability. The results of the DINAMIT study were replicated in a separate randomized trial, the IRIS trial (Immediate Risk Stratification Improves Survival), which enrolled patients with high-risk criteria early after acute myocardial infarction (ie, LVEF ≤40%, increased heart rate, and nonsustained VT),[38] and failed to show a survival benefit with prophylactic ICD therapy. Another marker of altered cardiac autonomic function, HRT, has been studied extensively as a predictor of SCD beyond LVEF. HRT is defined by instantaneous changes of heart rate induced by a premature ventricular beat, which typically consists of a brief heart rate acceleration followed by a gradual heart rate deceleration.[39] The onset and slope of the variations in heart rate are calculated to determine the HRT metric. A recent pooled analysis of studies evaluating the role of HRT in predicting SCD showed HRT to be particularly useful in postinfarct patients with an LVEF of greater than 30%.[39]

Another promising noninvasive risk marker that may add value to LVEF alone is T-wave alternans, which is directly linked to cellular arrhythmia mechanisms arising from abnormal calcium cycling. Several studies have reported that patients with reduced LVEF and negative T-wave alternans are at considerable lower risk of SCD, although such data have not been consistently replicated and larger randomized trials are warranted to verify these findings.[40]

Implantable Cardioverter–Defibrillator Therapy in Underrepresented Subgroups and Role of Comorbidities

When analyzing the baseline clinical features of patients included in major randomized trials of ICD therapy, it becomes evident that important subgroups of patients have been largely underrepresented in these trials. These underrepresented subgroups include women, elderly patients (aged >75 years), non-white patients, and patients with frailty and/or a high burden of associated comorbidities, such as advanced renal failure. The extent to which the results of major trials can be extrapolated to underrepresented subgroups of patients remains incompletely defined.

In this regard, studies investigating the presence of gender differences in the benefit of prophylactic ICD therapy have reported mixed results.[41–44] A metaanalysis of primary prevention ICD studies focused on the endpoints of total mortality, appropriate ICD therapies (defined as interventions on sustained VT or VF), and net ICD survival benefit in women compared with men.[45] The pooled analysis included a total of 7229 patients with severe LV dysfunction (74% with ischemic cardiomyopathy). Women constituted 23% of the total patient population, and suffered from more advanced forms of congestive heart failure and more comorbidities. Quantitative data synthesis, adjusted for baseline confounders and covariates, showed no difference in overall mortality in women compared with men (HR, 0.96; 95% CI, 0.67–1.39; $P = .84$), and significantly fewer appropriate ICD therapies in women (HR, 0.63; 95% CI, 0.49–0.82; $P<.001$; **Fig. 3**). These data strongly suggest significant gender differences in arrhythmic risk associated with severe LV dysfunction, supporting the concept that SCD may have a smaller impact on total mortality in women with such a disease condition.[45]

Similarly, to date there is no consistent evidence supporting a conclusive benefit of ICD therapy in elderly patients with severe LV dysfunction.[26,28,46–48] In primary prevention ICD trials, the mean age of enrolled patients was in the mid-60 year range, with more than 50% actually having an age of less than 60 years.[6,8,25,37,49] In contrast, in real-world practice, nearly 70% of ICDs are implanted in patients greater than 60 years old, with more than 40% in patients greater than 70 years old.[50] A primary prevention indication accounts for two-thirds of such devices.

Gender Differences in ICD Survival Benefit

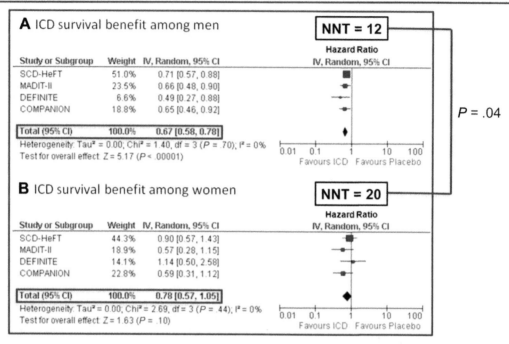

Fig. 3. Evidence for gender-specific differences in the benefit of implantable cardioverter–defibrillator (ICD) therapy. Compared with standard medical therapy (labeled as "placebo" in the Forest plot), ICD are associated with a significant reduction in all-cause mortality only in men (A) compared with women (B). COMPANION, Comparison of Medical Therapy, Pacing, and Defibrillation in Heart Failure; DEFINITE, Defibrillators in Non-Ischemic Cardiomyopathy Treatment Evaluation; HR, hazard ratio; MADIT, Multicenter Automatic Defibrillator Implantation trial; NNT, number needed to treat to prevent 1 death event; SCD-HeFT, Sudden Cardiac Death in Heart Failure trial. (*From* Santangeli P, Pelargonio G, Dello Russo A, et al. Gender differences in clinical outcome and primary prevention defibrillator benefit in patients with severe left ventricular dysfunction: a systematic review and meta-analysis. Heart Rhythm 2010;7:876–82.)

In a pooled analysis of randomized controlled trials, Santangeli and colleagues[51] included data from 5 trials (MADIT-II, DEFINITE, DINAMIT, SCD-HeFT, and IRIS) with a total of 5783 patients (44% elderly, defined as age >65 years). The primary analysis, which excluded the 2 trials enrolling patients early after acute myocardial infarction (DINAMIT and IRIS), found that prophylactic ICD therapy reduced mortality in younger patients (HR, 0.65; 95% CI, 0.50–0.83; P<.001). A smaller survival benefit was found in elderly patients (HR, 0.75; 95% CI, 0.61–0.91) that was not confirmed when MADIT-II patients older than 70 years were excluded or when data from DINAMIT and IRIS were included. Therefore, based on data from major device trials, prophylactic ICD therapy may be less beneficial for elderly patients with severe LV dysfunction compared with younger patients. As mentioned, these results

are in keeping with the recent subgroup analysis from the DANISH study that, despite not meeting the primary endpoint in the overall study cohort, showed a possible interaction between age and the benefit of ICD therapy in patients with nonischemic heart failure.[23]

Patients with severe LV dysfunction typically also present associated comorbidities (diabetes, peripheral arterial disease, chronic kidney disease) that may impact non-SCD mortality, thus potentially diminishing the benefit of ICD therapy. In the MADIT II study, the number of ICDs needed to prevent one death was nearly 40% higher in patients with diabetes compared with patients without diabetes (15 vs 11 ICDs, respectively).[52] Similar data arise from large observational studies on the role of ICD therapy in patients with significant renal dysfunction,[53,54] with a substantial increase in the risk of all-cause mortality proportional to the severity of the underlying kidney dysfunction. In these patients, a greater burden of nonarrhythmic mortality owing to associated comorbidities may negate a mortality benefit with ICD therapy.[55]

SUMMARY

Multiple randomized, controlled trials have unequivocally demonstrated that ICDs are highly effective in preventing SCD. In patients who have already suffered a cardiac arrest, there is consistent evidence supporting a benefit of ICD implantation to reduce mortality owing to recurrent cardiac arrest events. Thus far, the degree of LV dysfunction is the only parameter shown to identify primary prevention populations at higher risk of SCD, in which prophylactic implantation of ICDs may reduce the longitudinal risk of mortality. However, the clinical application of the current risk stratification approaches based on LVEF alone has failed to prevent the majority of SCD in the general population. Furthermore, the lack of specificity of LVEF for SCD has resulted in a significant number of potentially unnecessary ICD implants. Future cardiac implantable device studies should be focused on the discovery and validation of newer arrhythmic risk markers, to improve the predictive value of LVEF alone and improve SCD prevention in the general population.

REFERENCES

1. Zheng ZJ, Croft JB, Giles WH, et al. Sudden cardiac death in the United States, 1989 to 1998. Circulation 2001;104:2158–63.
2. Ford ES, Ajani UA, Croft JB, et al. Explaining the decrease in U.S. deaths from coronary disease, 1980-2000. N Engl J Med 2007;356:2388–98.
3. Ford ES, Capewell S. Proportion of the decline in cardiovascular mortality disease due to prevention versus treatment: public health versus clinical care. Annu Rev Public Health 2011;32:5–22.
4. Nabel EG, Braunwald E. A tale of coronary artery disease and myocardial infarction. N Engl J Med 2012;366:54–63.
5. Chugh SS, Reinier K, Teodorescu C, et al. Epidemiology of sudden cardiac death: clinical and research implications. Prog Cardiovasc Dis 2008; 51:213–28.
6. Bardy GH, Lee KL, Mark DB, et al. Amiodarone or an implantable cardioverter-defibrillator for congestive heart failure. N Engl J Med 2005;352:225–37.
7. Moss AJ, Hall WJ, Cannom DS, et al. Improved survival with an implanted defibrillator in patients with coronary disease at high risk for ventricular arrhythmia. Multicenter Automatic Defibrillator

8. Moss AJ, Zareba W, Hall WJ, et al. Prophylactic implantation of a defibrillator in patients with myocardial infarction and reduced ejection fraction. N Engl J Med 2002;346:877–83.
9. Tung R, Zimetbaum P, Josephson ME. A critical appraisal of implantable cardioverter-defibrillator therapy for the prevention of sudden cardiac death. J Am Coll Cardiol 2008;52:1111–21.
10. Germano JJ, Reynolds M, Essebag V, et al. Frequency and causes of implantable cardioverter-defibrillator therapies: is device therapy proarrhythmic? Am J Cardiol 2006;97:1255–61.
11. Myerburg RJ, Kessler KM, Castellanos A. Sudden cardiac death: epidemiology, transient risk, and intervention assessment. Ann Intern Med 1993;119: 1187–97.
12. Myerburg RJ. Sudden cardiac death: exploring the limits of our knowledge. J Cardiovasc Electrophysiol 2001;12:369–81.
13. Deo R, Epstein AE. Moving further upstream in the prevention of cardiac arrest and its complications. J Am Coll Cardiol 2016;67:1991–3.
14. Kudenchuk PJ, Cobb LA, Copass MK, et al. Amiodarone for resuscitation after out-of-hospital cardiac arrest due to ventricular fibrillation. N Engl J Med 1999;341:871–8.
15. Dorian P, Cass D, Schwartz B, et al. Amiodarone as compared with lidocaine for shock-resistant ventricular fibrillation. N Engl J Med 2002;346:884–90.
16. Kudenchuk PJ, Brown SP, Daya M, et al. Amiodarone, lidocaine, or placebo in out-of-hospital cardiac arrest. N Engl J Med 2016;374:1711–22.
17. Kuck KH, Cappato R, Siebels J, et al. Randomized comparison of antiarrhythmic drug therapy with implantable defibrillators in patients resuscitated from cardiac arrest : the Cardiac Arrest Study Hamburg (CASH). Circulation 2000;102:748–54.
18. The Antiarrhythmics versus Implantable Defibrillators (AVID) Investigators. A comparison of antiarrhythmic-drug therapy with implantable defibrillators in patients resuscitated from near-fatal ventricular arrhythmias. N Engl J Med 1997;337: 1576–83.
19. Connolly SJ, Gent M, Roberts RS, et al. Canadian implantable defibrillator study (CIDS): a randomized trial of the implantable cardioverter defibrillator against amiodarone. Circulation 2000;101: 1297–302.
20. Connolly SJ, Hallstrom AP, Cappato R, et al. Meta-analysis of the implantable cardioverter defibrillator secondary prevention trials. AVID, CASH and CIDS studies. Antiarrhythmics vs Implantable Defibrillator Study. Cardiac Arrest Study Hamburg. Canadian Implantable Defibrillator Study. Eur Heart J 2000; 21:2071–8.

Implantation Trial Investigators. N Engl J Med 1996;335:1933–40.

21. Epstein AE, DiMarco JP, Ellenbogen KA, et al. ACC/AHA/HRS 2008 guidelines for device-based therapy of cardiac rhythm abnormalities: a report of the American College of Cardiology/American Heart Association Task Force on practice guidelines (writing committee to revise the ACC/AHA/NASPE 2002 guideline update for implantation of cardiac pacemakers and antiarrhythmia devices): developed in collaboration with the American Association for Thoracic Surgery and Society of Thoracic Surgeons. Circulation 2008;117:e350–408.

22. Domanski MJ, Sakseena S, Epstein AE, et al. Relative effectiveness of the implantable cardioverter-defibrillator and antiarrhythmic drugs in patients with varying degrees of left ventricular dysfunction who have survived malignant ventricular arrhythmias. AVID Investigators. Antiarrhythmics versus implantable defibrillators. J Am Coll Cardiol 1999; 34:1090–5.

23. Kober L, Thune JJ, Nielsen JC, et al. Defibrillator implantation in patients with nonischemic systolic heart failure. N Engl J Med 2016;375:1221–30.

24. Bansch D, Antz M, Boczor S, et al. Primary prevention of sudden cardiac death in idiopathic dilated cardiomyopathy: the Cardiomyopathy Trial (CAT). Circulation 2002;105:1453–8.

25. Kadish A, Dyer A, Daubert JP, et al. Prophylactic defibrillator implantation in patients with nonischemic dilated cardiomyopathy. N Engl J Med 2004; 350:2151–8.

26. Desai AS, Fang JC, Maisel WH, et al. Implantable defibrillators for the prevention of mortality in patients with nonischemic cardiomyopathy: a meta-analysis of randomized controlled trials. JAMA 2004;292:2874–9.

27. Bristow MR, Saxon LA, Boehmer J, et al. Cardiac-resynchronization therapy with or without an implantable defibrillator in advanced chronic heart failure. N Engl J Med 2004;350:2140–50.

28. Curtis LH, Al-Khatib SM, Shea AM, et al. Sex differences in the use of implantable cardioverter-defibrillators for primary and secondary prevention of sudden cardiac death. JAMA 2007;298: 1517–24.

29. Hernandez AF, Fonarow GC, Liang L, et al. Sex and racial differences in the use of implantable cardioverter-defibrillators among patients hospitalized with heart failure. JAMA 2007;298:1525–32.

30. Shah B, Hernandez AF, Liang L, et al, Get With The Guidelines Steering Committee. Hospital variation and characteristics of implantable cardioverter-defibrillator use in patients with heart failure: data from the GWTG-HF (Get with the Guidelines-Heart Failure) registry. J Am Coll Cardiol 2009;53:416–22.

31. Al-Khatib SM, Hellkamp A, Curtis J, et al. Non-evidence-based ICD implantations in the United States. JAMA 2011;305:43–9.

32. La Rovere MT, Bigger JT Jr, Marcus FI, et al. Baroreflex sensitivity and heart-rate variability in prediction of total cardiac mortality after myocardial infarction. ATRAMI (autonomic tone and reflexes after myocardial infarction) Investigators. Lancet 1998;351:478–84.

33. Gorgels AP, Gijsbers C, de Vreede-Swagemakers J, et al. Out-of-hospital cardiac arrest–the relevance of heart failure. The Maastricht Circulatory Arrest Registry. Eur Heart J 2003;24:1204–9.

34. Buxton AE, Lee KL, Hafley GE, et al. Relation of ejection fraction and inducible ventricular tachycardia to mode of death in patients with coronary artery disease: an analysis of patients enrolled in the multicenter unsustained tachycardia trial. Circulation 2002;106:2466–72.

35. Huikuri HV, Tapanainen JM, Lindgren K, et al. Prediction of sudden cardiac death after myocardial infarction in the beta-blocking era. J Am Coll Cardiol 2003;42:652–8.

36. Ghuran A, Reid F, La Rovere MT, et al. Heart rate turbulence-based predictors of fatal and nonfatal cardiac arrest (The autonomic tone and reflexes after myocardial infarction substudy). Am J Cardiol 2002;89:184–90.

37. Hohnloser SH, Kuck KH, Dorian P, et al. Prophylactic use of an implantable cardioverter-defibrillator after acute myocardial infarction. N Engl J Med 2004; 351:2481–8.

38. Steinbeck G, Andresen D, Seidl K, et al. Defibrillator implantation early after myocardial infarction. N Engl J Med 2009;361:1427–36.

39. Disertori M, Mase M, Rigoni M, et al. Heart rate turbulence is a powerful predictor of cardiac death and ventricular arrhythmias in postmyocardial infarction and heart failure patients: a systematic review and meta-analysis. Circ Arrhythm Electrophysiol 2016;9 [pii:e004610].

40. De Ferrari GM, Sanzo A. T-wave alternans in risk stratification of patients with nonischemic dilated cardiomyopathy: can it help to better select candidates for ICD implantation? Heart Rhythm 2009;6: S29–35.

41. Russo AM, Day JD, Stolen K, et al. Implantable cardioverter defibrillators: do women fare worse than men? Gender comparison in the INTRINSIC RV trial. J Cardiovasc Electrophysiol 2009;20:973–8.

42. Russo AM, Poole JE, Mark DB, et al. Primary prevention with defibrillator therapy in women: results from the sudden cardiac death in heart failure trial. J Cardiovasc Electrophysiol 2008;19:720–4.

43. Russo AM, Stamato NJ, Lehmann MH, et al. Influence of gender on arrhythmia characteristics and outcome in the multicenter UnSustained tachycardia trial. J Cardiovasc Electrophysiol 2004;15:993–8.

44. Zareba W, Moss AJ, Jackson Hall W, et al. Clinical course and implantable cardioverter defibrillator

therapy in postinfarction women with severe left ventricular dysfunction. J Cardiovasc Electrophysiol 2005;16:1265–70.

45. Santangeli P, Pelargonio G, Dello Russo A, et al. Gender differences in clinical outcome and primary prevention defibrillator benefit in patients with severe left ventricular dysfunction: a systematic review and meta-analysis. Heart Rhythm 2010;7:876–82.

46. DerSimonian R, Laird N. Meta-analysis in clinical trials. Control Clin Trials 1986;7:177–88.

47. Duray G, Richter S, Manegold J, et al. Efficacy and safety of ICD therapy in a population of elderly patients treated with optimal background medication. J Interv Card Electrophysiol 2005;14: 169–73.

48. Drici MD, Burklow TR, Haridasse V, et al. Sex hormones prolong the QT interval and downregulate potassium channel expression in the rabbit heart. Circulation 1996;94:1471–4.

49. Cochrane Handbook for systematic reviews of interventions, Version 5.1.0. The Cochrane Collaboration, 2017. Available at: http://handbook-5-1.cochrane.org. Accessed September 1, 2017.

50. Buxton AE, Lee KL, Hafley GE, et al. Limitations of ejection fraction for prediction of sudden death risk in patients with coronary artery disease: lessons from the MUSTT study. J Am Coll Cardiol 2007;50: 1150–7.

51. Santangeli P, Di Biase L, Dello Russo A, et al. Meta-analysis: age and effectiveness of prophylactic implantable cardioverter-defibrillators. Ann Intern Med 2010;153:592–9.

52. Wittenberg SM, Cook JR, Hall WJ, et al. Comparison of efficacy of implanted cardioverter-defibrillator in patients with versus without diabetes mellitus. Am J Cardiol 2005;96:417–9.

53. Bogdan S, Nof E, Eisen A, et al. Clinical outcomes in patients with severe renal dysfunction including dialysis following defibrillator implantation. Am J Nephrol 2015;42:295–304.

54. Hess PL, Hellkamp AS, Peterson ED, et al. Survival after primary prevention implantable cardioverter-defibrillator placement among patients with chronic kidney disease. Circ Arrhythm Electrophysiol 2014; 7:793–9.

55. Steinberg BA, Al-Khatib SM, Edwards R, et al. Outcomes of implantable cardioverter-defibrillator use in patients with comorbidities: results from a combined analysis of 4 randomized clinical trials. JACC Heart Fail 2014;2:623–9.

Primary Prevention Implantable Cardiac Defibrillator Trials
What Have We Learned?

Jakub Sroubek, MD, PhD, Alfred E. Buxton, MD*

KEYWORDS

- ICD • Primary prevention • Sudden cardiac death • Ischemic cardiomyopathy
- Nonischemic cardiomyopathy

KEY POINTS

- To date, a total of nine randomized controlled primary prevention ICD trials have been published and support the notion that patients with reduced left ventricular systolic function derive net mortality benefit from ICD therapy.
- However, this benefit is not uniformly distributed. ICDs most consistently improve outcomes in individuals with ischemic heart disease, who are greater than or equal to 40 days post acute MI.
- The role of ICDs in other patients, including those with nonischemic cardiomyopathies, is much less certain. In some individuals, ICDs may lower the rate of arrhythmic deaths at the price of disproportionately increasing the number of nonarrhythmic deaths.
- Current guidelines are inadequate for selection of appropriate ICD candidates, because risk stratification is not used. Although there are many ways of predicting all-cause mortality, specific assessment of arrhythmic sudden cardiac death risk remains a challenge.

INTRODUCTION

Reduced left-ventricular systolic function (generally meaning an ejection fraction [EF] ≤40%) is found in a heterogenous group of disorders. In general, reduced EF is associated with increased mortality, regardless of the underlying anatomic substrate. Although many deaths in cardiomyopathy patients are "expected" and are attributed to a clinically well-delineated process, such as progressive pump-failure or myocardial ischemia, numerous cardiomyopathy deaths are unexpected and sudden. These sudden cardiac deaths (SCDs) have traditionally been thought to be a consequence of ventricular tachyarrhythmias, arrhythmias known to be highly prevalent in this patient population.

Until three decades ago, limited efforts could be made to address out-of-hospital ventricular arrhythmias, either by directly attempting to prevent the arrhythmias (eg, using antiarrhythmic medications or surgical ablation) or indirectly by treating the underlying disorders (eg, through treatment of the underlying cardiac disorders using heart failure medical regimens or revascularization). The introduction of the implantable cardiac defibrillator (ICD) in the 1980s meant that ventricular arrhythmias could be treated effectively as they occurred with high probability of preventing cardiac arrest.

Disclosure Statement: Dr A.E. Buxton has research grants from Medtronic and Biosense-Webster.
Cardiovascular Division, Department of Medicine, Clinical Electrophysiology Laboratory, Beth Israel Deaconess Medical Center, Harvard Medical School, Baker 4, 185 Pilgrim Road, Boston, MA 02215, USA
* Corresponding author.
E-mail address: abuxton@bidmc.harvard.edu

cardiacEP.theclinics.com

Subsequent decades of experience with these devices have demonstrated that the ICD can reduce (but not eliminate) risk of SCD and total mortality, in selected patient groups. As a result of technological evolution, the ICD has matured from a bulky, experimental device to one of the mainstays in the ever-expanding armamentarium of contemporary cardiomyopathy treatments.

Despite the perceived benefit that the introduction of the ICD has had for many patients, these devices are not a risk-free panacea suitable for each and every individual with left ventricular (LV) dysfunction. Although the role of ICDs in secondary SCD prevention[1] is well-established and rarely challenged, their appropriate place in primary SCD prevention strategies is much less clear. Identifying the right individuals who will benefit from a primary prevention device, and pinpointing the proper timing of ICD implantation, remains a challenge.

To date, nine large, randomized trials have examined the utility of primary prevention ICDs in patients with either ischemic cardiomyopathy[2–8] or nonischemic cardiomyopathy (NICM)[7,9,10] with reduced LVEF (**Tables 1–3**). They have raised as many questions as they have provided answers. Awareness of the results of these pivotal studies and the controversies that they have provoked is therefore important for any electrophysiologist seeking to provide optimal, individualized care for patients with cardiomyopathy. Before discussing each of these trials in detail, it is worth summarizing the key conclusions that are drawn from the literature as a whole:

- Overall, the use of ICDs reduces all-cause mortality in patients with reduced LVEF.
- Not all patients with reduced LVEF derive equal benefit from ICDs.
- The greatest mortality benefit is seen in patients with infarct-related cardiomyopathy.
- That said, this benefit is only seen if ICDs are implanted greater than or equal to 40 days after index myocardial infarction (MI).
- Earlier ICD implantation in these patients may not be helpful or may actually cause harm.
- The least mortality benefit is seen in patients with NICM with reduced LVEF, presumably because of the lower incidence of sustained, life-threatening ventricular arrhythmias in this population.
- Reduced LVEF is currently the prime benchmark in societal guidelines for ICD use because it was used as the central entry criterion for all relevant clinical trials; however, low LVEF is primarily associated with increased all-cause mortality and has no direct physiologic link to specific arrhythmias, although it certainly modifies the rate of SCD.

PRIMARY PREVENTION IMPLANTABLE CARDIOVERTER-DEFIBRILLATORS IN ISCHEMIC CARDIOMYOPATHY, 1990s

In the 1970s and 1980s, the understanding of mortality in patients with ischemic cardiomyopathy was derived from several key observations, reflected in the Multicenter Post Infraction Research Group (MPRG) study.[11] First, it was well established that survivors of acute MI had a very high overall out-of-hospital mortality rate. Second, it was recognized that many post-MI deaths were sudden (ie, SCDs) and therefore presumed caused by ventricular arrhythmias. Third, certain high-risk clinical features, such as low LVEF or frequent ventricular ectopy, portended worse prognosis. However, it should be said that there was insufficient evidence to parse out which of these risk factors were specific predictors of SCD risk as opposed to being mere markers of increased overall mortality.

These observations generated several questions: Can ICDs reduce the rate of SCD in post-MI patients? If so, would a lower SCD rate translate into lower all-cause mortality? Will this benefit be generalizable to the entire post-MI population or do we need to develop some sort of a risk stratification algorithm to identify a subset of individuals where ICDs are most cost-effective? Is there a reasonable alternative to ICDs, such as antiarrhythmic drugs (AADs)? This last question was particularly relevant because early ICDs (1980–1994) were epicardial devices that depended on surgical (thoracotomy) insertion associated with nonnegligible periprocedural risks.

The Multicenter Automatic Defibrillator Implantation Trial (MADIT-I)[2] was the first major published effort to address these questions. This study, conducted across 32 centers (mostly in the United States), enrolled MI-survivors with reduced LVEF ($\leq$35%), who had spontaneous nonsustained ventricular tachycardia (NSVT) at least 3 weeks after an index MI and who developed sustained VT/ventricular fibrillation in response to programmed electrical stimulation (PES) that was not suppressible with procainamide. These individuals were randomized to ICD therapy (n = 95) versus conventional therapy (n = 101). Although the use of AADs was not protocol-mandated in either study arm, the control group was prescribed amiodarone much more frequently (45%–75% at 1 month and trial end, respectively) than the ICD cohort (2%–7% at 1 month and trial end, respectively). During an average follow-up period of 27 months, there were 39 all-cause deaths in the control arm compared with 15 all-cause deaths in the ICD arm, yielding a hazard ratio (HR) of 0.46 (95% confidence interval [CI], 0.26–0.92; P = .009) in favor of ICD use.

Table 1
Primary prevention ICD trials, patient enrollment

Study (Publication Year)	Enrollment Period	Major Inclusion Criteria			Major Exclusion Criteria
		Major Clinical Criteria	LVEF	Major Electrophysiologic Criteria	
CABG-Patch[3] (1997)	Aug 1990–Apr 1996	Upcoming CABG (ICD implant done concurrently with CABG)	≤35%	Abnormal signal-averaged ECG	Poorly controlled diabetes Serum creatinine >3.0 mg/dL Concomitant valve surgery
MADIT-I[2] (1996)	Dec 1990–Mar 1996	MI ≥3 wk prior	≤35%	NSVT Underwent PES (at clinicians' discretion) PES positive and not suppressible by AADs	NYHA class IV CABG <2 mo prior PCI <3 mo prior
MUSTT[4] (1999)	Nov 1990–Oct 1996	Known CAD Required screening for exercise-induced ischemia and treatment, if appropriate	≤40%	NSVT PES positive	NYHA class IV
MADIT-II[5] (2002)	Jul 1997–Jan 2002	MI ≥1 mo prior	≤30%	Frequent ectopy (criterion relaxed mid-trial)	NYHA class IV Advanced cerebrovascular disease CABG/PCI <3 mo prior
DINAMIT[6] (2004)	Apr 1998–Jun 2002	MI in the last 6–40 d	≤35%	Abnormal heart rate variability ≥3 d after MI	NYHA class IV Recent or upcoming CABG Upcoming 3-vessel PCI
IRIS[8] (2009)	Jun 1999–Oct 2007	MI in the last 5–31 d	≤40%	Patients with LVEF >40% could also be enrolled if they had NSVT ≥150 bpm	NYHA class IV (if drug refractory) Indication for CABG
SCD-HeFT[7] (2005)	Sep 1997–Jul 2001	Ischemic or nonischemic cardiomyopathy	≤35%	None	NYHA class I and IV
DEFINITE[9] (2004)	Jul 1998–Jun 2002	Symptomatic, nonischemic cardiomyopathy	≤35%	Presence of NSVT or frequent PVCs	NYHA class IV EP testing in the past 3 mo
DANISH[10] (2016)	Feb 2008–Jun 2014	Symptomatic, nonischemic cardiomyopathy NYHA class IV allowed if CRT device implanted NT-proBNP >200 pg/mL	≤35%	None	End-stage renal disease on hemodialysis Permanent atrial fibrillation, resting HR >100 bpm

Abbreviations: AAD, antiarrhythmic drug; CABG, coronary artery bypass graft; CAD, coronary artery disease; CRT, cardiac resynchronization therapy; ECG, electrocardiogram; EP, electrophysiology; HR, heart rate; MI, myocardial infarction; NSVT, nonsustained ventricular tachycardia; NT-proBNP, N-terminal pro–brain natriuretic peptide; NYHA, New York Heart Association; PCI, percutaneous coronary intervention; PES, programmed electrical stimulation; PVC, premature ventricular contraction.

Table 2
Primary prevention ICD trials, patient characteristics

Study (Publication Year)	Notable Patient Characteristics	Study Arms	Follow-up	Possible Confounders
CABG-Patch[3] (1997)	Mean LVEF 27% Low ACE inhibitor use (54%–68%) Low β-blocker use (16%–24%) Low lipid-lowering drug use (8%–23%) Low AAD use (27%–37%) Frequent CHF exacerbation: Pulmonary rales (20%–25%) S3 gallop (11%–14%) High mean LV end-diastolic pressures (21–22 mm Hg)	ICD: 446 (52; 11.7% crossed over) Control: 454 (18; 4.0% crossed over)	32 mo (mean)	None Notably, rate of perioperative complications was similar in both arms
MADIT-I[2] (1996)	Mean LVEF 25%–27% Low ACE inhibitor use (5%–27%) Low β-blocker use (51%–60%) Pulmonary congestion in 18%–20%	ICD: 95 (7; 7.4% crossed over) Control: 101 (11; 10.9% crossed over)	27 mo (mean)	Amiodarone use more frequent in control group β-Blocker use more frequent in ICD group
MUSTT[4] (1999)	Median LVEF 29%–30% Intermediate ACE inhibitor use (72%–77%) Intermediate β-blocker use (29%–51%)	EP-guided AAT: 351 (103, 29% received AAD; 202, 58% received an ICD; 46, 13% crossed over) No AAT: 353 (35, 10% received AAD; 11, 3% received ICD)	39 mo (median)	β-Blocker use more frequent in no AAT group ICD implanted in 202 (58%) of EP-guided AAT patients
MADIT-II[5] (2002)	Mean LVEF 23% Intermediate ACE inhibitor use (68%–72%) Intermediate β-blocker use (70%) Intermediate lipid-lowering drug use (64%–67%)	ICD: 742 (32; 4.3% crossed over) Control: 490 (22; 4.5% crossed over)	20 mo (mean)	None
DINAMIT[6] (2004)	Mean LVEF 28% Frequent anterior MI (72.1%) Average time from MI to randomization 18 d Intermediate revascularization rate (62.0%–62.7%) High ACE inhibitor use (94.4%–94.9%) High β-blocker use (86.5%–87.0%) Intermediate lipid-lowering drug use (76.8%–79.5%)	ICD: 332 (22; 6.6% crossed over) Control: 342 (20; 5.8% crossed over)	30 mo (mean)	Amiodarone more frequent in control patients

Trial	Characteristics	Enrollment (crossover)	Follow-up	Notes
IRIS[8] (2009)	Mean LVEF 34.5%–34.6% Frequent anterior MI (64.2%–66.8%) Average time from MI to randomization 13 ± 7 d High ACE inhibitor use (81.5%–82.3%) High β-blocker use (85.7%–89.1%) Intermediate revascularization rate, if STEMI (71.5%–72.7%)	ICD: 445 (45; 10.1% crossed over) Control: 453 (39; 8.6% crossed over)	37 mo (mean)	Diabetes more common in ICD arm LBBB more common in ICD arm
SCD-HeFT[7] (2005)	Median LVEF 24%–25% High ACE inhibitor/angiotensin receptor inhibitor use (85%–98%) Intermediate β-blocker use (69%–82%) Intermediate lipid-lowering drug use (38%–48%) Frequent warfarin use (32%–37%)	ICD: 829 (113; 14%) received amiodarone at some point; 50, 6% crossed-out) Amiodarone: 845 (44; 5.2% became open-label) Placebo: 847 (81; 9.6% crossed over to amiodarone) 188 (11%) drug-receiving patients received ICD	45.5 mo (median)	β-Blocker use slightly more frequent in patients not on amiodarone
DEFINITE[9] (2004)	Mean LVEF 21.4% Frequent ACE inhibitor/angiotensin receptor inhibitor use (>85%) Frequent β-blocker use (84.9%) Amiodarone discouraged (5.2%)	ICD: 229 (4; 1.7% crossed over) Control: 229 (23; 10% crossed over)	29.0 mo (mean)	Patients in the ICD arm had shorter CHF history (2.39 y) than control subjects (3.27 y), P = .04 There were 11 (4.8%) CRT devices implanted in the ICD arm
DANISH[10] (2016)	Median LVEF 25% Idiopathic heart disease in 76% Frequent ACE inhibitor/angiotensin receptor blocker use (96%–97%) Frequent β-blocker use (92%) Intermediate aldosterone receptor antagonist use (57%–59%) Frequent CRT use (58%)	ICD: 556 (44; 7.9% crossed over) Control: 560 (27; 4.8% crossed over)	67.6 mo (median)	None

Abbreviations: AAD, antiarrhythmic drug; AAT, antiarrhythmic therapy; ACE, angiotensin-converting enzyme; CHF, congestive heart failure; CRT, cardiac resynchronization therapy; EP, electrophysiology; LBBB, left bundle branch block; MI, myocardial infarction; STEMI, ST-segment elevation myocardial infarction.

Table 3
Primary prevention ICD trials, results

Study (Publication Year)	Primary Findings	Notable Secondary Findings
CABG-Patch[3] (1997)	ICD: 101 (23%) all-cause deaths Control: 95 (21%) all-cause deaths HR, 1.07 (95% CI, 0.81–1.42), NS	Multiple covariates analyzed, similar results
MADIT-I[2] (1996)	ICD: 15 (16%) all-cause deaths Control: 39 (39%) all-cause deaths HR, 0.46 (95% CI, 0.26–0.82), P = .009	Limited subset analyses in the setting of small trial size
MUSTT[4] (1999)	EP-guided AAT: 90 (26%) cardiac arrests/deaths from arrhythmia No AAT: 68 (19%) cardiac arrests/deaths from arrhythmia 5-y RR, 0.73 (95% CI, 0.53–0.99), P = .04	Similar rate of all-cause deaths in both arms Within the EP-guided AAT arm, there were differences in outcomes based on ICD use: ICD recipients: 12 (6%) cardiac arrests/deaths from arrhythmia Patients without and ICD: 56 (38%) cardiac arrests/deaths from arrhythmia 5-y RR, 0.24 (95% CI, 0.13–0.43) All-cause deaths were also lower in ICD recipients Compared with a registry of PES-negative patients, who otherwise met all other enrollment criteria (n = 1397), PES-positive patients assigned to no AAT (n = 353) had higher cardiac arrests/deaths from arrhythmia and all-cause deaths
MADIT-II[5] (2002)	ICD: 105 (14.2%) all-cause deaths Control: 97 (19.8%) all-cause deaths HR, 0.69 (95% CI, 0.51–0.93), P = .016	Greatest mortality benefit of ICDs in patients with QRS >150 ms ICD survival benefit most dramatic >12 mo
DINAMIT[6] (2004)	ICD: 62 (18.7%) all-cause deaths Control: 58 (17.0%) all-cause deaths HR, 1.08 (95% CI, 0.76–1.55), P = .66	Arrhythmic deaths less frequent in ICD patients Nonarrhythmic deaths more frequent in ICD patients
IRIS[8] (2009)	ICD: 116 (26.1%) all-cause deaths Control: 117 (25.8%) all-cause deaths HR, 1.04 (95% CI, 0.81–1.35), P = .15	SCDs less frequent in ICD patients Nonsudden deaths more frequent in ICD patients
SCD-HeFT[7] (2005)	ICD: 182 (22%) all-cause deaths Amiodarone: 240 (28%) all-cause deaths Placebo: 244 (28%) all-cause deaths Amiodarone vs placebo: HR, 1.06 (97.5% CI, 0.86–1.30), P = .53 ICD vs non-ICD: HR, 0.77 (97.5% CI, 0.62–0.96), P = .007	All-cause mortality benefit of ICDs limited to NYHA II patients In ischemic CHF (n = 1310), HR of 0.79 (97.5% CI, 0.60–1.04), P = .05 In nonischemic CHF (n = 1211), HR of 0.73 (97.5% CI, 0.50–1.07) P = .06
DEFINITE[9] (2004)	ICD: 28 (12.2%) all-cause deaths Control: 40 (17.4%) all-cause deaths HR, 0.65 (95% CI, 0.40–1.06), P = .08	Most convincing all-cause death benefit from ICDs seen in patients with NYHA class III symptoms, patients with LVEF ≥20%, and in men There were fewer SCDs in the ICD arm
DANISH[10] (2016)	ICD: 120 (21.6%) all-cause deaths Control: 131 (23.4%) all-cause deaths HR, 0.87 (95% CI, 0.68–1.12), P = .28	All-cause deaths lower in ICD arm in patients <68 y All-cause deaths lower in ICD arm if NT-proBNP <1177 There were fewer SCDs in the ICD arm Benefit of ICDs after 5 y of follow-up uncertain

Abbreviations: AAT, antiarrhythmic therapy; CHF, congestive heart failure; CI, confidence interval; EP, electrophysiology; HR, hazard ratio; NS, not statistically significant; NT-proBNP, N-terminal pro–brain natriuretic peptide; NYHA, New York Heart Association; PES, programmed electrical stimulation; RR, relative risk.

Several features of this study limit its generalizability to contemporary practice. Perhaps most importantly, the background therapies of infarct-related cardiomyopathies used in this trial were not on par with today's standards: only 5% to 27% and 51% to 60% of enrolled patients were treated with β-blockers and angiotensin-converting enzyme (ACE) inhibitors, respectively (the use of lipid-lowering drugs was not reported). Similarly, no more than two-thirds of trial participants underwent coronary revascularization and most were smokers (73%–79%). The ICD devices used were early models with unsophisticated programming, half of which required thoracotomy for insertion. Second, the enrolled population was overall sick, with a mean LVEF 25% to 27%. Although New York Heart Association (NYHA) class IV patients were excluded from the study, 18% to 20% of participants exhibited signs of pulmonary congestion at the time of enrollment. Finally, an important selection bias plagued the MADIT-I trial: decision as to which patients should be selected for PVS occurred prerandomization and was left entirely up to clinicians' discretion.

The Coronary Artery Bypass Graft Trial (CABG-Patch) was a concurrent but much larger trial that randomized 900 participants across 37 sites (again, mostly in the United States).[3] The study enrolled patients with ischemic cardiomyopathy with LVEF less than 36%, all of whom were destined to undergo CABG surgery at the time of randomization; this is in stark contrast to MADIT-I, where not all patients were revascularized and if they were, a mandatory 2 to 3 months waiting period had to be observed before randomization. The CABG-Patch participants underwent a form of electrophysiologic risk-stratification (an abnormal signal-averaged electrocardiogram was required) and they were randomized either to an ICD (n = 446) or to conventional therapy (n = 454). Similarly to MADIT-I, most patients were smokers (76%–79%); few used β-blockers (16.0%–24.0%); and they were generally quite sick as judged by low mean LVEF of 27%, high mean LV end-diastolic pressure of 21 to 22 mm Hg, and a frequent clinical evidence of decompensated heart failure (pulmonary rales in 20%–25% and audible S3 gallop in 11%–14% of patients). However, unlike in MADIT-I, the CABG-Patch participants were usually not treated with AADs (63.3%–72.9% were not on an AAD).

Over an average follow-up period of 32 months, there were 101 all-cause deaths in the ICD cohort compared with 95 all-cause deaths in the control arm of the CABG-Patch trial; this minor difference in outcomes failed to reach statistical significance with an HR of 1.07 (95% CI, 0.81–1.42). The negative result persisted despite extensive covariate analyses. Causes of death were not reported, making it impossible to say whether ICDs had any specific effect on SCD rates. Why the results of CABG-Patch were so different from MADIT-I is likely because of multiple factors, including very different trial subject populations and variable use of AADs.

Further evidence of the utility of ICDs in patients with ischemic cardiomyopathy arrived somewhat unexpectedly in the form of the Multicenter Unsustained Tachycardia Trial (MUSTT).[4] Unlike MADIT-I or CABG-Patch, MUSTT was not designed to test efficacy of any specific antiarrhythmic therapy, such as the ICD. Instead, it was designed to test the hypothesis that electrophysiology (EP) study-guided antiarrhythmic therapy (AADs and ICDs) can specifically reduce the risk of SCD (rather than all-cause mortality).[12] Participants from 85 centers (all in the United States and Canada) with known but revascularized (when appropriate) coronary artery disease (CAD), reduced LVEF (≤40%), and history of nonsustained VT were subjected to PES and only those with inducible arrhythmias were subsequently randomized to EP-guided antiarrhythmic therapy (n = 351, mostly receiving class I agents) versus no antiarrhythmic therapy (n = 353). Compared with MADIT-I and CABG-Patch, most MUSTT patients were treated with ACE inhibitors (72%–77%), although β-blocker use remained infrequent and unequally distributed (29% of patients randomized to EP-guided therapy vs 51% of control subjects). After a median follow-up of 39 months, there were significantly more arrhythmic events and deaths in the control arm (n = 90) compared with the EP-guided therapy arm (n = 68) with a 5-year relative risk of 0.73 (95% CI, 0.53–0.99; P = .04). This did not translate into a statistically significant difference in all-cause mortality.

A substudy analysis revealed that the observed difference in outcomes was entirely attributable to the use of ICDs.[13] The study protocol allowed for the introduction of ICDs in patients randomized to the antiarrhythmic therapy arm of the trial, provided that at least one AAD failed to suppress inducible arrhythmias; this occurred in 202 (58%) individuals. Patients treated with ICDs not only experienced a significantly lower rate of SCD but also exhibited lower overall mortality compared with all other patients in the trial (ie, all control-arm patients or patients receiving AAD therapy but not an ICD).

A separate analysis of the MUSTT data then compared the outcomes of patients in the trial's control arm (ie, patients with inducible VT, who were randomized to receive no antiarrhythmic therapy; n = 353) with a separately tracked registry of individuals that met all MUSTT inclusion criteria but had no reproducibly inducible sustained arrhythmias (n = 1397). The 5-year arrhythmic death rate was significantly lower in the latter group (24%) than in the former patient set (32%; unadjusted HR, 0.71; 95% CI, 0.56–0.90; P = .005). When adjusted for covariates that included the unequal use of β-blockers in the two groups, the noninducible individuals also turned out to experience lower 5-year all-cause mortality (44%) compared with the inducible patients (48%; adjusted HR, 0.77; 95% CI, 0.64–0.92; P = .005). The results of the MUSTT trial therefore not only supported the use of ICDs in select individuals, but also validated the use of PES as a risk stratification strategy in patients with coronary disease and LVEF less than or equal to 40%.

PRIMARY PREVENTION IMPLANTABLE CARDIOVERTER-DEFIBRILLATORS IN ISCHEMIC CARDIOMYOPATHY, 2000s

The Multicenter Automatic Defibrillator Implantation Trial II (MADIT-II)[5] was the first study to look at the utility of ICDs in a population of patients with CAD who had suffered an acute MI at least 1 month earlier that did not undergo any kind of electrophysiologic risk-stratification. Only individuals with severe LV systolic dysfunction (LVEF ≤30%) were enrolled; those who underwent any revascularization procedures in the last 3 months were excluded. Compared with the older trials, the studied population was quite ill (mean LVEF, 23%), but was generally exposed to modern congestive heart failure (CHF) therapies (ACE inhibitors, β-blockers, and statins were used more frequently); also, most participants were revascularized. Although the protocol was supposed to have excluded patients with NYHA class IV heart failure symptoms, 5% of the study population was, in fact, NYHA class IV. Patients were randomized to ICD therapy (n = 742) and standard therapy (n = 490). During the modest mean follow-up period of 20 months, 105 (14.2%) and 97 (19.8%) of ICD and control patients died, respectively; this translated into a statistically significant all-cause mortality HR of 0.69 (95% CI, 0.51–0.93; P = .016), noticeably less than that observed in MADIT and MUSTT. Patients with wide QRS complex (QRS >150 ms) benefited the most from ICD use. A post hoc analysis of the trial data revealed that overall mortality benefit of ICDs was primarily driven by reduced SCD rate (HR, 0.33; 95% CI, 0.20–0.53; P<.0001); nonsudden deaths were not meaningfully affected by the use of ICDs.[14] Note that the difference in number of deaths between the treatment and control arms in this trial was 8 (vs 62 in MUSTT).

Another clue supporting the idea that patients with impaired LVEF, irrespective of electrophysiologic risk-stratification, may benefit from primary prevention ICDs came from the Sudden Cardiac Death in Heart Failure Trial (SCD-HeFT).[7] This study was unique in that, for the first time, it enrolled participants with reduced LVEF (≤35%) of ischemic and nonischemic cause (approximately 50% each). Also, the trial only included patients with NYHA class II and III symptoms (all the previous trials intended to exclude NYHA class IV patients, but allowed individuals without symptomatic heart failure to participate). Participants (n = 2521) were randomized to three arms: (1) conservatively programmed ICD (shock-only treatments delivered at HR >187 bpm; n = 847), (2) amiodarone (n = 845), and (3) placebo (n = 847) and followed for 45.5 months (median) during which a high rate of crossovers occurred. With 182 (22%) deaths in the ICD arm, 240 (28%) deaths in the amiodarone arm, and 244 (28%) deaths in the placebo arm, the ICD showed clear survival benefit compared with the other interventions (HR, 0.77; 97.5% CI, 0.62–0.96; P = .007), especially in patients with milder symptoms (in NYHA class II patients, HR was 0.54; 97.5% CI, 0.40–0.74). The mortality benefit of ICDs was most convincing in patients with ischemic cardiomyopathy (HR, 0.79; 97.5% CI, 0.60–1.04; P = .05). Amiodarone provided no survival benefit compared with placebo. A post hoc analysis of the trial data suggested that the overall mortality benefit of ICDs was primarily driven by a reduction in sudden tachyarrhythmic deaths (HR, 0.40; 95% CI, 0.27–0.59; P<.001) but that ICD use did not significantly affect the rate of noncardiac and heart failure deaths.[15]

It is worth noting that the relative risk reduction in MADIT-II and SCD-HeFT trials (31% and 23%) were much lower than in the trials that used PES for risk stratification (54% in MADIT-I and 55% in MUSTT). This may have been a result of absence of patient risk stratification in the newer trials and inclusion of patients with nonischemic disease in SCD-HeFT.

Taken together, the results of MADIT-II and SCD-HeFT led to the idea that ICDs improved all-cause mortality even when patients were selected solely based on a low LVEF (≤30% and ≤35%, respectively), making PES (as explored in MADIT-I and MUSTT) seem superfluous in this patient population. However, it is important to realize that low LVEF is only a "blunt" all-cause mortality risk-stratification instrument; there is no direct physiologic basis by which low LVEF specifically associates with a higher risk for ventricular tachyarrhythmias. Consequently, many patients with very low LVEF have high risk of *any* death even if they remain free of arrhythmias; in them, ICD therapy represents a costly intervention with much lower benefit. Conversely, the (arbitrary) LVEF less than or equal to 35% cutoff may leave many individuals specifically at-risk for lethal arrhythmias untreated. Thus, despite the demonstration in the MADIT-II and SCD-HeFT trials that a modest reduction in mortality is achieved by implanting ICDs solely on the basis of reduced EF, a significant mortality benefit is achieved by using PES in addition to EF in identifying patients likely to benefit from the ICD.

The Alternans Before Cardioverter Defibrillator (ABCD) trial[16] was designed to further characterize the utility of electrophysiologic measures as predictors of SCD. This 43-center (United States, Europe, and Israel) study enlisted 556 individuals with LVEF less than or equal to 40% attributable to ischemic disease. Patients with acute MI or revascularization within 28 days were excluded. There was no randomized intervention. Instead, all participants underwent PES (using the MUSTT protocol) and all were subjected to µV T-wave alternans (MTWA) testing before being encouraged to undergo ICD implantation. A total of 495 (87%) patients received an ICD that was programmed for shock-only treatment of VT/VT with rates greater than 171 bpm. Over the median follow-up period of 1.6 years, 65 (14%) patients reached the primary end point, defined as appropriate ICD therapy or SCD. Patients with abnormal MTWA and positive PES experienced a significantly higher annual event rate (12.6%) compared with patients with normal EP testing (2.3%). Moreover, MTWA and PES proved to be mutually complementary tests, each with low positive predictive value (9.5% and 11.1% at 1 year, respectively) but reasonable negative predictive value (95.3% and 95.1% at 1 year, respectively). Despite these encouraging results, enthusiasm to adopt MTWA as a mainstay risk-stratification tool was dampened by the observation that this modality's predictive capacity was limited to a mere 6 months; in other words, the study found that abnormal MTWA predicted SCD or appropriate ICD therapy for the future 6 months but was not able to accurately forecast risk beyond 12 months. Conversely, PES could predict adverse events even into the distant future.

Like MUSTT, the ABCD trial thus provided a rationale for continued use of PES, especially in patients not fitting the MADIT-II or SCD-HeFT profile (ie, those with ischemic cardiomyopathy and LVEF in the 35%–40% range). However, several limitations of ABCD need to be highlighted. First, the follow-up period was less than 2 years. Second, this was not a randomized trial, but rather an observational study; thus, by design, it could not directly prove that ICDs actually prevented SCD. Third, it is worthwhile noting that patients with permanent atrial fibrillation or those on AAD therapy were excluded (to allow for meaningful MTWA testing) and that despite the trial's intention to enroll patients with ischemic cardiomyopathy, only 369 (65%) individuals had LV dysfunction attributable to CAD. Lastly, there were a total of 71 (13%) individuals, who elected not to undergo ICD implantation; not surprisingly, this happened disproportionately more often with patients, whose EP testing was negative. Such disparity may have introduced an observation bias, whereby lower event rates may have been reported in patients without an ICD.

With the exception of CABG-Patch, all the trials discussed up to this point explored the utility of ICDs in patients in whom index MI or revascularization generally took place weeks or months before device implantation. Yet, it has been known for years that many post-MI all-cause deaths in patients with low LVEF occur in the first 6 months following the ischemic event.[17] More recently, a subanalysis of the Valsartan in Acute Myocardial Infarction Trial (VALIANT)[18] tracked 14,609 patients with a recent MI and reduced LVEF ($\leq$40%). Over a median follow-up of 24.7 months, there were 1067 (7%) SCDs or resuscitated cardiac arrests. Importantly, these events were much more frequent in the first 30 days post-MI (a monthly event rate of 1.4%; 95% CI, 1.2%–1.6%) than in the 1 to 6 months post-MI period (a monthly event rate of 0.50%; 95% CI, 0.45%–0.55%) or any time after that. If the first month after MI is the most vulnerable period for SCD and if most SCDs can truly be attributed to ventricular arrhythmias, it might follow that earlier postischemia ICD implants will prevent more deaths.

Two trials directly tested this hypothesis: The Defibrillator in Acute Myocardial Infarction Trial (DINAMIT)[6] and the Immediate Risk-stratification Improves Survival (IRIS) study.[8] Both studies enrolled patients with MI within 40 days that had LV dysfunction (LVEF $\leq$35% in DINAMIT and LVEF $\leq$40% in IRIS, although the latter trial also included individuals with LVEF >40% as long as they had evidence of NSVT or frequent ectopy). The DINAMIT study additionally required that enrolled subjects exhibited abnormal heart rate variability or a high mean heart rate (>80 bpm) on a 24-hour monitor. Patients were randomized either to usual care (n = 342 in DINAMIT and n = 453 in IRIS) or to ICD therapy (n = 332 in DINAMIT and n = 445 in IRIS), with more aggressive ICD programming in DINAMIT (treating all arrhythmias >175 bpm) as compared with IRIS (only treating rates >200 bpm). By design, the mean time from MI to randomization was short (18 days in DINAMIT and 13 days in IRIS). In both trials, the all-cause mortality rates in the two arms were nearly identical. Both trials made the same sobering observation: although the rate of arrhythmic deaths or SCD was lower in ICD recipients (HR, 0.42; 95% CI, 0.22–0.82; P = .009 in DINAMIT; and HR, 0.55; 95% CI, 0.31–1.00; P = .049 in IRIS), ICD implantation was associated with an increase in other types of deaths (HR, 1.75; 95% CI, 1.11–2.76; P = .02 for nonarrhythmic deaths in DINAMIT; and HR, 1.92; 95% CI, 1.29–2.84; P = .001 for non-SCDs in IRIS). Thus, in each trial, there was no survival benefit associated with ICD implantation.

To date, there is no universally accepted explanation for these observations but an abundance of proposed theories exists. One possibility is that ICD shocks may actually cause impaired healing following recent MI. Alternatively, some ventricular arrhythmias may themselves be survivable but may act as markers for a separate, fatal underlying process. For example, massive myocardial reinfarction could generate shockable ventricular fibrillation but could still result in death because of pump failure, regardless of the presence of an ICD. Similarly, the very notion that most SCDs are caused by arrhythmias may be flawed. This last concept derives credence from a review of 398 available pathology reports from deceased VALIANT participants.[19] Of the 105 individuals who died suddenly or unexpectedly, 51 had specific pathologic findings that could explain their demise (most often recurrent acute MI or myocardial rupture; n = 44). Even more surprisingly, the mean time from index MI to SCD was significantly longer in patients with no pathology findings (306 ± 246 days) compared with those with acute MI or rupture (137 ± 194 days). The study inferred that a mere 20% of all clinical SCDs in the first month after MI were caused by an exclusively arrhythmic cause; conversely, as many as 75% of SCD victims greater than 3 months after index MI had unremarkable pathology and thus probably succumbed to an arrhythmia. Regardless of the explanation for the ineffectiveness of ICDs in the early post-MI period, the results of the DINAMIT and IRIS trials have influenced current practice guidelines to discourage ICD use in the early post-MI period.

PRIMARY PREVENTION IMPLANTABLE CARDIOVERTER-DEFIBRILLATORS IN NONISCHEMIC CARDIOMYOPATHY

If the role of ICDs in patients with ischemic disease is difficult to define, then it is even harder to delineate in the treatment of NICM. Patients with NICM also suffer from a higher overall mortality than the general population, but less so than patients with ischemic disease.[20] In addition, NICM is not a single disease, but rather a mix of disorders that produce the same clinical syndrome. These properties make studying the utility of ICDs in NICM difficult, a feat attempted by only three trials.

The Defibrillators in Non-Ischemic Cardiomyopathy Evaluation (DEFINITE)[9] enrolled 458 patients with NICM (LVEF <36%) from across the United States; patients with familial cardiomyopathies associated with high SCD risk were excluded. Although enrollment criteria stipulated that patients have symptomatic heart failure, 99 (21.6%) exhibited NYHA class I functional status. Patients were randomized to usual therapy (n = 229) versus ICD (n = 229); over a mean follow-up period of 29.0 ± 14.4 months, there were fewer all-cause deaths (n = 28) and arrhythmic deaths (n = 3) in the ICD cohort than in the control group (40 all-cause deaths, 14 arrhythmic deaths). Although the all-cause mortality difference was not statistically significant, the HR for arrhythmic deaths was 0.20 (95% CI, 0.06–0.71; P = .006). Subgroup analyses presented some puzzling findings that included the observation that men and patients with NYHA class III symptoms derived all-cause mortality benefit from ICDs, in contrast to findings from the SCD-HeFT trial.

Approximately 50% of the SCD-HeFT trial[7] participants had NICM (n = 1211). As in DEFINITE, ICD-recipients with NICM died less frequently than control subjects, but this difference again failed to reach statistical significance (HR, 0.73; 97.5% CI, 0.50–1.07; P = .06). Unlike in DEFINITE, the net mortality benefit in (all) SCD-HeFT subjects was seen in those with NYHA class II symptoms. Of note, ICD use did reduce the rate of sudden tachyarrhythmic deaths in all NICM patients enrolled in the trial (HR, 0.34; 95% CI, 0.17–0.70; no P value reported), without affecting noncardiac or heart failure deaths.[15]

The Danish Study to Assess the Efficacy of ICDs in Patients with Non-Ischemic Heart Failure on Mortality (DANISH)[10] was published a full 11 years after SCD-HeFT. This, by far the most modern and comprehensive primary prevention ICD trial in patients with NICM, enrolled 1116 patients with LVEF less than or equal to 35% and elevated N-terminal pro–brain natriuretic peptide levels. Most participants had idiopathic NICM (76%) and nearly all were treated with β-blockers and ACE inhibitors/angiotensin receptor blockers; the use of mineralocorticoid receptor antagonist (57%–59%) and cardiac resynchronization therapy (58%) was also frequent, attesting to the state-of-the-art CHF management used in this trial. As in most other similar studies, patients were randomized to ICD therapy versus usual care. Over the median follow-up period of 67.6 months (49–85 months), there were 120 (21.6%) all-cause deaths in the ICD arm and 131 (23.4%) all-cause deaths in the control arm, a difference that was not statistically significant. As in DEFINITE, there was a statistically significant reduction of SCDs in ICD recipients (HR, 0.50; 95% CI, 0.31–0.82; $P = .005$). Subgroup analyses revealed an all-cause mortality benefit in ICD recipients who were either young (<59 years) or who exhibited evidence of lower N-terminal pro–brain natriuretic peptide less than 1177 pg/ml.

EVIDENCE THAT BENEFIT FROM IMPLANTABLE CARDIOVERTER-DEFIBRILLATORS IS NOT UNIFORMLY DISTRIBUTED IN TESTED POPULATIONS

The chief risk-stratifying agent used in most of the discussed trials was reduced LVEF. Yet, there is no direct physiologic evidence that low EF generates arrhythmias; in fact, all evidence suggests that that low LVEF is simply a marker for all-cause mortality. Low LVEF increases the risk of nonarrhythmic death just as much as it increases the risk of arrhythmic death. This raises the possibility that the net mortality benefit of ICDs (observed in MADIT-I, MADIT-II, MUSTT, and SCD-HeFT) may have been distributed unevenly across the studied populations. Indeed, prespecified subgroup analyses in the original trials identified patient strata that benefited from ICD use much more than others (eg, NYHA class II patients in SCD-HeFT or individuals with wide QRS in MADIT-II). Several post hoc trial substudies have addressed this important question in more detail.

A MUSTT substudy analyzed 674 trial participants.[21] This included 200 patients with inducible arrhythmias randomized to no antiarrhythmic therapy and 474 patients drawn from the trial's registry arm (ie, those with no inducible arrhythmias). The total 2-year mortality rate and arrhythmic death and cardiac arrest rate of this population were 22% and 14%, respectively. Multivariate analysis revealed that the risk factor profiles for arrhythmic death/cardiac arrest were similar but not identical to the risk factors for total mortality. For example, age and history of atrial fibrillation were predictors of all-cause mortality, but were not significantly associated with arrhythmic outcomes. Similarly, EF was the most potent predictor of all death but turned out to be only a comparatively weak predictor of lethal arrhythmias. Conversely, inducible VT

and history of heart failure were more predictive of arrhythmic death and cardiac arrest compared with all cause death. These observations led to the development of a risk-stratification model designed to identify patients with a low all-cause mortality/arrhythmic mortality ratio as the optimal candidates for ICD therapy.

Efforts were also made to risk-stratify participants of the MADIT-II trial.[22] A multivariate analysis of 1172 trial patients allowed for the development of a point-based total-mortality prediction model (consisting of 1 point each: NYHA class >II, atrial fibrillation, QRS duration >120 ms, age >70 years, and BUN >26 mg/dL). As expected, total mortality rose monotonically with increasing number of risk factors. However, not all patients derived the same benefit from ICD use. Patients with 1 or 2 points were more likely to survive if they had an ICD (HR, 0.40; 95% CI, 0.22–0.72; $P = .002$; and HR, 0.42; 95% CI, 0.25–0.70; $P<.001$, respectively). However, patients on either extreme of the risk spectrum (ie, those with either 0 points or ≥3 points) experienced no mortality benefit from ICD implantation. Thus, ICDs only benefited individuals with intermediate risk factor profiles.

Another work investigated the utility of the Seattle Heart Failure Model (SHFM, a multivariate predictor of all-cause mortality)[23] in the SCD-HeFT trial population.[24] Patients with higher SHFM scores derived less total mortality benefit from ICD implantation than did individuals with lower SHFM scores; in fact, patients in the highest SHFM quintile derived no benefit at all. However, it should be noted that this interaction only reached statistical significance in the second lowest quintile (4-year relative risk, 0.48; 95% CI, 0.26–0.89; $P = .019$). Also important to remember is that in contrast to MUSTT and MADIT-II, all patients in this analysis had clinical heart failure.

These findings present compelling evidence that not all patients with reduced LVEF actually benefit from ICDs. They also suggest that the "sickest" patients with multiple comorbidities are the ones who derive the least benefit from these devices. However, the discussed risk-stratification algorithms have yet to be tested prospectively in a randomized controlled trial, and they have not yet earned endorsement by societal guidelines.

SUMMARY

Despite three decades of experience and nine formal trials, the utility of ICDs in primary prevention is nowhere near clear. It is likely that patients with systolic LV dysfunction and a nonacute history of ischemia generally benefit the most from an ICD, particularly if PES induces arrhythmias. But even in these patients, it is hard to distinguish those with an isolated high risk of arrhythmia from those with high overall mortality. The role of ICDs in the NICM population is even murkier given the relative paucity of data; it is possible that certain substrata of NICM patients (eg, young individuals) also derive net benefit from device implantation. However, ICDs may have a neutral or even negative effect on all other patients with cardiomyopathy.

The fundamental challenge going forward is the development of adequate risk-stratification tools that can identify patients specifically at risk for SCD, if ICDs are to be used in a cost-effective manner. It should be stressed that, contrary to a frequently held belief, most of the broadly adopted risk stratification tools are not specific for SCD. Impaired LVEF is a prime example of a "blunt" mortality marker that has no ability to explicitly predict SCD. However, even many of the more sophisticated tools, including MTWA or heart rate variability, are also only good at pointing out "sick" patients, without specifically predicting arrhythmic risk. Patients who are identified using these imperfect tools certainly do tend to have a higher arrhythmia burden resulting in more SCDs, but also suffer from a proportionally elevated risk of succumbing to other pathologic processes. Even if ICDs successfully terminate arrhythmias in these patients, they may have no impact on overall mortality and may actually cause harm. Currently the only well-established SCD-specific risk stratification tool is PES, but better noninvasive modalities are badly needed. In addition to using more specific risk-stratification algorithms, future ICD trials should strive to better sort out the cause of death of deceased participants. To this end, investigators could use implantable loop recorders in the study control arms and advocate for routine use of postmortem examinations.

REFERENCES

1. Zipes DP, Wyse DG, Friedman PL, et al. A comparison of antiarrhythmic-drug therapy with implantable defibrillators in patients resuscitated from near-fatal ventricular arrhythmias. The Antiarrhythmics Versus Implantable Defibrillators (AVID) investigators. N Engl J Med 1997;337(22):1576–83.
2. Moss AJ, Hall WJ, Cannom DS, et al. Improved survival with an implanted defibrillator in patients with coronary disease at high risk for ventricular arrhythmia. Multicenter automatic defibrillator implantation trial investigators. N Engl J Med 1996;335(26):1933–40.
3. Bigger JT. Prophylactic use of implanted cardiac defibrillators in patients at high risk for ventricular arrhythmias after coronary-artery bypass graft surgery. Coronary artery bypass graft (CABG) patch trial investigators. N Engl J Med 1997;337(22):1569–75.
4. Buxton AE, Lee KL, Fisher JD, et al. A randomized study of the prevention of sudden death in patients with coronary artery disease. Multicenter unsustained tachycardia trial investigators. N Engl J Med 1999;341(25):1882–90.
5. Moss AJ, Zareba W, Hall WJ, et al. Prophylactic implantation of a defibrillator in patients with myocardial infarction and reduced ejection fraction. N Engl J Med 2002;346(12):877–83.
6. Hohnloser SH, Kuck KH, Dorian P, et al. Prophylactic use of an implantable cardioverter-defibrillator after acute myocardial infarction. N Engl J Med 2004;351(24):2481–8.
7. Bardy GH, Lee KL, Mark DB, et al. Amiodarone or an implantable cardioverter-defibrillator for congestive heart failure. N Engl J Med 2005;352(3):225–37.
8. Steinbeck G, Andresen D, Seidl K, et al. Defibrillator implantation early after myocardial infarction. N Engl J Med 2009;361(15):1427–36.
9. Kadish A, Dyer A, Daubert J, et al. Prophylactic defibrillator implantation in patients with nonischemic dilated cardiomyopathy. N Engl J Med 2004;350(21):2151–8. Available at: papers2://publication/uuid/8FCACC70-7501-410B-B95E-B16232EC7ABF.
10. Køber L, Thune JJ, Nielsen JC, et al. Defibrillator implantation in patients with nonischemic systolic heart failure. N Engl J Med 2016;375(13):1221–30.
11. The Multicenter Research Group. Risk stratification and survival after myocardial infarction. N Engl J Med 1983;309(6):331–6.
12. Buxton AE, Marchlinski FE, Waxman HL, et al. Prognostic factors in nonsustained ventricular tachycardia. Am J Cardiol 1984;53(9):1275–9.
13. Buxton AE, Lee KL, DiCarlo L, et al. Electrophysiologic testing to identify patients with coronary artery disease who are at risk for sudden death. Multicenter unsustained tachycardia trial investigators. N Engl J Med 2000;342(26):1937–45.
14. Greenberg H, Case RB, Moss AJ, et al. Analysis of mortality events in the Multicenter Automatic Defibrillator Implantation Trial (MADIT-II). J Am Coll Cardiol 2004;43(8):1459–65.
15. Packer DL, Prutkin JM, Hellkamp AS, et al. Impact of implantable cardioverter-defibrillator, amiodarone, and placebo on the mode of death in stable patients with heart failure: analysis from the sudden cardiac death in heart failure trial. Circulation 2009;120(22):2170–6.
16. Costantini O, Hohnloser SH, Kirk MM, et al. The ABCD (Alternans before Cardioverter Defibrillator) Trial. Strategies using T-wave alternans to improve

efficiency of sudden cardiac death prevention. J Am Coll Cardiol 2009;53(6):471–9.

17. Bigger JTJ, Fleiss JL, Kleiger R, et al. The relationships among ventricular arrhythmias, left ventricular dysfunction, and mortality in the 2 years after myocardial infarction. Circulation 1984;69(2):250–8.

18. Solomon SD, Zelenkofske S, McMurray JJV, et al. Sudden death in patients with myocardial infarction and left ventricular dysfunction, heart failure, or both. N Engl J Med 2005;352(25):2581–8.

19. Pouleur AC, Barkoudah E, Uno H, et al. Pathogenesis of sudden unexpected death in a clinical trial of patients with myocardial infarction and left ventricular dysfunction, heart failure, or both. Circulation 2010;122(6):597–602.

20. Strickberger SA, Hummel JD, Bartlett TG, et al. Amiodarone versus implantable cardioverter-defibrillator: randomized trial in patients with nonischemic dilated cardiomyopathy and asymptomatic nonsustained ventricular tachycardia - AMIOVIRT. J Am Coll Cardiol 2003;41(10):1707–12.

21. Buxton AE, Lee KL, Hafley GE, et al. Limitations of ejection fraction for prediction of sudden death risk in patients with coronary artery disease. Lessons from the MUSTT study. J Am Coll Cardiol 2007; 50(12):1150–7.

22. Goldenberg I, Vyas AK, Hall WJ, et al. Risk stratification for primary implantation of a cardioverter-defibrillator in patients with ischemic left ventricular dysfunction. J Am Coll Cardiol 2008;51(3): 288–96.

23. Levy WC, Mozaffarian D, Linker DT, et al. The Seattle heart failure model: prediction of survival in heart failure. Circulation 2006;113(11):1424–33.

24. Levy WC, Lee KL, Hellkamp AS, et al. Maximizing survival benefit with primary prevention implantable cardioverter-defibrillator therapy in a heart failure population. Circulation 2009;120(10):835–42.

The Subcutaneous Defibrillator

Jonathan Weinstock, MD*, Christopher Madias, MD

KEYWORDS

- Defibrillator • Subcutaneous • Sudden death • Ventricular fibrillation

KEY POINTS

- The transvenous implantable cardioverter-defibrillator (ICD) has been shown in multiple studies to be effective in prevention of sudden cardiac death in select populations.
- The Achilles heel of traditional ICD technology has been the transvenous lead.
- The subcutaneous ICD provides effective sudden death protection, while avoiding lead-related complications of traditional transvenous systems.
- The subcutaneous ICD is a reasonable option for patients with an ICD indication who do not need bradycardia pacing or cardiac resynchronization therapy.

INTRODUCTION

Sudden cardiac death as a result of arrhythmic arrest is the leading cause of cardiovascular mortality worldwide.[1] Since being introduced in the 1980s, the implantable cardioverter-defibrillator (ICD) has been shown in numerous clinical trials to impart a survival benefit in both a primary and secondary prevention setting.[2–5]

Conventional transvenous ICDs have significant procedural and long-term risks, most of which result from placement of a lead in the venous system and the right ventricle. The procedural and short-term risks include pneumothorax, pericardial effusion, cardiac tamponade, lead dislodgement, and venous occlusion.[6] Long-term risks include device/lead infection and lead malfunction. In large retrospective analyses, transvenous lead survival is highly variable but has been reported as low as 60% at 8 years.[7] Transvenous lead survival is susceptible to design limitations and to the stressors of the anatomic environment in which the lead is implanted, including perpetual cardiac motion.

Lead failure is more likely to occur in younger ICD patients owing to a longer, more active life. Lead extraction is often used as a result of lead failure and is necessitated in the setting of lead infection, compounding the risks of either situation alone.[8]

The fully subcutaneous ICD (S-ICD, Boston Scientific, Marlborough, MA) has been developed in an attempt to avoid the drawbacks of transvenous ICD systems. Eliminating transvenous leads averts the procedural risk associated with venous and cardiac access, removes the device from cardiac mechanical stress, and obviates the potential risks associated with future transvenous lead extraction. The concept of the S-ICD is particularly attractive for patients with limited or no vascular access, in those who are at high risk or who have had prior intravascular infections, and in younger patients. The S-ICD was approved for use by the European Union in 2009 and by the US Food and Drug Administration in 2012. This article reviews the efficacy, safety, and inherent limitations of the S-ICD.

The authors have nothing to disclose.
Division of Cardiology, Cardiac Arrhythmia Center, Tufts Medical Center, 800 Washington Street, Boston, MA 02111, USA
* Corresponding author.
E-mail address: jweinstock1@tuftsmedicalcenter.org

THE SUBCUTANEOUS DEFIBRILLATOR

Although there have been 3 progressive iterations of the S-ICD, with reduction in size and modification of other features, the basic functioning of the device and implant considerations remain the same. The S-ICD system consists of a pulse generator and single electrode, which has an 8-cm shock coil toward the distal end, flanked by 2 sensing poles (**Fig. 1**). The device and electrode are implanted based on anatomic landmarks, with fluoroscopy optional to confirm optimal electrode placement. A subcutaneous pocket for the device is created in the left midaxillary line, at the fifth or sixth intercostal space, ideally at the level of the apex of the left ventricle. The electrode is then tunneled subcutaneously in 2 directions, from a small incision just left of the xyphoid process. The first tunnel is created medially from the pocket to the xyphoid incision and the second cranially along the left side of the sternum. The electrode is sutured to subcutaneous tissue at the xyphoid incision. In the final position, the electrode will lie leftward of the sternum, with the coil and both sensing poles directed vertically along the parasternal plane (**Fig. 2**). The proximal end of the electrode is then connected to the S-ICD generator, which is secured in the pocket with a stay suture. The initial implanting technique included a third small incision at the cranial parasternal position to allow for tunneling of the electrode and for placement of a stay suture at the distal tip. Many operators have eliminated the third incision, opting instead for a 2-incision technique, with adequate electrode stability and safety.[9] Positioning the

electrode along the right sternal border is occasionally necessitated to improve sensing and/or the defibrillation threshold (DFT).

Sensing in the S-ICD is achieved via one of 3 vectors: between the proximal sensing pole and generator (primary vector), the distal sensing pole and generator (secondary vector), or the distal to proximal sensing poles (alternate vector). At the time of implant, the device automatically chooses the optimal sensing vector based on the greatest R wave to T wave ratio. The choice of sensing vector can be overridden manually if there is a clinically favored vector.

Routine evaluation of patients in whom an S-ICD is being considered includes screening a modified surface electrocardiogram (ECG) for the potential of T-wave oversensing. Surface ECG tracings are obtained from surface leads placed at the approximate location of the 3 sensing positions of the system. A plastic overlay (**Fig. 3**) is then applied to the surface tracing, which evaluates adequate R wave to T wave ratios, and eliminates vectors in which the potential for oversensing is high. This exercise is performed with patients in both a supine and standing position. Importantly, one of the 3 sensing vectors has to be acceptable in both positions for an implant to proceed.

Contrary to a recent shift away from DFT testing with transvenous devices,[10] DFT testing is routinely performed at the time of S-ICD implantation. Initial studies of the S-ICD deemed a 15J safety margin as adequate when performing DFT testing. In the event of DFT testing failure, shock polarity can be reversed and retested. Fluoroscopic assessment and revision of the electrode and generator positions might be necessary to achieve an adequate DFT safety margin. Eventual success can often be achieved with repositioning the generator as posterior as possible and confirming that it is at the same level as the apex of the left ventricle. Occasionally, repositioning the electrode along the right sternal border might also be required.[11]

Two arrhythmia zones are programmable in the S-ICD within the range of 170 to 240 beats per minute. In the shock zone, analysis is based on the rate alone. In the conditional lower rate zone, additional discrimination is applied in an attempt to avoid inappropriate shocks for supraventricular tachycardia (SVT). When a ventricular arrhythmia is detected that falls within a therapy zone, the device will deliver an 80J biphasic shock, which will automatically reverse polarity if the initial shock fails. An example of the stored electrograms from an appropriate shock for ventricular fibrillation is shown in **Fig. 4**. The device will deliver up to 5 shocks per arrhythmia episode. The output of 80J is nonprogrammable outside of DFT testing.

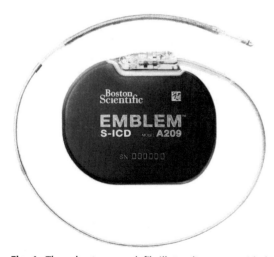

Fig. 1. The subcutaneous defibrillator. (Image provided courtesy of Boston Scientific. © 2017 Boston Scientific Corporation or its affiliates. All rights reserved.)

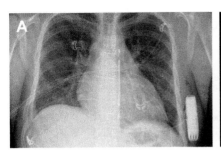
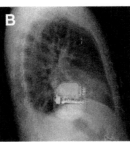

Fig. 2. (*A*, *B*) Posteroanterior and lateral chest radiograph of an implanted S-ICD system.

The S-ICD is capable of providing postshock pacing via a 200-mA transthoracic pulse for 30 seconds after the shock if a longer than 3.5-second pause is detected. Importantly, the device cannot provide long-term bradycardia pacing or antitachycardia pacing (ATP).

SUBCUTANEOUS IMPLANTABLE CARDIOVERTER-DEFIBRILLATOR EFFICACY

The data for the efficacy and safety of the S-ICD are derived entirely from nonrandomized studies. The initial studies sought to evaluate the ideal configuration of the S-ICD, concluding that the now familiar position of the electrode resulted in the lowest DFT.[12] The S-ICD was equally effective compared with a transvenous device in the same patients in terminating ventricular fibrillation (VF) with a comparatively higher DFT (36.6 ±19.8J vs 11.1 ±8.5J). In addition, this study evaluated the permanent implantation in a pilot study of 6 and then 55 patients. In those patients, VF was detected accurately in all cases of DFT testing and successfully treated with 65J in 2 DFT tests, in 98% of patients.[12]

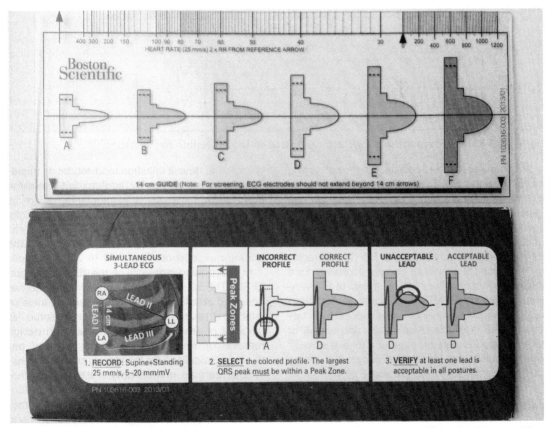

Fig. 3. The surface ECG S-ICD screening tool. (Image provided courtesy of Boston Scientific. © 2017 Boston Scientific Corporation or its affiliates. All rights reserved.)

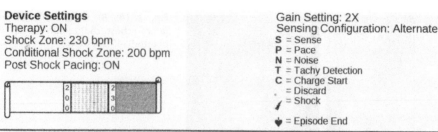

Device Settings
Therapy: ON
Shock Zone: 230 bpm
Conditional Shock Zone: 200 bpm
Post Shock Pacing: ON

Gain Setting: 2X
Sensing Configuration: Alternate
S = Sense
P = Pace
N = Noise
T = Tachy Detection
C = Charge Start
 = Discard
 = Shock

 = Episode End

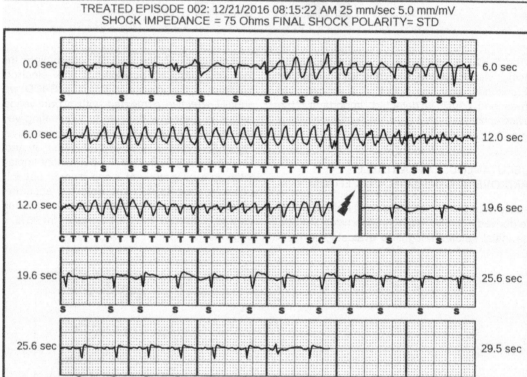

TREATED EPISODE 002: 12/21/2016 08:15:22 AM 25 mm/sec 5.0 mm/mV
SHOCK IMPEDANCE = 75 Ohms FINAL SHOCK POLARITY= STD

Fig. 4. An S-ICD stored report from a successfully treated episode of ventricular fibrillation.

Data have now been published on the safety and efficacy of the S-ICD in diverse populations of ischemic and nonischemic cardiomyopathies and genetic cardiac disorders, for both primary and secondary prevention. The largest such series is pooled data from the Investigational Device Exemption (IDE) study and the EFFORTLESS registry, examining 882 patients who were followed for a mean of 651 days after implant. A total of 111 ventricular tachycardia (VT)/VF episodes were treated in 59 patients. A single shock was successful in terminating VF in 90.1% of episodes, and 98.2% of VT/VF episodes were terminated after 5 shocks.[10] Other studies show similar efficacy both during DFT testing and follow-up (**Table 1**).[12–20]

PROCEDURAL COMPLICATIONS

The most frequently encountered procedure-related complications of the S-ICD include pocket hematoma, device infection, and electrode migration. As stated previously, lead-related complications of transvenous ICD implants, such as pneumothorax, cardiac tamponade, and vascular complications, are entirely avoided. In general, the incidence of complications decreases with operator experience.[21]

In the pooled analysis of the IDE study and EFFORTLESS registry, pocket hematomas occurred in 0.4% of patients. Superficial/incision infection treated conservatively occurred in 0.3% of patients, and infection requiring device removal or revision occurred in 1.7% of patients.[13] Guidelines for the management of transvenous cardiac rhythm device infection do not apply to the S-ICD, as the consequences of infection and failure of conservative management are less concerning. Device infection and erosion can often be treated successfully with antibiotics and pocket/electrode revision.[22]

Table 1
Summary of major trials of safety and efficacy of the subcutaneous implantable cardioverter-defibrillator

Author, year	Number of Patients	Mean Age (y)	Follow-up	ICM (%)	NICM (%)	Other Cardiac Disease (%)	Primary Prevention (%)	Success with DFT Testing (%)	Appropriate Detection with DFT Testing (%)	Conversion Rate of Events in Follow-up (%)	Inappropriate Shocks (%)	Complications Requiring Intervention (%)
Burke et al,[13] 2015	882	50.3	651 d	37.8	31.8	30.4	69.9	99.2	NA	98.2	13.1	9.6
Lambiase et al,[14] 2014	472	49	558 d	37	9.1	53.9	63	99.7	NA	100	7	6.4
Weiss et al,[15] 2013	314	51.9	330 d	NA	NA	NA	79.4	100	99.8	95.2	13	1.3
Köbe et al,[16] 2013	69	45	217 d	15.9	36.2	47.9	59.4	95.5	NA	100	4	4
Jarman & Todd,[17] 2013	111	33	12.7 mo	14	5	81	50	100	100	100	15	16
Aydin et al,[18] 2012	40	42	229 d	22.5	22.5	55	42.5	97.5	NA	100	5	13
Olde Nordkamp et al,[19] 2012	118	50	18 mo	38	18.5	43.5	60	100	NA	100	13	14
Dabiri Abkenari et al,[20] 2011	31	53	286 d	58	13	29	67.7	100	100	100	16	10
Bardy et al,[12] 2010	55	56	10 mo	67	18	15	78	98	100	100	9	11

Abbreviations: ICM, ischemic cardiomyopathy; NA, not available; NICM, nonischemic cardiomyopathy.

Removal of the device and electrode is a relatively low-risk procedure in contrast to transvenous lead extraction. Electrode migration was an issue with early S-ICD implants but was mitigated with the introduction of a suture sleeve at the site of the xyphoid incision.[19] The 2-incision technique maintains the xyphoid suture sleeve but eliminates the upper incision and fixation point, with no increase in lead migration rate.[9]

INAPPROPRIATE SHOCKS

Inappropriate shocks are detrimental from a quality-of-life perspective and might have deleterious effects on cardiac function and mortality.[23] The first step in avoiding inappropriate shocks is careful patient screening with the use of the manufacturer-developed screening tool, which is designed to decrease the possibility of double QRS counting and T wave oversensing. When applied to patients who had transvenous ICDs but otherwise would be candidates for S-ICD implantation, 8% of patients failed screening.[24] In a similar study that required qualifying in 2 vectors as passing criteria, 14.8% of patients failed screening. Notably, a wide QRS complex was associated with failure of screening.[25]

The rate of inappropriate shocks in studies of the S-ICD ranges between 4% and 16% despite the mandatory use of the surface ECG screening tool. The causes of inappropriate shocks can be grouped into (1) SVT, (2) oversensing of physiologic cardiac electrical events due to large T waves and P waves or wide QRS complexes or from a reduction in QRS amplitude leading to a decrease in the R to T wave ratio, or (3) sensing of noncardiac events (myopotentials, electromagnetic interference). Programming a conditional zone in the S-ICD to allow for SVT discrimination has been shown to dramatically reduce the rate of inappropriate shocks without a reduction in the appropriate shock rate.[26]

In the EFFORTLESS S-ICD registry, 48 of the 581 patients experienced a total of 101 inappropriate shocks. The most common cause (73%) was cardiac signal oversensing. Fifteen of the 18 episodes of shocks for SVT occurred with rates in the shock zone (not subject to discrimination), with the remaining 3 being errors of discrimination. Among the episodes of cardiac signal oversensing, 64% occurred during regular SVT, most of which were likely sinus tachycardia. Patient characteristics associated with inappropriate shocks included atrial fibrillation and hypertrophic cardiomyopathy. Inappropriate shocks in patients with hypertrophic cardiomyopathy were most often due to T-wave oversensing. Freedom from inappropriate shocks was predicted by the selection of the primary sensing vector when compared with the secondary and alternate vectors. Interventions after an inappropriate shock that were effective in reducing recurrence included reprogramming of the sensing vector or changes in the conditional zone and shock zone rates.[27] Medication changes might be needed to treat rapidly conducting SVT; in 2 registry patients, ablation was performed. In patients in whom oversensing occurs during elevated heart rates, treadmill testing can help guide optimal sensing vector selection.[28] The use of exercise testing for the surface ECG screening preprocedure is suggested by some investigators in patients with inherited cardiomyopathies, such as hypertrophic cardiomyopathy, who exhibit repolarization abnormalities that might change with increased heart rates.[29]

SUBCUTANEOUS IMPLANTABLE CARDIOVERTER-DEFIBRILLATOR LIMITATIONS

Because of the inability to provide bradycardia pacing, the S-ICD is not appropriate for patients with a pacing indication or for those who require cardiac resynchronization therapy. In addition, the S-ICD is unable to provide ATP. In patients who have exhibited prior episodes of recurrent monomorphic ventricular tachycardia (MMVT), the S-ICD is not recommended. Notably, in the pooled data from the IDE and EFFORTLESS registries in which patients with prior MMVT were excluded, only one patient underwent subsequent implant of a transvenous ICD because of the need for ATP. Only 1.4% of patients had more than 1 documented episode of MMVT.[13] These data combined with the questionable value of ATP in the primary prevention population[30] strongly argue that besides patients with previous recurrent MMVT, the lack of ATP in the S-ICD should not be a factor in selecting appropriate patients for this technology.

The concomitant presence of unipolar pacing from another implanted device is a contraindication to S-ICD implantation; however, bipolar pacing is not an obligatory contraindication. Although not a favored approach, there have been several case reports and case series of the safe, combined use of both the S-ICD and bipolar permanent pacemakers[31] in specific circumstances. The safe use of the S-ICD has also been reported in single cases with other implanted electrical devices, such as deep brain stimulators.[32] There has been no systematic study of the simultaneous use of a left ventricular assist devices (LVAD), and the case report literature is inconsistent with some reports of inappropriate shocks and others with no interaction or the ability to avoid interaction with reprograming the sensing vector or adjustment of the LVAD speed.[33,34]

COMPARISON WITH TRANSVENOUS IMPLANTABLE CARDIOVERTER-DEFIBRILLATOR

There are currently no randomized data available looking at a direct comparison between safety and efficacy of transvenous ICDs and the S-ICD. Indirect comparisons of efficacy and safety in large studies suggest a favorable performance of the S-ICD. In the IDE study, there was a 92.1% rate of conversion of spontaneous VT/VF with the first S-ICD shock,[15] which is higher than the 83% observed rate in the Sudden Cardiac Heart Failure Trial (SCD-Heft).[35] To achieve Food and Drug Administration approval, the IDE study documented a 180-day freedom from the primary safety end point of 99% and any implant-related complication of 92%, well more than similar end points used in the approval of transvenous devices.[30] A retrospective analysis of 3717 S-ICD implants in the US National Cardiovascular Database Registry revealed similar DFT testing success rates and in-hospital complication rates between S-ICD patients and single- and dual-chamber transvenous ICD patients.[36]

The SVT discrimination accuracy of the S-ICD was directly tested against algorithms in transvenous devices in the START study. Both devices exhibited 99% to 100% accuracy in detection of ventricular arrhythmias. The S-ICD exhibited 98.0% accuracy in SVT determination, compared with 76.7% for single-chamber and 68.0% for dual-chamber transvenous devices.[37]

In a Dutch retrospective study of 140 patients who received an S-ICD and 140 matched patients who received a transvenous ICD, the overall complication rate was not significantly different (14% S-ICD vs 18% transvenous ICD). The transvenous ICD group had more lead-related complications, whereas the S-ICD group had significantly more non–lead-related complications. The incidence of ICD therapy (shocks plus ATP) was significantly more in the transvenous ICD group, but there was no difference in the incidence of appropriate and inappropriate shocks.[38]

A randomized study of the S-ICD versus transvenous systems is ongoing. The Prospective, Randomized Comparison of Subcutaneous and Transvenous Implantable Cardioverter-Defibrillator Therapy (PRAETORIAN) study is enrolling 700 patients with an indication for an ICD, randomized in a 1:1 fashion to transvenous ICD or S-ICD. The primary end point is inappropriate shocks and complications, and secondary end points are shock efficacy and mortality.[39]

SUMMARY

The S-ICD represents a potential shift in sudden death prevention away from traditional transvenous systems. Data so far suggest that the S-ICD provides comparable sudden death protection with the major advantage of avoiding the lead-related complications of traditional transvenous systems. The S-ICD should be considered in patients with an ICD indication who do not have a pacing indication or prior history of recurrent MMVT. The device is particularly well suited to patients with limited or no venous access, patients at high risk for infection, or younger patients who will require long-term arrhythmia protection. Ongoing studies and the PRAETORIAN trial will provide data on long-term efficacy and safety of the S-ICD and aid clinicians in decisions of optimal patient selection.

REFERENCES

1. Estes NAM. Predicting and preventing sudden cardiac death. Circulation 2011;124(5):651–6.
2. Moss AJ, Zareba W, Hall WJ, et al. Prophylactic implantation of a defibrillator in patients with myocardial infarction and reduced ejection fraction. N Engl J Med 2002;346(12):877–83.
3. Moss AJ, Hall WJ, Cannom DS, et al. Improved survival with an implanted defibrillator in patients with coronary disease at high risk for ventricular arrhythmia. N Engl J Med 1996;335(26):1933–40.
4. Bardy GH, Lee KL, Mark DB, et al. Amiodarone or an implantable cardioverter–defibrillator for congestive heart failure. N Engl J Med 2005;352(3):225–37.
5. Antiarrhythmics versus Implantable Defibrillators (AVID) Investigators. A comparison of antiarrhythmic-drug therapy with implantable defibrillators in patients resuscitated from near-fatal ventricular arrhythmias. N Engl J Med 1997;337(22):1576–84.
6. van Rees JB, de Bie MK, Thijssen J, et al. Implantation-related complications of implantable cardioverter-defibrillators and cardiac resynchronization therapy devices. J Am Coll Cardiol 2011;58(10):995–1000.
7. Kleemann T, Becker T, Doenges K, et al. Annual rate of transvenous defibrillation lead defects in implantable cardioverter-defibrillators over a period of >10 years. Circulation 2007;115(19):2474–80.
8. Wilkoff BL, Love CJ, Byrd CL, et al. Transvenous lead extraction: Heart Rhythm Society expert consensus on facilities, training, indications, and patient management: this document was endorsed by

the American Heart Association (AHA). Heart Rhythm 2009;6(7):1085–104.

9. Knops RE, Olde Nordkamp LRA, de Groot JR, et al. Two-incision technique for implantation of the subcutaneous implantable cardioverter-defibrillator. Heart Rhythm 2013;10(8):1240–3.

10. Healey JS, Hohnloser SH, Glikson M, et al. Cardioverter defibrillator implantation without induction of ventricular fibrillation: a single-blind, non-inferiority, randomised controlled trial (SIMPLE). Lancet 2015;385(9970):785–91.

11. Frommeyer G, Zumhagen S, Dechering DG, et al. Intraoperative defibrillation testing of subcutaneous implantable cardioverter-defibrillator systems—a simple issue? J Am Heart Assoc 2016; 5(3):e003181.

12. Bardy GH, Smith WM, Hood MA, et al. An entirely subcutaneous implantable cardioverter–defibrillator. N Engl J Med 2010;363(1):36–44.

13. Burke MC, Gold MR, Knight BP, et al. Safety and efficacy of the totally subcutaneous implantable defibrillator: 2-year results from a pooled analysis of the IDE study and EFFORTLESS registry. J Am Coll Cardiol 2015;65(16):1605–15.

14. Lambiase PD, Barr C, Theuns DAMJ, et al. Worldwide experience with a totally subcutaneous implantable defibrillator: early results from the EFFORTLESS S-ICD registry. Eur Heart J 2014; 35(25):1657–65.

15. Weiss R, Knight BP, Gold MR, et al. Safety and efficacy of a totally subcutaneous implantable-cardioverter defibrillator. Circulation 2013;128(9):944–53.

16. Köbe J, Reinke F, Meyer C, et al. Implantation and follow-up of totally subcutaneous versus conventional implantable cardioverter-defibrillators: a multicenter case-control study. Heart Rhythm 2013;10(1): 29–36.

17. Jarman JWE, Todd DM. United Kingdom national experience of entirely subcutaneous implantable cardioverter-defibrillator technology: important lessons to learn. Europace 2013;15(8):1158–65.

18. Aydin A, Hartel F, Schlüter M, et al. Shock efficacy of subcutaneous implantable cardioverter-defibrillator for prevention of sudden cardiac death clinical perspective. Circ Arrhythm Electrophysiol 2012; 5(5):913–9.

19. Olde Nordkamp LRA, Dabiri Abkenari L, Boersma LVA, et al. The entirely subcutaneous implantable cardioverter-defibrillator: initial clinical experience in a large Dutch cohort. J Am Coll Cardiol 2012;60(19):1933–9.

20. Dabiri Abkenari L, Theuns DAMJ, Valk SDA, et al. Clinical experience with a novel subcutaneous implantable defibrillator system in a single center. Clin Res Cardiol 2011;100(9):737–44.

21. Knops RE, Brouwer TF, Barr CS, et al. The learning curve associated with the introduction of the subcutaneous implantable defibrillator. Europace 2016;18(7):1010–5.

22. Brouwer TF, Driessen AHG, Olde Nordkamp LRA, et al. Surgical management of implantation-related complications of the subcutaneous implantable cardioverter-defibrillator. JACC Clin Electrophysiol 2016;2(1):89–96.

23. Daubert JP, Zareba W, Cannom DS, et al. Inappropriate implantable cardioverter-defibrillator shocks in MADIT II: frequency, mechanisms, predictors, and survival impact. J Am Coll Cardiol 2008; 51(14):1357–65.

24. Groh CA, Sharma S, Pelchovitz DJ, et al. Use of an electrocardiographic screening tool to determine candidacy for a subcutaneous implantable cardioverter-defibrillator. Heart Rhythm 2014;11(8): 1361–6.

25. Randles DA, Hawkins NM, Shaw M, et al. How many patients fulfil the surface electrocardiogram criteria for subcutaneous implantable cardioverter-defibrillator implantation? Europace 2014;16(7): 1015–21.

26. Gold MR, Weiss R, Theuns DAMJ, et al. Use of a discrimination algorithm to reduce inappropriate shocks with a subcutaneous implantable cardioverter-defibrillator. Heart Rhythm 2014;11(8): 1352–8.

27. Nordkamp LRAO, Brouwer TF, Barr C, et al. Inappropriate shocks in the subcutaneous ICD: incidence, predictors and management. Int J Cardiol 2015; 195:126–33.

28. Kooiman KM, Knops RE, Olde Nordkamp L, et al. Inappropriate subcutaneous implantable cardioverter-defibrillator shocks due to T-wave oversensing can be prevented: implications for management. Heart Rhythm 2014;11(3):426–34.

29. Weinstock J, Bader YH, Maron MS, et al. Subcutaneous implantable cardioverter defibrillator in patients with hypertrophic cardiomyopathy: an initial experience. J Am Heart Assoc 2016;5(2): e002488.

30. Poole JE, Gold MR. Who should receive the subcutaneous implanted defibrillator? response to Jeanne E. Poole, MD, and Michael R. Gold, MD, PhD. Circ Arrhythm Electrophysiol 2013;6(6):1236–45.

31. Huang J, Patton KK, Prutkin JM. Concomitant use of the subcutaneous implantable cardioverter defibrillator and a permanent pacemaker. Pacing Clin Electrophysiol 2016;39(11):1240–5.

32. Bader Y, Weinstock J. Successful implantation of a subcutaneous cardiac defibrillator in a patient with a preexisting deep brain stimulator. HeartRhythm Case Rep 2015;1:241–4.

33. Pfeffer TJ, König T, Duncker D, et al. Subcutaneous implantable cardioverter-defibrillator shocks after left ventricular assist device implantation. Circ Arrhythm Electrophysiol 2016;9(11) [pii:e004633].

34. Saeed D, Albert A, Westenfeld R, et al. Left ventricular assist device in a patient with a concomitant subcutaneous implantable cardioverter defibrillator. Circ Arrhythm Electrophysiol 2013;6(3):e32–3.

35. Blatt JA, Poole JE, Johnson GW, et al. No benefit from defibrillation threshold testing in the SCD-HeFT (Sudden Cardiac Death in Heart Failure Trial). J Am Coll Cardiol 2008;52(7):551–6.

36. Friedman DJ, Parzynski CS, Varosy PD, et al. Trends and in-hospital outcomes associated with adoption of the subcutaneous implantable cardioverter defibrillator in the United States. JAMA Cardiol 2016;1(8):900.

37. Gold MR, Theunes DA, Knight BP, et al. Head-to-head comparison of arrhythmia discrimination performance of subcutaneous and transvenous ICD arrhythmia detection algorithms: the START study. J Cardiovasc Electrophysiol 2012;23(4):359–66.

38. Brouwer TF, Yilmaz D, Lindeboom R, et al. Long-term clinical outcomes of subcutaneous versus transvenous implantable defibrillator therapy. J Am Coll Cardiol 2016;68(19):2047–55.

39. Olde Nordkamp LRA, Knops RE, Bardy GH, et al. Rationale and design of the PRAETORIAN trial: a prospective, RAndomizEd comparison of subcuTaneOus and tRansvenous ImplANtable cardioverter-defibrillator therapy. Am Heart J 2012; 163(5):753–60.e2.

Future Directions
Management of Sudden Cardiac Death

Robert W. Neumar, MD, PhD

KEYWORDS

- Cardiac arrest • Cardiopulmonary resuscitation • Postcardiac arrest • Bystander CPR
- Automated external defibrillator • Targeted temperature management • Coronary angiography
- Percutaneous coronary intervention

KEY POINTS

- Incidence of emergency medical service (EMS)-treated out-of-hospital cardiac arrest is approximately 57 per 100,000 population per year in the United States.
- Of EMS-treated out-of-hospital cardiac arrest patients, 9% survive hospital discharge with good neurologic function.
- Optimizing the structure and performance of the system of care for out-of-hospital cardiac arrest is fundamental to improving outcomes.
- A more robust scientific and technological pipeline is needed to optimize the detection and treatment of out-of-hospital cardiac arrest.

INTRODUCTION

Despite current and future advances in preventing sudden cardiac arrest, there will always be a need to optimize early recognition and treatment when cardiac arrest does occur. For out-of-hospital cardiac arrest (OHCA), this requires a complex system of care made up of bystanders, 911 dispatchers, emergency medical service (EMS) providers, and hospital-based providers.[1,2] The structure and performance of these systems of care vary greatly, and each system is only as strong as the weakest link in its chain of survival. In 2015, the Institute of Medicine (IOM) published a report entitled "Strategies to Improve Cardiac Arrest Survival: A Time to Act."[3] This report outlined 8 strategies to improve sudden cardiac arrest survival in the United States (**Box 1**).

The IOM report clearly defines the contemporary challenges in the treatment of cardiac arrest, and provides a strategic framework for improving outcomes. This article highlights the key strategies proposed in the IOM report, reflects on the challenges faced in implementing them, and discusses what might be the most innovative and impactful solutions. Although the IOM report focuses on both OHCA and in-hospital cardiac arrest, this article will focus only on OHCA.

NATIONAL CARDIAC ARREST REGISTRY

National data on the incidence of cardiac arrest are extremely limited. The most fundamental challenge is the inconsistency in definitions used to define the disease. The International Liaison Committee on Resuscitation defines cardiac arrest as the cessation of cardiac mechanical activity as confirmed by the absence of signs of circulation.[4] Because cardiac arrest is the final common pathway of human death, this definition alone does not

Disclosure Statement: PhysioControl: Equipment support for laboratory and clinical research.
Department of Emergency Medicine, University of Michigan Medical School, 1500 East Medical Center Drive, Room TC B1220, Ann Arbor, MI 48109, USA
E-mail address: neumar@umich.edu

Card Electrophysiol Clin 9 (2017) 785–790
http://dx.doi.org/10.1016/j.ccep.2017.08.008
1877-9182/17/© 2017 Elsevier Inc. All rights reserved.

cardiacEP.theclinics.com

Box 1
Recommendations from the 2015 Institute of Medicine report Strategies to Improve Cardiac Arrest Survival: A Time to Act

1. Establish a national cardiac arrest registry
2. Foster a culture of action through public awareness and training
3. Enhance the capabilities and performance of EMS systems
4. Set national accreditation standards related to cardiac arrest for hospitals and health care systems
5. Adopt continuous quality improvement programs
6. Accelerate research on pathophysiology, new therapies, and translation of science for cardiac arrest
7. Accelerate research on the evaluation and adoption of cardiac arrest therapies
8. Create the National Cardiac Arrest Collaborative

From Committee on the Treatment of Cardiac Arrest: Current status and future directions; Board on Health Sciences Policy; Institute of Medicine; Graham R, McCoy MA, Schultz AM, editors. Strategies to improve cardiac arrest survival: a time to act. Washington (DC): National Academies Press (US); 2015. Available at: https://www.ncbi.nlm.nih.gov/books/NBK305685/. Accessed September 26, 2017; with permission.

discern sudden or unexpected cardiac arrest from the approximately 2.6 million annual deaths in the United States (824 deaths per 100,000 population).[5] The World Health Organization (WHO) defines sudden cardiac death as unexpected, unexplained death within 1 hour of symptom onset for witnessed events, or within 24 hours of last observed alive and symptom-free, for unwitnessed events.[6] Although this definition attempts to select for sudden unexpected death, symptom duration before death is not routinely collected in EMS records and would likely be inaccurate if it was collected and reported. It would also be difficult to reliably associate specific symptoms with subsequent cardiac arrest in many cases. Although the WHO reported that cardiovascular disease was the number one cause of death in 2015 (17.7 million), they did not report on the incidence of sudden cardiac death. The Centers for Disease Control and Prevention (CDC) Wide-ranging Online Data for Epidemiologic Research (WONDER) database uses 4-digit *International Statistical Classification of Diseases and Related Health Problems*, 10th revision, (ICD-10) codes and 113 cause-of-death recode to determine the cause and location of death. In this database, there were 350,000 annual cases with any mention of cardiac arrest, of which 140,000 occurred in an in-patient facility, leaving approximately 210,000 potentially occurring outside the hospital.[7] The National Institutes of Health-Funded Resuscitation Outcomes Consortium was a North American multicenter clinical research network that collected OHCA incidence and outcome data in defined geographic populations from 2005 to 2015. This group defined cardiac arrests based on whether they were EMS-assessed and whether they were EMS-treated. EMS-assessed included patients who were evaluated by organized EMS personnel and treated (shock delivered or chest compressions by EMS personnel) or not treated by EMS personnel. EMS-treated included only those that were assessed and treated by EMS personnel.[8] In the final year of the Resuscitation Outcomes Consortium (June 2014–May 2015), the incidence of EMS-assessed OHCA was 110.8 per 100,000 population (95% CI 108.9–112.6/100,000) and EMS-treated OHCA was 57.3 per 100,000 population (56.0–58.7/100,000).[7] Extrapolating these results to the entire US population would indicate that there are 356,000 EMS-assessed and 184,000 EMS-treated cardiac arrests annually. These numbers are significantly higher than the CDC estimate. The discrepancy highlights the limitation of reporting OHCA incidence and outcomes based on only EMS-treated patients, which underestimates the incidence, overestimates the survival rate, and is subject to variability when the proportion of EMS-assessed patients that are treated changes. The Cardiac Arrest Registry to Enhance Survival (CARES) is the largest active OHCA registry in the United States. Participation is voluntary. In 2016, CARES collected data on 61,647 EMS-treated OHCAs in the United States. Of these, 20% had an initial cardiac rhythm of ventricular fibrillation or ventricular tachycardia, 41% received bystander cardiopulmonary resuscitation (CPR), 29% had return of spontaneous circulation long enough to be admitted to the hospital, and 9% survived to hospital discharge with good neurologic function. Although the CARES registry has the limitation of collecting data only on EMS-treated patients, it does provide a valuable resource of individual EMS agencies to benchmark the performance of their system of care and annually evaluate the impact of quality improvement programs on process measures and outcomes.

Because preventing sudden cardiac arrest is the most cost-effective strategy, it will be essential to develop mechanisms to accurately monitor and report the incidence of sudden cardiac arrest. However, the fundamental challenge will be to define the patient population that will be included by using characteristics that can be reliably collected and reported nationwide. An effective registry will also need to collect and report data on both process measures and outcomes to facilitate quality improvement measures across the entire system of care. This approach provides the opportunity for local systems to monitor their own processes and outcome variables, and compare them to local, regional, and national benchmarks. Each system can identify its own weakest links and steer resources toward quality improvement measures that will have the greatest potential impact on outcomes. The IOM has recommended a single National Surveillance Program to monitor and report incidence, processes of care, and patient-centered outcomes at a local, state, and national level. Creation of this registry is foundational to advancing the field of cardiac arrest resuscitation.

FOSTERING A CULTURE OF ACTION

Cardiac arrest is arguably the most life-threatening human condition. It is also the only critical illness that requires an untrained or minimally trained bystander or family member to (1) accurately make the diagnosis, (2) activate the medical response system, and (3) provide the most important initial therapy, which is CPR. Moreover, every minute these actions are delayed significantly decreases the patient's chance of survival. Making the diagnosis is fundamentally challenging based on the continued confusion among lay public and press about the difference between and heart attack and cardiac arrest. Patients with sudden cardiac arrest often have agonal gasping for several minutes, which can delay recognition that the condition is truly cardiac arrest. Due to this and the unreliability of checking pulses, the current American Heart Association (AHA) recommendation is to start CPR if someone suddenly becomes unresponsive and is not breathing normally. Although this strategy increases the risk of starting chest compressions on someone who is not in cardiac arrest (ie, seizure), the benefit of early recognition, EMS activation, and initiation of chest compression is believed to outweigh the risk of initiating chest compressions in those not in cardiac arrest. Existing data clearly demonstrate that patients receiving bystander CPR are twice as likely to survive as those that do not receive bystander CPR.[9] Formal CPR training courses for the lay public have had an important impact on bystander CPR rates. It is estimated that the AHA and Red Cross train or retrain more than 30 million people each year. This approach also has its limitations, creating a culture in which it is believed that someone has to be trained and certified to respond to a cardiac arrest. In addition, many who take

courses are reluctant to respond in a real cardiac arrest situation because they are concerned they will not do it right. A major advance has been the change to hands-only CPR, which has been demonstrated to be as effective as chest compression plus mouth-to-mouth ventilation when used by bystanders. This greatly simplifies training and overcomes potential reluctance to perform mouth-to-mouth breathing due to concerns of disease transmission. Hands-only CPR has also opened the way for Internet-based brief instructional video and just-in-time CPR instruction by 911 dispatchers. These approaches have great potential to increase bystander CPR rates in a way that translates into improved outcomes.[10,11] More sophisticated approaches include crowdsourcing strategies in which people who are willing to respond to a cardiac arrest in a public place are notified on their smart phone of the arrest location and the nearest automated external defibrillator (AED). Although this approach has been reported to increase bystander CPR rates in some settings, the impact on outcomes remains to be determined.[12] One major limitation is that most OHCAs do not occur in a public setting and thus are not affected by these systems.[13] Although yet to be realized, innovation in this space has great potential to affect outcomes. Success in creating a culture of action will be realize when it becomes newsworthy if someone experiences a cardiac arrest in a public setting and does not get bystander CPR and AED applied before EMS arrives.

OPTIMIZING EMERGENCY MEDICAL SERVICE SYSTEM CAPABILITIES AND PERFORMANCE

EMS system performance can have a tremendous impact on OHCA survival. Specific strategies include just-in-time CPR instruction and coaching by 911 dispatchers, crowdsourcing notification of nearby responders, strategic AED deployment, and optimizing the quality of EMS resuscitation. Supplying first responders, such as firefighters and police, with an AED can significantly decrease time to initial defibrillation.[14] Other potential ways to deploy AEDs include rideshare drivers or drones.[15] High-performance CPR by EMT and paramedic responders involves a pit crew approach to delivering basic and advanced life support measures in a way that optimizes CPR quality (**Box 2**).[16] Debriefing provider teams to provide feedback on process and physiologic parameters recorded by the defibrillator is an essential component in optimized EMS care. As more sophisticated modalities emerge to monitor the physiologic response to CPR, the ultimate goal will be goal-directed CPR strategy based on noninvasive physiologic monitoring of brain and myocardial blood flow during chest compressions.

A major barrier to improving overall outcomes is the high proportion of OHCAs that are unwitnessed. Survival rate for unwitnessed OHCA is 4.7% compared with 16.9% for bystander-witnessed OHCA.[17] System optimization will have little impact on the unwitnessed subpopulation due to delay in detection and initiation of therapy. An example of detecting and treating unwitnessed OHCA in high-risk patients are automated implantable cardioverter-defibrillators, or wearable defibrillators. However, these strategies are not feasible for the general population with a much lower risk of OHCA. Alternatively, physiologic surveillance devices that transmit data to smart phones could potentially detect sudden cardiac arrest, sound an audible alarm to potential responders in the vicinity, and call 911 with Global Positioning System (GPS) coordinates.[18] This could markedly reduce the proportion of OHCAs that are unwitnessed, which would have a measurable impact on outcomes.

OPTIMIZING HOSPITAL PERFORMANCE

Cardiac arrest resuscitation does not end when a patient is transported to the emergency department or admitted to the intensive care unit. There is compelling evidence that the quality of care provided in the emergency department and intensive care unit after return of spontaneous circulation affects patient outcomes. Variability in postcardiac arrest treatment and outcomes between hospitals is 1 piece of evidence.[19] Hypothermic-targeted temperature management improves outcomes based on

prospective, randomized clinical trials.[20,21] Early coronary angiography and percutaneous coronary intervention for postarrest patients with ST-elevation myocardial infarction (STEMI) or high suspicion of acute myocardial infarction is strongly associated with improved outcomes.[22] Both of these interventions have been given a level 1 recommendation in the most recent AHA Guidelines for CPR and Emergency Cardiovascular Care but are variably implemented.[23] Optimization of hemodynamics, ventilation, oxygenation, blood glucose, and seizure management are all supported by some clinical evidence.[24] Cardiac arrest centers, similar to trauma and stroke centers, have been proposed and implemented in some states as preferred destination hospitals for patients who achieve return of spontaneous circulation after OHCA or who are transported with ongoing resuscitation.[25] However, this involves bypassing the nearest hospital, which could delay delivery of a higher level of care or increase the risk of repeated arrest before hospital arrival. In addition to a more consistent implementation of postcardiac arrest care, cardiac arrest centers could be equipped to provide advanced therapies such as extracorporeal CPR for refractory cardiac arrest or coronary angiography and percutaneous coronary intervention with ongoing CPR. Cardiac arrest receiving centers should have adequate intensive care unit capacity that meets the standards for care for treatment and prognostication. The IOM has proposed national accreditation standards related to cardiac arrest for hospitals and health care systems.[3] Public reporting of cardiac arrest outcomes should be required for receiving hospitals.

ACCELERATING RESEARCH

The 2015 IOM report called for accelerated research on pathophysiology, new therapies, and translation of science for cardiac arrest, as well as the evaluation and adoption of cardiac arrest therapies. Between 1995 and 2014, there were only 81 published randomized, controlled trials (~4 per year) focused on OHCA, 80% of which were performed outside the United States.[26] Between 2007 and 2016, National Institute of Health funding for cardiac arrest research declined from $35.4 million per year to 28.5 million per year when adjusted for inflation.[27] This equates to a research investment of $91 per annual death for cardiac arrest compared with $2200 per annual death for stroke and $2100 per annual death for heart disease. This limited amount of research and research funding is reflected in the quality of evidence supporting treatment guidelines. **Table 1** illustrates the level of evidence used to create the most recent 2015 AHA guidelines for CPR and

Table 1
Level of evidence supporting 2015 American Heart Association guidelines for cardiopulmonary resuscitation and emergency cardiovascular care

Level of Evidence	Description	Number of Recommendations	Percent
A	High quality evidence	3	1%
B-R	Moderate-quality evidence with randomized studies	50	15%
B-NR	Moderate-quality evidence with non-randomized studies	46	15%
C-LD	Limited data	145	46%
C-EO	Expert opinion	73	23%

Data from Neumar RW, Shuster M, Callaway CW, et al. Part 1: Executive summary: 2015 American Heart Association guidelines update for cardiopulmonary resuscitation and emergency cardiovascular care. Circulation 2015;132 (18 Suppl 2):S316; with permission.

emergency cardiovascular care.[28] Most striking is that more than two-thirds of the 315 treatment recommendations are based on limited data or expert opinion. These results highlight the persistent knowledge gap in resuscitation science that can only be addressed through accelerated research efforts as called for by the IOM.

One major challenge to accelerating research efforts is the limited pipeline of investigators focused on cardiac arrest resuscitation. The most recent data show that there are only 60 National Institute of Health-funded cardiac arrest principal investigators in the United States, 25% of which are on trainee grants.[27] This number has been stagnant for the last decade. Accelerating research in cardiac arrest resuscitation will require a significant financial and training investment to simultaneously jumpstart both scientific investigation and the career development of cardiac arrest scientists.

STRUCTURED COLLABORATION

The 2015 IOM report proposed the creation of a National Cardiac Arrest Collaborative (NCAC) that would bring together national stakeholders to move the field forward. The initial meeting of NCAC occurred in Bethesda, MD, on May 11, 2017. At that time, leaders from stakeholder organizations decided to initially focus on increasing public and provider awareness and creating a culture of action. The NCAC ultimate goal is to facilitate implementation of all recommendations in the 2015 IOM report.[3]

SUMMARY

Sudden cardiac arrest is a major pubic heath challenge responsible for 1 in 5 deaths in the United States.[3] In 2010, The American Heart Association Emergency Cardiovascular Care Committee set

an impact goal of doubling cardiac arrest survival by 2020.[29] Since that time, the survival rate for EMS treated OHCA in the United States has increased from an estimated 7.9% to 10.8% in 2016.[9,29] Although progress has been made, there remains tremendous potential to improve outcomes. Key strategies outlined by the IOM include a national registry, creating a culture of action, optimizing the system of care, investing in research across the translational spectrum, and collaboration among key stakeholders.[3] Implementation of these strategies has the potential to save thousands of lives annually.

REFERENCES

1. Neumar RW, Barnhart JM, Berg RA, et al. Implementation strategies for improving survival after out-of-hospital cardiac arrest in the United States: consensus recommendations from the 2009 American Heart Association Cardiac Arrest Survival Summit. Circulation 2011;123(24):2898–910.
2. Kronick SL, Kurz MC, Lin S, et al. Part 4: systems of care and continuous quality improvement: 2015 American Heart Association guidelines update for cardiopulmonary resuscitation and emergency cardiovascular care. Circulation 2015;132(18 Suppl 2):S397–413.
3. Committee on the Treatment of Cardiac Arrest: Current status and future directions; Board on Health Sciences Policy; Institute of Medicine; Graham R, McCoy MA, Schultz AM, editors. Strategies to improve cardiac arrest survival: a time to act. Washington (DC): National Academies Press (US); 2015. Available at: https://www.ncbi.nlm.nih.gov/books/NBK305685/. Accessed September 26, 2017.
4. Perkins GD, Jacobs IG, Nadkarni VM, et al. Cardiac arrest and cardiopulmonary resuscitation outcome reports: update of the Utstein Resuscitation Registry Templates for out-of-hospital cardiac arrest: a statement for healthcare professionals from a task force

of the International Liaison Committee on Resuscitation (American Heart Association, European Resuscitation Council, Australian and New Zealand Council on Resuscitation, Heart and Stroke Foundation of Canada, InterAmerican Heart Foundation, Resuscitation Council of Southern Africa, Resuscitation Council of Asia); and the American Heart Association Emergency Cardiovascular Care Committee and the Council on Cardiopulmonary, Critical Care, Perioperative and Resuscitation. Circulation 2015; 132(13):1286–300.

5. WHO. Sudden cardiac death: report of a WHO scientific group. Presented at a meeting held in Geneva (Switzerland) from 24-27 October, 1984.

6. Sudden Cardiac Death. 1985.

7. Benjamin EJ, Blaha MJ, Chiuve SE, et al. Heart disease and stroke statistics-2017 update: a report from the American Heart Association. Circulation 2017;135(10):e146–603.

8. Morrison LJ, Nichol G, Rea TD, et al. Rationale, development and implementation of the resuscitation outcomes Consortium Epistry-Cardiac arrest. Resuscitation 2008;78(2):161–9.

9. Non-Traumatic National Summary Report. Cardiac Arrest Registry to Enhance Survival (CARES); 2016.

10. Bobrow BJ, Spaite DW, Vadeboncoeur TF, et al. Implementation of a Regional Telephone Cardiopulmonary Resuscitation Program And Outcomes After Out-Of-Hospital Cardiac Arrest. JAMA Cardiol 2016;1(3):294–302.

11. Dumas F, Rea TD, Fahrenbruch C, et al. Chest compression alone cardiopulmonary resuscitation is associated with better long-term survival compared with standard cardiopulmonary resuscitation. Circulation 2013;127(4):435–41.

12. Ringh M, Rosenqvist M, Hollenberg J, et al. Mobile-phone dispatch of laypersons for CPR in out-of-hospital cardiac arrest. N Engl J Med 2015; 372(24):2316–25.

13. Brooks SC, Simmons G, Worthington H, et al. The PulsePoint Respond mobile device application to crowdsource basic life support for patients with out-of-hospital cardiac arrest: challenges for optimal implementation. Resuscitation 2016;98:20–6.

14. Malta Hansen C, Kragholm K, Pearson DA, et al. Association of bystander and first-responder intervention with survival after out-of-hospital cardiac arrest in North Carolina, 2010-2013. JAMA 2015;314(3): 255–64.

15. Boutilier JJ, Brooks SC, Janmohamed A, et al. Optimizing a Drone Network to deliver automated external defibrillators. Circulation 2017;135(25): 2454–65.

16. Meaney PA, Bobrow BJ, Mancini ME, et al. Cardiopulmonary resuscitation quality: [corrected] improving cardiac resuscitation outcomes both inside and outside the hospital: a consensus

statement from the American Heart Association. Circulation 2013;128(4):417–35.

17. Non-Traumatic National Survival Report. Cardiac Arrest Registry to Enhances Survival (CARES); 2016.

18. Rickard J, Ahmed S, Baruch M, et al. Utility of a novel watch-based pulse detection system to detect pulselessness in human subjects. Heart Rhythm 2011;8(12):1895–9.

19. Carr BG, Kahn JM, Merchant RM, et al. Inter-hospital variability in post-cardiac arrest mortality. Resuscitation 2009;80(1):30–4.

20. Bernard SA, Gray TW, Buist MD, et al. Treatment of comatose survivors of out-of-hospital cardiac arrest with induced hypothermia. N Engl J Med 2002; 346(8):557–63.

21. Hypothermia after Cardiac Arrest Study Group. Mild therapeutic hypothermia to improve the neurologic outcome after cardiac arrest. N Engl J Med 2002; 346(8):549–56.

22. Kern KB, Lotun K, Patel N, et al. Outcomes of comatose cardiac arrest survivors with and without ST-segment elevation myocardial infarction: importance of coronary angiography. JACC Cardiovasc Interv 2015;8(8):1031–40.

23. Callaway CW, Donnino MW, Fink EL, et al. Part 8: post-cardiac arrest care: 2015 American Heart Association guidelines update for cardiopulmonary resuscitation and emergency cardiovascular care. Circulation 2015;132(18 Suppl 2):S465–82.

24. Callaway CW, Soar J, Aibiki M, et al. Part 4: Advanced Life Support: 2015 International Consensus on Cardiopulmonary Resuscitation and Emergency Cardiovascular Care Science With Treatment Recommendations. Circulation 2015; 132(16 Suppl 1):S84–145.

25. Nichol G, Aufderheide TP, Eigel B, et al. Regional systems of care for out-of-hospital cardiac arrest: a policy statement from the American Heart Association. Circulation 2010;121(5):709–29.

26. Sinha SS, Sukul D, Lazarus JJ, et al. Identifying important gaps in randomized controlled trials of adult cardiac arrest treatments: a systematic review of the published literature. Circ Cardiovasc Qual Outcomes 2016;9(6):749–56.

27. Coute RA, Panchal AR, Mader TJ, et al. National Institutes of Health-Funded Cardiac Arrest Research: a 10-year trend analysis. J Am Heart Assoc 2017;6(7).

28. Neumar RW, Shuster M, Callaway CW, et al. Part 1: Executive Summary: 2015 American Heart Association guidelines update for cardiopulmonary resuscitation and emergency cardiovascular care. Circulation 2015;132(18 Suppl 2):S315–67.

29. Neumar RW. Doubling cardiac arrest survival by 2020: achieving the American Heart Association impact goal. Circulation 2016;134(25):2037–9.

Moving?

Make sure your subscription moves with you!

To notify us of your new address, find your **Clinics Account Number** (located on your mailing label above your name), and contact customer service at:

Email: journalscustomerservice-usa@elsevier.com

800-654-2452 (subscribers in the U.S. & Canada)
314-447-8871 (subscribers outside of the U.S. & Canada)

Fax number: 314-447-8029

Elsevier Health Sciences Division
Subscription Customer Service
3251 Riverport Lane
Maryland Heights, MO 63043

*To ensure uninterrupted delivery of your subscription, please notify us at least 4 weeks in advance of move.

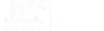

Printed and bound by CPI Group (UK) Ltd, Croydon, CR0 4YY

03/10/2024

01040383-0005